Moderate Preterm, Late Preterm and Early Term Births

Editors

LUCKY JAIN
TONSE N.K. RAJU

CLINICS IN PERINATOLOGY

www.perinatology.theclinics.com

Consulting Editor
LUCKY JAIN

December 2013 • Volume 40 • Number 4

ELSEVIER

1600 John F. Kennedy Boulevard • Suite 1800 • Philadelphia, Pennsylvania, 19103-2899

http://www.theclinics.com

CLINICS IN PERINATOLOGY Volume 40, Number 4
December 2013 ISSN 0095-5108, ISBN-13: 978-0-323-26120-3

Editor: Kerry Holland
Developmental Editor: Stephanie Carter

Clinics in Perinatology (ISSN 0095-5108) is published quarterly by Elsevier Inc., 360 Park Avenue South, New York, NY 10010-1710. Months of issue are March, June, September, and December. Business and Editorial Offices: 1600 John F. Kennedy Blvd., Ste. 1800, Philadelphia, PA 19103-2899. Customer Service Office: 3251 Riverport Lane, Maryland Heights, MO 63043. Periodicals postage paid at New York, NY and additional mailing offices. Subscription prices are $285.00 per year (US individuals), $445.00 per year (US institutions), $340.00 per year (Canadian individuals), $545.00 per year (Canadian institutions), $420.00 per year (foreign individuals), $545.00 per year (foreign institutions), $135.00 per year (US students), and $195.00 per year (Canadian and foreign students). Foreign air speed delivery is included in all Clinics subscription prices. All prices are subject to change without notice. **POSTMASTER:** Send address changes to *Clinics in Perinatology*, Elsevier Health Sciences Division, Subscription Customer Service, 3251 Riverport Lane, Maryland Heights, MO 63043. **Customer Service: Telephone: 1-800-654-2452** (U.S. and Canada); **1-314-447-8871** (outside U.S. and Canada). **Fax: 1-314-447-8029. E-mail: journalscustomerservice-usa@elsevier.com** (for print support); **journalsonlinesupport-usa@elsevier.com** (for online support).

Reprints. For copies of 100 or more, of articles in this publication, please contact the Commercial Reprints Department, Elsevier Inc., 360 Park Avenue South, New York, NY 10010-1710. Tel. 212-633-3874; Fax: 212-633-3820; E-mail: reprints@elsevier.com.

Clinics in Perinatology is also pubilshed in Spanish by McGraw-Hill Interamericana Editores S.A., P.O. Box 5-237, 06500 Mexico D.F., Mexico.

Clinics in Perinatology is covered in *MEDLINE/PubMed (Index Medicus) Current Contents, Excepta Medica, BIOSIS and ISI/BIOMED.*

Printed in the United States of America.

Contributors

CONSULTING EDITOR

LUCKY JAIN, MD, MBA
Richard W. Blumberg Professor and Executive Vice Chairman, Department of Pediatrics, Emory University School of Medicine; Executive Medical Director, Children's Physician Group, Emory Children's Center, Children's Healthcare of Atlanta, Atlanta, Georgia

EDITORS

LUCKY JAIN, MD, MBA
Richard W. Blumberg Professor and Executive Vice Chairman, Department of Pediatrics, Emory University School of Medicine; Executive Medical Director, Children's Physician Group, Emory Children's Center, Children's Healthcare of Atlanta, Atlanta, Georgia

TONSE N.K. RAJU, MD, DCH
Medical Officer and Program Director, Chief, Pregnancy and Perinatology Branch, *Eunice Kennedy Shriver* National Institute of Child Health and Human Development, National Institutes of Health, Bethesda, Maryland

AUTHORS

CANDE V. ANANTH, PhD, MPH
Department of Obstetrics and Gynecology, College of Physicians and Surgeons; Department of Epidemiology, Joseph L. Mailman School of Public Health, Columbia University, New York, New York

VINOD K. BHUTANI, MD, FAAP
Professor of Pediatrics, Division of Neonatal-Developmental Medicine, Department of Pediatrics, Lucile Packard Children's Hospital, Stanford University School of Medicine, Stanford, California

SEAN F. EDMUNDS, MD
Department of Obstetrics and Gynecology, University of Utah School of Medicine, Salt Lake City, Utah

JANET L. ENGSTROM, PhD, RN, CNM, WHNP-BC
Professor of Women, Children and Family Nursing, College of Nursing, Rush University Medical Center, Chicago, Illinois; Associate Dean for Research, Department of Research, Frontier Nursing University, Hyden, Kentucky

GABRIEL J. ESCOBAR, MD
Perinatal Research Unit, Division of Research; Systems Research Initiative, Division of Research, Kaiser Permanente Northern California, Oakland, California

ALEXANDER M. FRIEDMAN, MD
Department of Obstetrics and Gynecology, College of Physicians and Surgeons, Columbia University, New York, New York

CYNTHIA GYAMFI-BANNERMAN, MD
Department of Obstetrics and Gynecology, College of Physicians and Surgeons, Columbia University, New York, New York

ROBIN L. HAYNES, PhD
Principal Associate, Department of Pathology, Boston Children's Hospital, Harvard Medical School, Boston, Massachusetts

JAY D. IAMS, MD
Division of Maternal Fetal Medicine, The Ohio State University Medical Center, Columbus, Ohio

LUCKY JAIN, MD, MBA
Richard W. Blumberg Professor and Executive Vice Chairman, Department of Pediatrics, Emory University School of Medicine; Executive Medical Director, Children's Physician Group, Emory Children's Center, Children's Healthcare of Atlanta, Atlanta, Georgia

HANNAH C. KINNEY, MD
Professor of Pathology, Department of Pathology, Boston Children's Hospital, Harvard Medical School, Boston, Massachusetts

MICHAEL W. KUZNIEWICZ, MD, MPH
Assistant Professor, Perinatal Research Unit, Division of Research, Kaiser Permanente Northern California, Oakland; Division of Neonatology, University of California, San Francisco, San Francisco, California

ABBOT R. LAPTOOK, MD
Professor of Pediatrics, Medical Director, Department of Pediatrics, Women and Infants Hospital of Rhode Island, The Warren Alpert Medical School of Brown University, Providence, Rhode Island

ASHLEY DARCY MAHONEY, PhD, NNP-BC
Assistant Professor, Nell Hodgson Woodruff School of Nursing, Neonatal Nurse Practitioner, Emory University, Atlanta, Georgia; South Dade Neonatology, Miami, Florida

PAULA MEIER, PhD, RN, FAAN
Professor of Pediatrics and Professor of Women, Children and Family Nursing, NICU Director for Clinical Research and Lactation, Division of Neonatology, Department of Pediatrics, College of Nursing, Rush University Medical Center, Chicago, Illinois

SARAH-JANE PARKER, BA
Perinatal Research Unit, Division of Research, Kaiser Permanente Northern California, Oakland, California

ALOKA L. PATEL, MD
Associate Professor of Pediatrics, Division of Neonatology, Department of Pediatrics, Rush University Medical Center, Chicago, Illinois

RICHARD A. POLIN, MD
Professor of Pediatrics, Columbia University College of Physicians and Surgeons, New York, New York

TONSE N.K. RAJU, MD, DCH
Medical Officer and Program Director, Chief, Pregnancy and Perinatology Branch, *Eunice Kennedy Shriver* National Institute of Child Health and Human Development, National Institutes of Health, Bethesda, Maryland

RAKESH SAHNI, MD
Professor of Clinical Pediatrics, Columbia University College of Physicians and Surgeons, New York, New York

ALINA SCHNAKE-MAHL, BA
Systems Research Initiative, Division of Research, Kaiser Permanente Northern California, Oakland, California

ROBERT M. SILVER, MD
Department of Obstetrics and Gynecology, University of Utah School of Medicine, Salt Lake City, Utah

ROBERT A. SINKIN, MD, MPH
Charles Fuller Professor of Neonatology, Division Head, Neonatology, Department of Pediatrics, University of Virginia Children's Hospital, University of Virginia, Charlottesville, Virginia

LYNN A. SLEEPER, ScD
Chief Scientist, Center for Statistical Analysis and Research, New England Research Institutes, Watertown, Massachusetts

JONATHAN R. SWANSON, MD
Assistant Professor of Pediatrics, Department of Pediatrics, University of Virginia Children's Hospital, University of Virginia, Charlottesville, Virginia

ANDREA N. TREMBATH, MD, MPH
Division of Neonatology, Department of Pediatrics, UH Rainbow Babies and Children's Hospital, Cleveland, Ohio

BETTY VOHR, MD
Professor of Pediatrics, Alpert Medical School of Brown University, Department of Pediatrics, Women and Infants Hospital, Providence, Rhode Island

JOSEPH J. VOLPE, MD
Bronson Crothers Professor of Neurology, Department of Neurology, Boston Children's Hospital, Harvard Medical School, Boston, Massachusetts

MATTHEW B. WALLENSTEIN, MD
Division of Neonatal-Developmental Medicine, Department of Pediatrics, Lucile Packard Children's Hospital, Stanford University School of Medicine, Stanford, California

MICHELE WALSH, MD, MSE
Division of Neonatology, Department of Pediatrics, UH Rainbow Babies and Children's Hospital, Cleveland, Ohio

KAREN WRIGHT, PhD, RN, NNP-BC
Assistant Professor of Women, Children and Family Nursing, College of Nursing, Rush University Medical Center, Chicago, Illinois

Contents

Foreword: The Tug of War Between Stillbirths and Elective Early Births xv

Lucky Jain

Preface: Late Preterm and Early Term Births xix

Lucky Jain and Tonse N.K. Raju

Epidemiology of Moderate Preterm, Late Preterm and Early Term Delivery 601

Cande V. Ananth, Alexander M. Friedman, and Cynthia Gyamfi-Bannerman

Moderate preterm, late preterm, and early term deliveries represent a major and growing public health concern. These deliveries are associated with significant financial burden and pose serious risks to mothers and newborns. Women who deliver at moderate and late gestational ages in one pregnancy are at increased risk of delivering at these gestational ages, or earlier, in a subsequent pregnancy. Births in moderate preterm and late preterm gestational ages are associated with significant infant morbidity and mortality. Efforts to reduce deliveries in moderate preterm and late preterm gestations and interventions designed to ameliorate the problems in infants delivered at the gestational ages may be targets worthy of future investigation.

Stillbirth Reduction Efforts and Impact on Early Births 611

Sean F. Edmunds and Robert M. Silver

A major justification for the intentional delivery of a pregnancy before 39 weeks' gestation is a reduction in stillbirth. However, there is a considerable downside to late preterm or early term deliveries. Infants born before 39 weeks' gestation are at increased risk for numerous complications and even death. Thus, it is critical to identify which medical problems and circumstances place the fetus at high enough risk for stillbirth so as to justify late preterm or early term birth. This article highlights information pertinent to the pros and cons of iatrogenic preterm birth in pregnancies at risk for stillbirth.

Early Births and Congenital Birth Defects: A Complex Interaction 629

Jonathan R. Swanson and Robert A. Sinkin

Congenital birth defects and early/premature birth are common complex conditions affecting populations throughout the world, the interaction of which accounts for a significant proportion of neonatal morbidity and mortality. The relationship between these two conditions is not well understood. Several congenital birth defects can directly lead to early delivery. In addition, certain fetal conditions may necessitate early or premature delivery, several of which are also associated with maternal conditions necessitating early birth. Further understanding of both the incidences and causes of congenital birth defects and of early and premature birth will facilitate establishment of strategies to improve neonatal mortality and morbidity.

Physiologic Underpinnings for Clinical Problems in Moderately Preterm and Late Preterm Infants   645

Rakesh Sahni and Richard A. Polin

This article highlights some of the important developmental characteristics that underpin common problems seen in moderate and late preterm infants. Preterm birth is associated with an increased prevalence of clinical problems caused by functional immaturities in a wide variety of organ systems, acquired problems, and problems associated with inadequate monitoring and/or follow-up plans. There are variations in the degree of maturation among infants of similar gestational ages because the developmental process is nonlinear. Therefore, different organ systems mature at rates and trajectories that are specific to their functions. A better understanding of these principles can help guide optimal treatment strategies.

Respiratory Disorders in Moderately Preterm, Late Preterm, and Early Term Infants   665

Ashley Darcy Mahoney and Lucky Jain

Even when it is just a few weeks before term gestation, early birth has consequences, resulting in higher morbidity and mortality. Respiratory issues related to moderate prematurity include delayed neonatal transition to air breathing, respiratory distress resulting from delayed fluid clearance (transient tachypnea of the newborn), surfactant deficiency (respiratory distress syndrome), and pulmonary hypertension. Management approaches emphasize appropriate respiratory support to facilitate respiratory transition and minimize iatrogenic injury. Studies are needed to determine the impact of respiratory distress coupled with mild-moderate prematurity on long-term outcome.

Jaundice and Kernicterus in the Moderately Preterm Infant   679

Matthew B. Wallenstein and Vinod K. Bhutani

Moderate preterm infants remain at increased risk for adverse outcomes, including acute bilirubin encephalopathy (ABE). Evidence-based guidelines for management of hyperbilirubinemia in preterm infants less than 35 weeks' gestational age are not yet optimized. High concentrations of unconjugated bilirubin can cause permanent posticteric neurologic sequelae (kernicterus). Clinical manifestations of ABE in preterm infants are similar to, but often more subtle than, those of term infants. This review outlines clinical strategies to operationalize management of hyperbilirubinemia in moderately preterm infants to meet recently published consensus-based recommendations.

Management of Breastfeeding During and After the Maternity Hospitalization for Late Preterm Infants   689

Paula Meier, Aloka L. Patel, Karen Wright, and Janet L. Engstrom

Among infants born moderately and late preterm or early term, the greatest challenge for breastfeeding management is the late preterm infant (LPI) who is cared for with the mother in the maternity setting. Breastfeeding failure among LPIs and their mothers is high. Evidence-based strategies are needed to protect infant hydration and growth, and the maternal milk supply, until complete feeding at breast can be established. This article reviews the evidence for lactation and breastfeeding risks in LPIs and their mothers and describes strategies for managing these immaturity-related feeding problems. Application to moderately and early preterm infants is made throughout.

Neuropathologic Studies of the Encephalopathy of Prematurity in the Late Preterm Infant

707

Robin L. Haynes, Lynn A. Sleeper, Joseph J. Volpe, and Hannah C. Kinney

It has been widely suggested that brain damage in survivors of late preterm deliveries is similar to that in early preterm infants, only less severe. This report addresses this concept through reanalysis of published neuropathologic data obtained according to late preterm in comparison with early preterm ages. Findings suggest that the spectrum of brain injury in the late preterm infant, as determined in an autopsy population, is similar to that found in early preterm infants, with potential differential susceptibility for different neuronal, glial, and vascular indices. Further research is needed to more clearly define developmental cellular susceptibilities in preterm populations.

Neurologic and Metabolic Issues in Moderately Preterm, Late Preterm, and Early Term Infants

723

Abbot R. Laptook

Common neurologic morbidities encountered in very preterm and extremely preterm infants (intracranial hemorrhage, white matter injury and periventricular leukomalacia, and apnea of prematurity) are much less common in moderately preterm and late preterm infants. The frequency of germinal matrix hemorrhage–intraventricular hemorrhage and white matter injury are reported to be low, but selection bias in neuroimaging surveillance prevents ascertainment of precise frequencies. The major neurologic morbidity of moderately and late preterm infants is feeding difficulty reflecting developmental integration of suck, swallow, and breathing.

Long-Term Outcomes of Moderately Preterm, Late Preterm, and Early Term Infants

739

Betty Vohr

At present, moderate preterm (MPT) infants born at 32 to 33 weeks' gestation and late preterm (LPT) infants born at 34 to 36 weeks' gestation make up the largest subgroup of preterm infants and contribute to more than 80% of premature births in the United States. There is increasing evidence that both MPT and LPT infants are at increased risk of neurologic impairments, developmental disabilities, school failure, and behavior and psychiatric problems. Population studies suggest that for each 1 week decrease in gestational age below 39 weeks, there are stepwise increases in adverse outcomes after adjusting for confounders.

Hospital Readmissions and Emergency Department Visits in Moderate Preterm, Late Preterm, and Early Term Infants

753

Michael W. Kuzniewicz, Sarah-Jane Parker, Alina Schnake-Mahl, and Gabriel J. Escobar

The increased vulnerability of late preterm infants is no longer a novel concept in neonatology, with many studies documenting excess morbidity and mortality in these infants during the birth hospitalization. Because outcomes related to gestational age constitute a continuum, it is important to analyze data from the gestational age groups that bookend late preterm infants infants–moderate preterm infants (31–32 weeks) and early term infants (37–38 weeks). This article evaluates hospital readmissions and emergency department visits in the first 30 days after discharge from birth hospitalization in a large cohort of infants greater than or equal to 31 weeks' gestation.

Quality Initiatives Related to Moderately Preterm, Late Preterm, and Early Term Births   777

Andrea N. Trembath, Jay D. Iams, and Michele Walsh

Most premature infants born in the United States each year are classified as either moderately preterm (MPT) or late preterm (LPT) infants. Unnecessary variation in care and lack of evidence-based practices may contribute to the morbidities of prematurity. Quality-improvement (QI) initiatives designed for neonates have primarily focused on extremely low-gestational-age newborns. However, the lessons learned in this group of infants could be applied to decreasing unnecessary variation among MPT and LPT infants. Practice variation in the timing of nonindicated preterm deliveries, the use of progesterone, respiratory care practices, feeding management, and discharge planning are particularly in need of QI.

Moderately Preterm, Late Preterm and Early Term Infants: Research Needs   791

Tonse N.K. Raju

In spite of increased appreciation that all preterm infants and early term infants are at higher risk for mortality and morbidities compared with their term counterparts, there are many knowledge gaps affecting optimal clinical care for this vulnerable population. This article presents a research agenda focusing on the systems biology, epidemiology, and clinical and translational sciences on this topic.

Index   799

PROGRAM OBJECTIVE

The goal of *Clinics in Perinatology* is to keep practicing perinatologists, neonatologists, obstetricians, practicing physicians and residents up to date with current clinical practice in perinatology by providing timely articles reviewing the state of the art in patient care.

TARGET AUDIENCE:

Perinatologists, neonatologists, obstetricians, practicing physicians, residents and healthcare professionals who provide patient care utilizing findings from *Clinics in Perinatology*.

LEARNING OBJECTIVES

Upon completion of this activity, participants will be able to:
1. Describe the epidemiology of moderate preterm, late preterm and early term delivery.
2. Discuss jaundice and kernicterus in the moderately preterm infant.
3. Identify long-term outcomes of moderately preterm, late pre-term and early term infants.

ACCREDITATION

The Elsevier Office of Continuing Medical Education (EOCME) is accredited by the Accreditation Council for Continuing Medical Education (ACCME) to provide continuing medical education for physicians.

The EOCME designates this enduringmaterial for a maximum of 15 *AMA PRA Category 1 Credit*(s)™. Physicians should claim only the credit commensurate with the extent of their participation in the activity.

All other health care professionals requesting continuing education credit for this enduring material will be issued a certificate of participation.

DISCLOSURE OF CONFLICTS OF INTEREST

The EOCME assesses conflict of interest with its instructors, faculty, planners, and other individuals who are in a position to control the content of CME activities. All relevant conflicts of interest that are identified are thoroughly vetted by EOCME for fair balance, scientific objectivity, and patient care recommendations. EOCME is committed to providing its learners with CME activities that promote improvements or quality in healthcare and not a specific proprietary business or a commercial interest.

The planning committee, staff, authors and editors listed below have identified no financial relationships or relationships to products or devices they or their spouse/life partner have with commercial interest related to the content of this CME activity:
Cande Ananth, PhD, MPH; Vinod Bhutani, MD; Nicole Congleton; Sean F. Edmunds, MD; Janet Engstrom, PhD; Gabriel Escobar, MD; Alexander Friedman, MD; Cynthia Gyamfi-Bannerman, MD; Robin Haynes, PhD; Kerry Holland; Brynne Hunter; Jay Iams, MD; Lucky Jain, MD, MBA; Hannah Kinney, MD; Michael W. Kuzniewicz, MD, MPH; Abbot Laptook, MD; Sandy Lavery; Jill McNair; Palani Murugesan; Sarah-Jane Parker; Aloka Patel, MD; Tonse Raju, MD, DCH; Alina Schnake-Mahl; Rakeshy Sahni; Robert Silver, MD; Robert Sinkin, MD, MPH; Lynn A. Sleeper, ScD; Jonathan R. Swanson, MD; Andrea N. Trembath, MD, MPH; Betty Vohr, MD; Joseph J. Volpe, MD; Matthew B. Wallenstein, MD; Michele Walsh, MD, FAAP; Karen L. Wright, PhD, NNP-BC.

The planning committee, staff, authors and editors listed below have identified financial relationships or relationships to products or devices they or their spouse/life partner have with commercial interest related to the content of this CME activity:
Ashley Darcy Mahoney, PhD, NNP-BC, RN is on speakers bureau for Ikaria, Inc.
Paula P. Meier, PhD, RN, FAAN has a research grant and is a consultant/advisor for Medela, Inc.
Richard Polin, MD is a consultant/advisor for Discovery Labs, Inc.

UNAPPROVED/OFF-LABEL USE DISCLOSURE

The EOCME requires CME faculty to disclose to the participants:
1. When products or procedures being discussed are off-label, unlabelled, experimental, and/or investigational (not US Food and Drug Administration (FDA) approved); and
2. Any limitations on the information presented, such as data that are preliminary or that represent ongoing research, interim analyses, and/or unsupported opinions. Faculty may discuss information about pharmaceutical agents that is outside of FDA-approved labelling. This information is intended solely for CME and is not intended to promote off-label use of these medications. If you have any questions, contact the medical affairs department of the manufacturer for the most recent prescribing information.

TO ENROLL

To enroll in the *Clinics in Perinatology* Continuing Medical Education program, call customer service at 1-800-654-2452 or sign up online at http://www.theclinics.com/home/cme. The CME program is available to subscribers for an additional annual fee of $212 USD.

METHOD OF PARTICIPATION

In order to claim credit, participants must complete the following:

1. Complete enrolment as indicated above.
2. Read the activity.
3. Complete the CME Test and Evaluation. Participants must achieve a score of 70% on the test. All CME Tests and Evaluations must be completed online.

CME INQUIRIES/SPECIAL NEEDS

For all CME inquiries or special needs, please contact elsevierCME@elsevier.com.

CLINICS IN PERINATOLOGY

FORTHCOMING ISSUES

March 2014
Advances in Neonatal Neurology
Praveen Ballabh, and Stephen Back,
Editors

June 2014
Neonatal Nutrition
Brenda Poindexter, and Heidi Karpen,
Editors

September 2014
Renal and Urologic Issues
Larry Greenbaum, and Michelle Rheault,
Editors

RECENT ISSUES

September 2013
Pain Management in the Peripartum Period
Randall P. Flick, and James R. Hebl, *Editors*

June 2013
Retinopathy of Prematurity
Graham E. Quinn, and Alistair R. Fielder,
Editors

March 2013
Necrotizing Enterocolitis
Patricia Wei Denning, and
Akhil Maheshwari, *Editors*

Foreword

The Tug of War Between Stillbirths and Elective Early Births

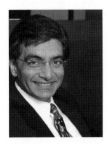

Lucky Jain, MD, MBA
Consulting Editor

In August of 1956, nearly four years before John F. Kennedy became president of the United States, Mrs Jacqueline Kennedy gave birth to a stillborn child. Arabella Kennedy was born lifeless at 36 weeks' gestation; this event had a deep and lasting impact on Mrs Kennedy. It also impacted the actions and approach of her health care team in subsequent pregnancies (and her two preterm deliveries) since the fear of another stillbirth was foremost on Mrs Kennedy's mind. This story, stripped of its celebrity overtones, is still played over and over again, all over the world. The tug of war between stillbirths and early deliveries continues!

In the many decades since then, we have seen a remarkable reduction in *perinatal mortality* rates. These gains, as shown in **Fig. 1**, have come from a reduction in *both* still-births and infant deaths.[1] A further reduction in perinatal mortality could be reliably achieved if the 6000 or so stillbirths each year in the United Stated beyond 39 weeks' gestation could be eliminated. However, that would require elective delivery of all women beyond 39 weeks' gestation, an action that would surely have untoward conse-quences of its own.[2] Although multifactorial in its origin, there is no doubt that the trend toward higher early term births has contributed to additional short-term and long-term neonatal morbidity.[3,4] This is particularly important for elective cesarean births whereby early birth coupled with lack of labor has led to a higher incidence of neonatal transi-tional problems.[5] Perinatal quality initiatives by many states and campaigns for public awareness have led to a measurable decrease in early term cesarean sections. In one recent study, Oshiro and coworkers[6] implemented a rapid-cycle process improve-ment program in 26 participating hospitals to decrease elective scheduled early term deliveries. Over a 12-month period, elective scheduled early term deliveries decreased from 27.8% in the 1st month to 4.8% in the 12th month (**Fig. 2**). Several other states have implemented similar programs and are reporting considerable success.

Clin Perinatol 40 (2013) xv–xviii
http://dx.doi.org/10.1016/j.clp.2013.08.002   **perinatology.theclinics.com**
0095-5108/13/$ – see front matter © 2013 Elsevier Inc. All rights reserved.

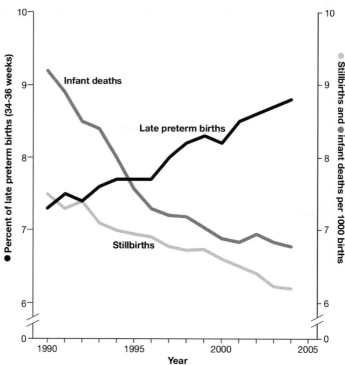

Fig. 1. Trends in late preterm birth, stillbirth, and infant mortality, United States, 1990–2004. The *left axis* shows trends in stillbirth and infant mortality rates; the *right axis* shows trends in late preterm births (34–36 wk). Late preterm birth rates are shown per 100 live births; stillbirth rates, per 1000 total births; and infant death rates, per 1000 live births. (Source: Linked birth and infant death data, National Center for Health Statistics.) (*From* Ananth C, Gyamfi C, Jain L. Characterizing risk profiles of infants who are delivered at late preterm gestations: does it matter? Am J Obstet Gynecol 2008;199:329–31; with permission.)

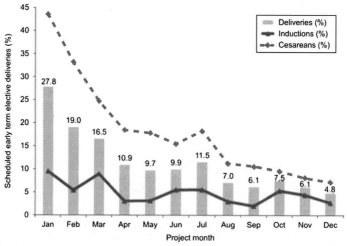

Fig. 2. Scheduled elective singleton early term deliveries by delivery type (%). For each delivery type, the number is the number of scheduled elective singleton early term deliveries and the denominator is the number of all scheduled singleton early term deliveries. (*From* Oshiro B, Kowalewski L, Sappenfield W, et al. A multistate quality improvement program to decrease elective deliveries before 39 weeks of gestation. Obstet Gynecol 2013;121:1025–31; with permission.)

Yet another vexing issue is the complex relationship between the increase in late preterm births and the seemingly symmetrical (and potentially causally related) decline in stillbirths shown in **Fig. 1**. In many countries, particularly the United States and Canada, there has been a significant rise in late preterm births over the last several decades. One study showed that for births between 34 and 36 weeks' gestation, labor induction doubled and cesarean sections increased by 50% between 1990 and 2006.[7] An inevitable question associated with this trend is the potential protective effect of indicated late preterm and early term births on the stillbirth rate. A glimpse into this association was provided in a recent commentary by Kramer and colleagues.[2] As these authors point out, the benefit of reducing stillbirths through early iatrogenic delivery appears to be a logical conclusion; however, this epidemiologic association is not backed by rigorous data. As in **Fig. 3**, a comparison of gestational age–specific stillbirth rates 1992–1994 versus 2003–2005 shows that nearly all of the reduction in stillbirths in the United States appears to be due to a reduction in stillbirths at 40 weeks or more; early scheduled births at less than 39 weeks should

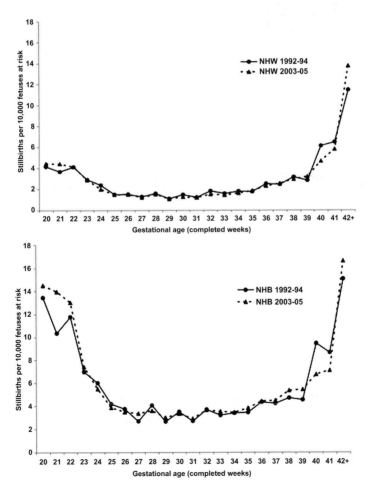

Fig. 3. The rise in late preterm obstetric intervention: has it done more good than harm? (*Adapted from* Kramer MS, Zhang X, Iams J. The rise in late preterm obstetric intervention: has it done more good than harm? Paediatr Perinat Epidemiol 2013;27:7–10; with permission.)

therefore get no credit for this observed improvement and may indeed have done more harm than good.

Dr Raju and I are delighted to have the opportunity (once again) to put together a comprehensive review of late preterm and early term births for the *Clinics in Perinatology*. The many well-written articles in this edition reflect a new level of understanding of this topic; they also reflect a remarkable level of collaborative work between obstetricians and neonatologists and their collective efforts to improve perinatal outcomes.

Lucky Jain, MD, MBA
Department of Pediatrics
Emory Children's Center
Emory University School of Medicine
2015 Uppergate Drive
Atlanta, GA 30322, USA

E-mail address:
ljain@emory.edu

REFERENCES

1. Ananth C, Gyamfi C, Jain L. Characterizing risk profiles of infants who are delivered at late preterm gestations: does it matter? Am J Obstet Gynecol 2008;199: 329–31.
2. Kramer MS, Zhang X, Iams J. The rise in late preterm obstetric intervention: has it done more good than harm? Paediatr Perinat Epidemiol 2013;27:7–10.
3. Ramachandrappa A, Rosenberg ES, Wagoner S, et al. Morbidity and mortality in late preterm infants with severe hypoxic respiratory failure on extra-corporeal membrane oxygenation. J Pediatr 2011;159:192–8.
4. Williams BL, Dunlop AL, Kramer M, et al. Perinatal origins of first grade academic failure: role of prematurity and maternal factors. Pediatrics 2013;131:693–700.
5. Tita A, Landon MB, Spong CY, et al, Eunice Kennedy Shriver NICHD Maternal-Fetal Medicine Units Network. Timing of elective repeat cesarean delivery at term and neonatal outcomes. N Engl J Med 2009;360:111–20.
6. Oshiro B, Kowalewski L, Sappenfield W, et al. A multistate quality improvement program to decrease elective deliveries before 39 weeks of gestation. Obstet Gynecol 2013;121:1025–31.
7. Martin JA, Kermeyer S, Osterman M, et al. Born a bit too early: recent trends in late preterm births. National Center for Health Statistics Data Brief 2009;(24):1–8.

Preface

Late Preterm and Early Term Births

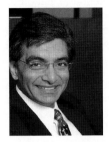 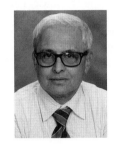

Lucky Jain, MD, MBA   Tonse N.K. Raju, MD, DCH
Editors

In 2006, we edited a special issue of *Clinics in Perinatology* on late preterm births[1]; this was a byproduct of the 2005 workshop on this topic organized by the *Eunice Kennedy Shriver* National Institute of Child Health and Human Development (NICHD). After reviewing the then available meager literature on "near-term infants," the panel concluded that the phrase be replaced with "late preterm" to underscore the fact that infants born between $34^{0/7}$ through $36^{6/7}$ weeks of gestation are immature and vulnerable and require close monitoring, evaluation, and follow-up. The workshop highlighted clinical care priorities and proposed a research agenda.[2,3]

Neither the NICHD workshop panel nor the authors of the 2006 *Clinics in Perinatology* special issue could have predicted the enormous impact these events had on the clinical practice and research concerning late preterm births. The special issue of the *Clinics in Perinatology* promptly sold out and publications began appearing in reputable journals highlighting problems related to late preterm infants. Much progress has been made in this field since then; the National Library of Medicine PubMed page search under "late preterm" will now yield over 300 publications, including original research, review articles, systematic reviews, editorial opinions, and practice guidelines.

The focus on the late preterm infant seems to have uncovered two other understudied gestational age groups, one on each side of the late preterm spectrum: studies related to "moderate preterm" and "early term" births,[4] further highlighted our lack of understanding of consequences of early birth, even if it is by 2 to 3 weeks and the importance of maintaining the gestational maturational continuum.

We are pleased that this issue of the *Clinics in Perinatology* has given us an opportunity to highlight advances in our collective knowledge on late preterm births with an added focus on the less studied moderate preterm group. Many review articles in this issue confirm that late preterm infants are a vulnerable subset of newborn infants and

Clin Perinatol 40 (2013) xix–xx
http://dx.doi.org/10.1016/j.clp.2013.07.013
0095-5108/13/$ – see front matter © 2013 Published by Elsevier Inc.

perinatology.theclinics.com

outline additional research priorities to rectify our knowledge gaps. Articles by leading experts cover epidemiology and recent trends in moderately preterm, late preterm, and early term births. In addition to an extensive discussion of clinical problems related to global immaturity, this issue provides comprehensive information about the causes of late preterm birth and their footprint on short-term and long-term outcomes.[5]

This is an exciting time in clinical medicine for quality improvement and standardized care. Joint efforts by obstetricians, perinatologists, and neonatologists everywhere are beginning to show a measurable effect on late preterm and early term births and have set up a model of care to be emulated for other complex clinical challenges.

Lucky Jain, MD, MBA
Emory University School of Medicine and
Children's Healthcare of Atlanta
2015 Uppergate Drive
Atlanta, GA 30322, USA

Tonse N.K. Raju, MD, DCH
Eunice Kennedy Shriver National Institute
of Child Health and Human Development
National Institutes of Health
6100 Executive Boulevard, Room 4B03, MSC 7510
Bethesda, MD 20892, USA

E-mail addresses:
ljain@emory.edu (L. Jain)
rajut@mail.nih.gov (T.N.K. Raju)

REFERENCES

1. Jain L, Raju TNK. Preface: Late preterm pregnancy and the newborn. Clin Perinatol 2006;33(4):xv–xvi.
2. Raju TN. The problem of late-preterm (near-term) births: a workshop summary. Pediatr Res 2006;60(6):775–6.
3. Engle WA. Morbidity and mortality in late preterm and early term newborns: a continuum. Clin Perinatol 2011;38:493–516.
4. Reddy UM, Bettegowda VR, Dias T, et al. Term pregnancy: a period of heterogeneous risk for infant mortality. Obstet Gynecol 2011;117:1279–87.
5. Spong CY, Mercer BM, D'Alton M, et al. Timing of indicated late-preterm and early-term birth. Obstet Gynecol 2011;118(2 Pt 1):323–33.

Epidemiology of Moderate Preterm, Late Preterm and Early Term Delivery

Cande V. Ananth, PhD, MPH[a,b,*], Alexander M. Friedman, MD[a],
Cynthia Gyamfi-Bannerman, MD[a]

KEYWORDS

- Preterm delivery • Late preterm delivery • Early term delivery • Epidemiology
- Trends

KEY POINTS

- Moderate preterm and late preterm deliveries and, to a lesser extent, early term deliveries, represent a major and growing public health concern.
- Infants delivered at these gestational ages are at considerably increased risk of mortality as well as respiratory and nonrespiratory morbidity.
- Equally, there is evidence that these infants may be at increased risk for long-term neurocognitive and behavioral problems and reduced school performance.
- Efforts to reduce the proportion of deliveries in moderate preterm and late preterm gestations and interventions designed to ameliorate the problems in infants delivered at these gestational ages may be targets worthy of future investigations.

INTRODUCTION

Moderate preterm, late preterm, and early term deliveries represent a major public health concern. Moderate preterm and late preterm deliveries—defined, respectively, as delivery between $32^{0/7}$ and $33^{6/7}$ weeks and between $34^{0/7}$ and $36^{6/7}$ weeks—are associated with adverse short-term and long-term outcomes and an increased health care burden.[1–3] Infants delivered at this gestational age are at disproportionately higher risk for major neonatal complications as well as hospital readmission, major morbidity, and death.[4–10] Infants born in the moderate preterm and late preterm periods are more likely to develop psychiatric disorders[11] and poor fetal growth[12] and experience mental and physical developmental delay.[13,14]

[a] Department of Obstetrics and Gynecology, College of Physicians and Surgeons, Columbia University, 622 West 168th Street, New York, NY 10032, USA; [b] Department of Epidemiology, Joseph L. Mailman School of Public Health, Columbia University, 722 West 168th Street, New York, NY 10032, USA
* Corresponding author. Department of Obstetrics and Gynecology, College of Physicians and Surgeons, Columbia University Medical Center, 622 West 168th Street, New York, NY 10032.
E-mail address: cande.ananth@columbia.edu

Clin Perinatol 40 (2013) 601–610
http://dx.doi.org/10.1016/j.clp.2013.07.001
0095-5108/13/$ – see front matter © 2013 Elsevier Inc. All rights reserved.

perinatology.theclinics.com

Early term delivery—defined as delivery between $37^{0/7}$ and $38^{6/7}$ weeks—is associated with increased risk for many of these same adverse outcomes compared with delivery at $39^{0/7}$ weeks or later. Infants born in the early term period are at increased risk of developing respiratory distress syndrome (RDS), newborn sepsis, and hypoglycemia and require neonatal intensive care unit (NICU) admission and prolonged hospitalization.[15,16] Early term delivery is also associated with increased risk for mortality, increased health care utilization, and adverse long-term outcomes, such as poor growth, learning disorders, and cerebral palsy.[17–19]

Birth prior to 39 weeks may occur as a result of (1) spontaneous early term or preterm labor; (2) prelabor spontaneous rupture of chorioamniotic membranes; (3) maternal and fetal pathology necessitating an iatrogenic delivery; or (4) delivery for nonindicated reasons (ie, because of patient or provider preference).[20] Recent research has validated several clinical strategies to prevent spontaneous preterm birth, including progesterone administration and cervical cerclage for at-risk subgroups.[21–24] National organizations, such as the American Congress of Obstetricians and Gynecologists and the March of Dimes, have led educational and policy initiatives to eliminate the practice of nonindicated delivery prior to 39 weeks' gestational age.[25–28] For many maternal medical and obstetric conditions, however, high-quality data are lacking regarding optimal timing of delivery, and recommendations are based on limited evidence or expert opinion.[20] For conditions that may lead to a catastrophic neonatal or maternal outcome, decision analyses may favor early delivery.[29,30] Some analyses have demonstrated that higher rates of late preterm delivery are associated with decreased stillbirth and neonatal death[31] and restrictions on early term delivery may be associated with increased rates of fetal death approaching term.[27]

Given the public health importance of delivery prior to 39 weeks' gestational age, the purpose of this review is to determine the prevalence and trends of moderate preterm, late preterm, and early term deliveries. In addition, this article presents data on the epidemiology of deliveries in the moderate preterm, late preterm, and early term gestation window as well as neonatal and infant mortality and morbidity.

PREVALENCE RATES AND TEMPORAL TRENDS OF MODERATE PRETERM, LATE PRETERM, AND EARLY TERM DELIVERIES

Increases in the prevalence of early term delivery have been modest relative to increases in the late preterm and early term periods. In 2008, deliveries at 32 to 33, 34 to 36, and 37 to 38 weeks accounted for 1.2%, 7.5%, and 29.7%, respectively, of all births in the United States (**Fig. 1**)—these proportions have all increased over the past 2 decades in the United States. In 1995, the proportions of deliveries at 32 to 33, 34 to 36, and 37 to 38 weeks were 1.1%, 6.2%, and 20.6%, respectively (**Fig. 2**). The absolute increases in deliveries in the moderate preterm and late preterm (34–36 weeks) periods were 0.1% and 1.3%, respectively, whereas early term delivery increased 9.1%. Evidence suggests these changes are primarily due to more frequent obstetric intervention, with an increase in the proportion of deliveries in one gestational age window leading to a reduction of another. The increase in delivery at 37 to 38 weeks' gestational age is the result of a shift away from delivery at 39 weeks or greater gestational age. National-level data suggest that similar trends across the developed world mirror those in the United States, with increased prevalence of late preterm birth. A meta-analysis of deliveries in the United States, Canada, and 26 other European countries found that the prevalence of moderate preterm and late preterm birth ($32^{0/7}$ to $36^{6/7}$ days) ranged from 4.4% to 10.0%.[31] Variation in

Gestational age distribution, 2008

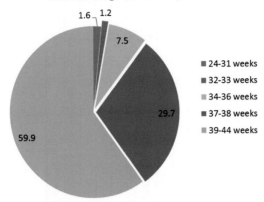

Fig. 1. Proportion of deliveries at 24–31, 32–33, 34–36, 37–38, and 39–44 weeks in the United States among live births in 2008.

reported prevalence of moderate preterm and late preterm delivery may be due in part to whether multiple gestations are included in analyses (**Table 1**).

RECURRENCE OF MODERATE PRETERM AND LATE PRETERM DELIVERIES

Data regarding the recurrence risks of moderate preterm and late preterm delivery are sparse whereas those related to early term delivery remain unexplored. Ananth and colleagues[32] published data on the recurrence of moderate preterm and late preterm delivery in a cohort of 153,000 women with the first 2 consecutive pregnancies in Missouri (1989–1997). Women who delivered at 32 to 33 and 34 to 36 weeks in their first pregnancy were more likely to deliver at the same gestation window in the subsequent pregnancy (**Table 2**). In addition, these increased recurrence risks

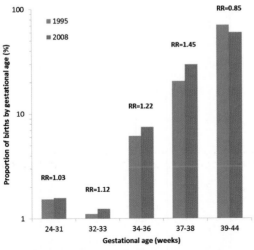

Fig. 2. Changes in the proportion of deliveries at 24–31, 32–33, 34–36, 37–38, and 39–44 weeks in the United States among singleton live births between 1995 and 2008.

Table 1
Reports detailing prevalence rates of moderate preterm, late preterm delivery, and early term delivery

Author	Study Year(s)	Country	Design	Prevalence Rates (%)		
				Moderate Preterm	Late Preterm	Early Term
Baroutis et al,[33] 2013	1980–2008	Greece	Cohort	1.1	7.5	NA
Norman et al,[34] 2009	1980–2004	Scotland	Cohort	6.6 (Moderate–late preterm)		NA
Lisonkova et al,[31] 2012	2004	US, Canada, Europe	Meta-analysis	4.4–10.0 (Moderate–late preterm)		NA
Martin et al,[35] 2009	1990–2006	United States	Cohort	1.6	9.1	28.9
Joseph et al,[36] 2002	1985–1997	Canada	Cohort	1.1	7.4	NA
Barros et al,[37] 2006	1985–2003	Central/South America	Cohort			
Ananth et al,[38] 2005	1989–2000	United States	Cohort	10.0–10.4 (Moderate–late preterm)		NA
Langhoff-Roos et al,[39] 2006	1995–2004	Finland	Cohort	5.4 (Moderate–late preterm)		NA

Abbreviation: NA, data not available.

Table 2
Recurrence of the timing of preterm delivery in the second pregnancy based on severity and clinical subtype of preterm delivery in the first pregnancy

Preterm Delivery in First Pregnancy	Preterm Delivery in the Second Singleton Pregnancy: Adjusted Odds Ratio (95% Confidence Interval)					
	28–31 wk		32–33 wk		34–36 wk	
	Spontaneous	Indicated	Spontaneous	Indicated	Spontaneous	Indicated
28–31 wk						
Spontaneous	6.1 (3.3, 11.5)	3.0 (1.6, 5.7)	3.8 (2.7, 5.4)	2.1 (1.0, 4.4)	2.9 (2.4, 3.5)	2.1 (1.4, 3.1)
Indicated	3.4 (1.7, 6.7)	15.3 (9.8, 24.0)	1.7 (0.7, 3.8)	12.8 (7.8, 20.9)	0.9 (0.6, 1.4)	9.6 (7.4, 12.6)
32–33 wk						
Spontaneous	5.8 (4.2, 8.0)	2.7 (1.5, 5.0)	5.9 (4.6, 7.2)	2.6 (1.4, 4.8)	3.0 (2.5, 3.5)	1.7 (1.2, 2.4)
Indicated	1.7 (0.6, 4.5)	8.2 (4.5, 14.7)	0.9 (0.3, 2.8)	11.9 (7.3, 19.3)	1.1 (0.7, 1.7)	10.2 (7.9, 13.1)
34–36 wk						
Spontaneous	3.0 (2.4, 3.6)	2.1 (1.6, 2.9)	3.1 (2.6, 3.6)	1.9 (1.4, 2.6)	3.0 (2.8, 3.2)	1.0 (0.8, 1.2)
Indicated	1.9 (1.2, 2.9)	5.3 (3.8, 7.5)	0.8 (0.4, 1.4)	6.2 (4.6, 8.5)	0.8 (0.6, 1.0)	5.8 (5.0, 6.7)

Odds ratios are adjusted for maternal age (second birth), education (second birth), marital status, race/ethnicity, smoking, and alcohol use, prepregnancy body mass index, and lack of or late initiation of prenatal care and interpregnancy interval.

Adapted from Ananth CV, Getahun D, Peltier MR, et al. Recurrence of spontaneous versus medically indicated preterm birth. Am J Obstet Gynecol 2006;195(3):648; with permission.

persisted based on the underlying clinical subtype of preterm delivery. For instance, if women delivered at 32 to 33 weeks spontaneously in the first pregnancy, the recurrence risk of delivering at 32 to 33 weeks in the next pregnancy was higher for spontaneous delivery than for indicated delivery at 32 to 33 weeks in the second pregnancy. This pattern persisted based in both severity of preterm delivery and the underlying precipitating events that led to delivery at preterm gestations.

RISK FACTORS FOR MODERATE PRETERM, LATE PRETERM, AND EARLY TERM DELIVERIES

A review of international epidemiologic data (see **Table 1**) on moderate preterm, late preterm, and early term delivery demonstrates several important trends. Although spontaneous late preterm deliveries account for the majority of births before 37 weeks' gestational age, indicated birth between $34^{0/7}$ and $36^{6/7}$ weeks has increased substantially over the past 3 decades and represents a significant contributing factor to the overall increase in preterm delivery rates. This relative increase of indicated moderate preterm and late preterm delivery may continue to increase because (1) obstetric management strategies to decrease preterm delivery affect spontaneous but not indicated preterm birth and (2) maternal medical (chronic) conditions and risk factors that predispose to indicated preterm birth are generally increasing. Secular trends in delivery between $37^{0/7}$ to $38^{6/7}$ weeks are generally less well described because early term birth has only recently been identified as a public health concern. The proportion of infants born within this group may be increasing, however, secondary to the same maternal health and pregnancy factors leading to indicated late preterm delivery.[31,33–39]

ADVERSE INFANT OUTCOMES ASSOCIATED WITH DELIVERY FROM 32 TO 38 WEEKS' GESTATION
Moderate Preterm Birth (32–33 Weeks)

Moderately preterm infants are at significantly increased risk for morbidity compared with babies born at later gestational ages.[40] A study of more than 65,000 infants showed respiratory and nonrespiratory morbidity were inversely related to gestational age, a trend persisting into the moderate preterm and late preterm period.[41] Moderately preterm infants are at increased risk for hospital readmission.[41] Boyce and colleagues[42] found that infants born from 33 to 36 weeks had similar rates of admission for severe respiratory syncytial virus infection compared with infants born at less than 32 weeks. Neonatal risk may be a result of both prematurity and the obstetric condition that led to delivery. Moderate preterm infants delivered in the setting of preterm premature rupture of membranes or a maternal or fetal indication experienced higher rates of neonatal mortality compared with those delivered after preterm labor with intact membranes.[43]

Late Preterm Birth (34–36 Weeks)

Late preterm birth is a major risk factor for neonatal morbidity. A study including more than 20,000 late preterm births found ventilator use and transient tachypnea of newborns more frequent in late preterm infants compared with term infants.[44] A study by Yoder and colleagues[45] found that respiratory morbidity from all causes decreased as gestational age increased: 34 weeks (22%), 35 weeks (8.5%), 36 weeks (3.9%), and 39 weeks (0.7%). In analysis of late preterm deliveries, the Consortium on Safe Labor found that RDS, transient tachypnea of the newborn, pneumonia, respiratory failure, surfactant use, and ventilator use increased as gestational age at delivery decreased. RDS was 40-fold higher at 34 weeks compared with 39 weeks, whereas NICU admission was 11 times more common at 34 weeks (67.4%) compared with 39 weeks (6.1%).[46] Major medical complications, including intraventricular hemorrhage, necrotizing enterocolitis, patent ductus arteriosus, and sepsis, are more common in late preterm than term infants. Late preterm neonates are at increased risk for infant mortality. Reddy[47] found neonatal mortality rates at 34, 35, and 36 weeks (7.1, 4.8, and 2.8 per 1000 deliveries, respectively) were increased compared with delivery at term.[47] Tomashek and colleagues[9] found late preterm infants had respective increases in early, late, and overall infant mortality by factors of 6, 2, and 3, respectively.

Early Term Birth (37–38 Weeks)

Early term birth is associated with increased respiratory morbidity. Data from the Consortium on Safe Labor[46] found that compared with delivery at 39 weeks, delivery at 37 weeks led to a 3.1-fold increase in RDS, a 2.5-fold increase in transient tachypnea of the newborn, a 1.7-fold increase in pneumonia, a 2.8-fold increase in respiratory failure, a 4.8-fold increase in surfactant use, and a 2.8-fold increase in ventilator use. Tita and colleagues[15] evaluated neonatal outcomes after term elective cesarean delivery in the absence of maternal or neonatal indications. More than a third (35.8%) of deliveries were performed prior to 39 weeks' gestation with an attributable risk of morbidity for delivery at 37 weeks of 48% compared with attributable risk of 27% at 38 weeks. Morbidity at $38^{4/7}$ to $38^{6/7}$ weeks remained significantly increased compared with delivery at 39 weeks. Clark and colleagues[16] evaluated early elective term delivery within the Hospital Corporation of America. Elective deliveries at 37 weeks and 38 weeks were associated with respective NICU admission rates of 17.8% and 8%. Delivery at or beyond 39 weeks resulted in significantly lower risk of NICU admission (4.6%).

Fetal lung maturity testing has not been shown to effectively predict respiratory morbidity in late preterm and early term infants and the use of fetal lung maturity testing is questionable for early term infants. Bates and colleagues[48] found that composite adverse neonatal outcomes were worse in infants delivered between 36 weeks and 38 weeks after mature fetal pulmonary indices compared with infants born at 39 and 40 weeks. Other studies have confirmed these findings.[49] Late preterm birth is a risk factor for neonatal and infant mortality. Reddy and colleagues[47] found that at 37 and 38 weeks, neonatal mortality rates were 1.7 per 1000 and 1.0 per 1000, respectively, and infant mortality rates were 4.1 per 1000 and 2.7 per 1000, respectively. These rates are significantly higher than for infants born at 39 weeks.[47]

SUMMARY

Moderate preterm and late preterm deliveries and, to a lesser extent, early term deliveries, represent a major and growing public health concern. Infants delivered at these gestational ages are at considerably increased risk of mortality as well as respiratory and nonrespiratory morbidity. Equally, there is evidence that these infants may be at increased risk long-term neurocognitive and behavioral problems and reduced school performance.[50–53] Efforts to reduce proportion of deliveries in moderate term and late preterm gestations and interventions designed to ameliorate the problems in infants delivered at these gestational ages may be targets worthy of future investigations.

REFERENCES

1. Gilbert WM, Nesbitt TS, Danielsen B. The cost of prematurity: quantification by gestational age and birth weight. Obstet Gynecol 2003;102(3):488–92.

2. Clements KM, Barfield WD, Ayadi MF, et al. Preterm birth-associated cost of early intervention services: an analysis by gestational age. Pediatrics 2007; 119(4):e866–74.
3. Petrou S, Mehta Z, Hockley C, et al. The impact of preterm birth on hospital inpatient admissions and costs during the first 5 years of life. Pediatrics 2003; 112(6 Pt 1):1290–7.
4. Shapiro-Mendoza CK, Tomashek KM, Kotelchuck M, et al. Effect of late-preterm birth and maternal medical conditions on newborn morbidity risk. Pediatrics 2008;121(2):e223–32.
5. Wang ML, Dorer DJ, Fleming MP, et al. Clinical outcomes of near-term infants. Pediatrics 2004;114(2):372–6.
6. Kramer MS, Demissie K, Yang H, et al. The contribution of mild and moderate preterm birth to infant mortality. Fetal and Infant Health Study Group of the Canadian Perinatal Surveillance System. JAMA 2000;284(7):843–9.
7. Escobar GJ, Joffe S, Gardner MN, et al. Rehospitalization in the first two weeks after discharge from the neonatal intensive care unit. Pediatrics 1999;104(1):e2.
8. Escobar GJ, Clark RH, Greene JD. Short-term outcomes of infants born at 35 and 36 weeks gestation: we need to ask more questions. Semin Perinatol 2006;30(1):28–33.
9. Tomashek KM, Shapiro-Mendoza CK, Davidoff MJ, et al. Differences in mortality between late-preterm and term singleton infants in the United States, 1995-2002. J Pediatr 2007;151(5):450–6, 456.e451.
10. Bastek JA, Sammel MD, Pare E, et al. Adverse neonatal outcomes: examining the risks between preterm, late preterm, and term infants. Am J Obstet Gynecol 2008;199(4):367.e361–8.
11. Rogers CE, Lenze SN, Luby JL. Late preterm birth, maternal depression, and risk of preschool psychiatric disorders. J Am Acad Child Adolesc Psychiatry 2013;52(3):309–18.
12. Santos IS, Matijasevich A, Domingues MR, et al. Late preterm birth is a risk factor for growth faltering in early childhood: a cohort study. BMC Pediatr 2009;9:71.
13. Woythaler MA, McCormick MC, Smith VC. Late preterm infants have worse 24-month neurodevelopmental outcomes than term infants. Pediatrics 2011; 127(3):e622–9.
14. Morse SB, Zheng H, Tang Y, et al. Early school-age outcomes of late preterm infants. Pediatrics 2009;123(4):e622–9.
15. Tita AT, Landon MB, Spong CY, et al. Timing of elective repeat cesarean delivery at term and neonatal outcomes. N Engl J Med 2009;360(2):111–20.
16. Clark SL, Miller DD, Belfort MA, et al. Neonatal and maternal outcomes associated with elective term delivery. Am J Obstet Gynecol 2009;200(2):156.e151–4.
17. Crump C, Sundquist K, Winkleby MA, et al. Early-term birth (37-38 weeks) and mortality in young adulthood. Epidemiology 2013;24(2):270–6.
18. Barros FC, Rossello JL, Matijasevich A, et al. Gestational age at birth and morbidity, mortality, and growth in the first 4 years of life: findings from three birth cohorts in Southern Brazil. BMC Pediatr 2012;12:169.
19. Zapolski TC, Guller L, Smith GT. Construct validation theory applied to the study of personality dysfunction. J Pers 2012;80(6):1507–31.
20. Spong CY, Mercer BM, D'Alton M, et al. Timing of indicated late-preterm and early-term birth. Obstet Gynecol 2011;118(2 Pt 1):323–33.
21. Fonseca EB, Celik E, Parra M, et al, Fetal Medicine Foundation Second Trimester Screening G. Progesterone and the risk of preterm birth among women with a short cervix. N Engl J Med 2007;357(5):462–9.

22. Owen J, Hankins G, Iams JD, et al. Multicenter randomized trial of cerclage for preterm birth prevention in high-risk women with shortened midtrimester cervical length. Am J Obstet Gynecol 2009;201(4):375.e371–8.

23. Hassan SS, Romero R, Vidyadhari D, et al. Vaginal progesterone reduces the rate of preterm birth in women with a sonographic short cervix: a multicenter, randomized, double-blind, placebo-controlled trial. Ultrasound Obstet Gynecol 2011;38(1):18–31.

24. Meis PJ, Klebanoff M, Thom E, et al. Prevention of recurrent preterm delivery by 17 alpha-hydroxyprogesterone caproate. N Engl J Med 2003;348(24):2379–85.

25. Donovan EF, Lannon C, Bailit J, et al. A statewide initiative to reduce inappropriate scheduled births at 36(0/7)-38(6/7) weeks' gestation. Am J Obstet Gynecol 2010;202(3):243.e241–8.

26. Oshiro BT, Henry E, Wilson J, et al. Decreasing elective deliveries before 39 weeks of gestation in an integrated health care system. Obstet Gynecol 2009; 113(4):804–11.

27. Ehrenthal DB, Hoffman MK, Jiang X, et al. Neonatal outcomes after implementation of guidelines limiting elective delivery before 39 weeks of gestation. Obstet Gynecol 2011;118(5):1047–55.

28. Ashton DM. Elective delivery at less than 39 weeks. Curr Opin Obstet Gynecol 2010;22(6):506–10.

29. Robinson BK, Grobman WA. Effectiveness of timing strategies for delivery of individuals with placenta previa and accreta. Obstet Gynecol 2010;116(4): 835–42.

30. Robinson BK, Grobman WA. Effectiveness of timing strategies for delivery of individuals with vasa previa. Obstet Gynecol 2011;117(3):542–9.

31. Lisonkova S, Sabr Y, Butler B, et al. International comparisons of preterm birth: higher rates of late preterm birth are associated with lower rates of stillbirth and neonatal death. BJOG 2012;119(13):1630–9.

32. Ananth CV, Getahun D, Peltier MR, et al. Recurrence of spontaneous versus medically indicated preterm birth. Am J Obstet Gynecol 2006;195(3):643–50.

33. Baroutis G, Mousiolis A, Mesogitis S, et al. Preterm birth trends in Greece, 1980-2008: a rising concern. Acta Obstet Gynecol Scand 2013;92(5):575–82.

34. Norman JE, Mackenzie F, Owen P, et al. Progesterone for the prevention of preterm birth in twin pregnancy (STOPPIT): a randomised, double-blind, placebo-controlled study and meta-analysis. Lancet 2009;373(9680):2034–40.

35. Martin JA, Kirmeyer S, Osterman M, et al. Born a bit too early: recent trends in late preterm births. NCHS Data Brief 2009;(24):1–8.

36. Joseph KS, Demissie K, Kramer MS. Obstetric intervention, stillbirth, and preterm birth. Semin Perinatol 2002;26(4):250–9.

37. Barros FC, Velez Mdel P. Temporal trends of preterm birth subtypes and neonatal outcomes. Obstet Gynecol 2006;107(5):1035–41.

38. Ananth CV, Joseph KS, Oyelese Y, et al. Trends in preterm birth and perinatal mortality among singletons: United States, 1989 through 2000. Obstet Gynecol 2005;105(5 Pt 1):1084–91.

39. Langhoff-Roos J, Kesmodel U, Jacobsson B, et al. Spontaneous preterm delivery in primiparous women at low risk in Denmark: population based study. BMJ 2006;332(7547):937–9.

40. Shapiro-Mendoza CK, Lackritz EM. Epidemiology of late and moderate preterm birth. Semin Fetal Neonatal Med 2012;17(3):120–5.

41. Rubaltelli FF, Bonafe L, Tangucci M, et al. Epidemiology of neonatal acute respiratory disorders. A multicenter study on incidence and fatality rates of

neonatal acute respiratory disorders according to gestational age, maternal age, pregnancy complications and type of delivery. Italian Group of Neonatal Pneumology. Biol Neonate 1998;74(1):7–15.

42. Boyce TG, Mellen BG, Mitchel EF Jr, et al. Rates of hospitalization for respiratory syncytial virus infection among children in medicaid. J Pediatr 2000;137(6): 865–70.

43. Chen A, Feresu SA, Barsoom MJ. Heterogeneity of preterm birth subtypes in relation to neonatal death. Obstet Gynecol 2009;114(3):516–22.

44. McIntire DD, Leveno KJ. Neonatal mortality and morbidity rates in late preterm births compared with births at term. Obstet Gynecol 2008;111(1):35–41.

45. Yoder BA, Gordon MC, Barth WH Jr. Late-preterm birth: does the changing obstetric paradigm alter the epidemiology of respiratory complications? Obstet Gynecol 2008;111(4):814–22.

46. Consortium on Safe Labor, Hibbard JU, Wilkins I, et al. Respiratory morbidity in late preterm births. JAMA 2010;304(4):419–25.

47. Reddy UM, Ko CW, Raju TN, et al. Delivery indications at late-preterm gestations and infant mortality rates in the United States. Pediatrics 2009;124(1):234–40.

48. Bates E, Rouse DJ, Mann ML, et al. Neonatal outcomes after demonstrated fetal lung maturity before 39 weeks of gestation. Obstet Gynecol 2010;116(6): 1288–95.

49. Kamath BD, Marcotte MP, DeFranco EA. Neonatal morbidity after documented fetal lung maturity in late preterm and early term infants. Am J Obstet Gynecol 2011;204(6):518.e511–8.

50. Williams BL, Dunlop AL, Kramer M, et al. Perinatal origins of first-grade academic failure: role of prematurity and maternal factors. Pediatrics 2013;131(4): 693–700.

51. Lipkind HS, Slopen ME, Pfeiffer MR, et al. School-age outcomes of late preterm infants in New York City. Am J Obstet Gynecol 2012;206(3):222.e221–6.

52. Odd DE, Emond A, Whitelaw A. Long-term cognitive outcomes of infants born moderately and late preterm. Dev Med Child Neurol 2012;54(8):704–9.

53. Kerstjens JM, de Winter AF, Sollie KM, et al. Maternal and pregnancy-related factors associated with developmental delay in moderately preterm-born children. Obstet Gynecol 2013;121(4):727–33.

Stillbirth Reduction Efforts and Impact on Early Births

Sean F. Edmunds, MD, Robert M. Silver, MD*

KEYWORDS

- Stillbirth • Placental insufficiency • Late preterm birth • Early term birth

KEY POINTS

- Despite the medical risks of intentional delivery of a pregnancy before 39 weeks' gestation, it is considered to be justified in some cases to reduce the risk of stillbirth.
- The stillbirth rate has decreased dramatically over the past 60 years, in part because of improved management of conditions associated with an increased risk for stillbirth.
- Examples of such conditions include hypertensive disorders of pregnancy, diabetes, intrauterine growth restriction, placental abnormalities, some birth defects, multiple gestation, and abnormal fetal testing.
- The optimal gestational age for delivery in many of these conditions is uncertain.
- There is no evidence that delivery before 39 weeks' gestation reduces the risk of recurrent stillbirth.

INTRODUCTION

The emotional impact of stillbirth, defined as death of the fetus at 20 or more weeks' gestation, is considerable for families and clinicians. In 2006 the United States reported 25,972 stillbirths, nearly equaling the number of reported infant deaths.[1] Stillbirth is responsible for around one-half of perinatal deaths and is almost 10 times more frequent than sudden infant death syndrome.[2,3]

The rate of stillbirth in the United States has dropped dramatically over the past 100 years, decreasing almost 100-fold. This trend has been due to major improvements in the care of conditions such as RhD alloimmunization, diabetes, and preeclampsia. There has been considerable emphasis on identifying pregnancies at risk for stillbirth and aggressively managing them to avoid stillbirth. In many cases this involves antenatal fetal testing such as nonstress tests, assessment of amniotic fluid index, biophysical profile, and Doppler velocimetry studies. Each of these tests

Department of Obstetrics & Gynecology, University of Utah School of Medicine, 30 North 1900 East 2B200 SOM, Salt Lake City, UT 84132, USA
* Corresponding author.
E-mail address: robert.silver@hsc.utah.edu

Clin Perinatol 40 (2013) 611–628
http://dx.doi.org/10.1016/j.clp.2013.07.002   perinatology.theclinics.com
0095-5108/13/$ – see front matter © 2013 Elsevier Inc. All rights reserved.

identifies fetuses at increased risk for stillbirth. However, they are only effective because such fetuses are then delivered before a stillbirth occurs. The rates of stillbirth have generally plateaued over the past 40 years, but there has been a slight decrease during the past 20 years, primarily attributable to a decrease in late stillbirths occurring after 28 weeks' gestation.[1]

Conversely, preterm birth carries important risks for the neonate, including long-term morbidity and neonatal death.[4–8] These issues are extensively reviewed elsewhere in this issue. This article reviews the pros and cons of late preterm and near term birth for the prevention of stillbirth, as well as generally accepted indications for such deliveries.

IMPLICATIONS OF LATE PRETERM OR EARLY TERM DELIVERY

As seen in **Fig. 1**, over the past 20 years in the United States there has been a decrease in stillbirth after 28 weeks. At the same time, there has been an increase in preterm delivery at 34 to 36 weeks' gestation (**Fig. 2**). Accordingly, there is seemingly well-founded speculation that these 2 trends are directly linked. Moreover, countries with high rates of preterm birth at 32 to 36 weeks' gestation have lower stillbirth and neonatal death rates at and beyond 32 weeks' gestation.[9]

Preterm or early delivery could theoretically limit stillbirth risk. It goes without question that all ongoing pregnancies carry a stillbirth risk, even after the pregnancy reaches term gestation. However, it is known that neonatal mortality and morbidity are increased with preterm and early term birth.[5–8] Thus, the goal of stillbirth reduction must be taken in the context of increased risks of prematurity.

We can gain a better understanding of the risk/benefit ratio of late preterm or early term delivery in reducing stillbirth by examining the prospective fetal mortality rate. By definition, this is the number of fetal deaths at a given gestational age plus fetal deaths that would occur at a later gestational age if the pregnancy remains undelivered per 1000 live births.[10] Accordingly, iatrogenic delivery would prevent stillbirth at that week as well as in subsequent weeks of gestation. Conversely, expectant management of the pregnancy allows for potential stillbirth in that given week, as well as in each subsequent week that delivery does not occur.[10,11] In simple terms, this is the "hazard risk" or "percentage of fetal deaths in ongoing pregnancy."

The prospective fetal mortality rate by gestational age (in weeks) in the United States in 2005 is shown in **Fig. 3**. At 34 to 37 weeks' gestation the mortality rate is 0.23 to

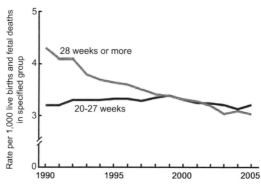

Fig. 1. Fetal mortality rates by period of gestation: United States, 1990 to 2005. (*From* MacDorman MF, Kirmeyer S. Fetal and perinatal mortality, United States, 2005. National vital statistics reports; vol 57 no 8. Hyattsville, MD: National Center for Health Statistics; 2009.)

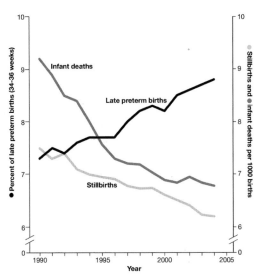

Fig. 2. Trends in late preterm birth, stillbirth, and infant mortality, United States, 1990 to 2004. (*From* Ananth CV, Gyamfi C, Jain L. Characterizing risk profiles of infants who are delivered at late preterm gestations: does it matter? Am J Obstet Gynecol 2008;199:330; with permission.)

0.29 per 1000 births. There is an increase at 38 weeks' gestation to 0.35 per 1000 births. At 39 weeks' gestation it is then 0.4 per 1000 births. A substantial increase does not occur until after 40 weeks' gestation.[10]

An assessment of fetal mortality rates in the United Kingdom between 1978 and 1985 is depicted in **Fig. 4**. As with the data from the United States, a substantial increase in mortality does not occur until after 39 weeks' gestation. Before this gestational age, the rate remains low and relatively stable. Reddy and colleagues[12] evaluated nonanomalous stillbirths in the United States between 2001 and 2002, stratified by maternal age (**Fig. 5**). The results were similar to those of the aforementioned

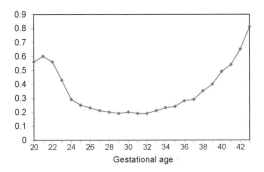

Note: The prospective fetal mortality rate is the number of fetal deaths at a given gestational age per 1,000 live births and fetal deaths at that gestational age or greater

Fig. 3. Prospective fetal mortality rate by single weeks of gestation; United States, 2005. (*From* MacDorman MF, Kirmeyer S. Fetal and perinatal mortality, United States, 2005. National vital statistics reports; vol 57 no 8. Hyattsville, MD: National Center for Health Statistics; 2009.)

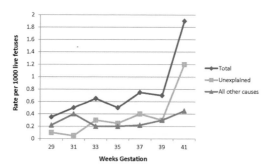

Fig. 4. Stillbirths in the 2 weeks period following each gestational age, per 100 fetuses undelivered at that gestational age. (*From* Yudkin PL, Wood L, Redman CW. Risk of unexplained stillbirth at different gestational ages. Lancet 1987;329:1192–4; with permission.)

studies. Although the same pattern was observed in all age groups, it was most profound in women older than 35 years. The pattern also is more pronounced in cases of unexplained stillbirths.[11]

Unfortunately, there have been few studies analyzing the risk of stillbirth while considering the "competing" risk of neonatal death (due to prematurity) over varying gestational ages. In Scotland, data from 1985 to 1996 were used to create a life-table analysis to determine the cumulative probability of perinatal death (stillbirth and neonatal death within 4 weeks of life combined) for deliveries performed between 37 and 43 weeks' gestation. The lowest cumulative risk for perinatal death occurred at 38 weeks' gestation.[13]

In summary, for the general population, the risk of ongoing stillbirth increases after 38 to 39 weeks' gestation. Of note, specific details regarding obstetric or medical factors are unavailable in these studies. It can be implied, however, that if attempts to

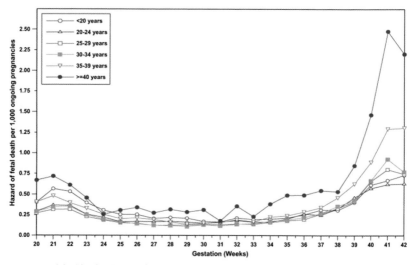

Fig. 5. Hazard (risk) of stillbirth for singleton births without congenital anomalies by gestational age, 2001 to 2002. (*From* Reddy UM, Ko CW, Willinger M. Maternal age and the risk of stillbirth throughout pregnancy in the United States. Am J Obstet Gynecol 2006;195:764–70; with permission.)

lower the stillbirth rate through indicated delivery are to be practiced, the greatest benefit is seen at 39 weeks' gestation or later. The risks associated with premature delivery at 34 to 38 weeks outweigh the risk of stillbirth before 39 weeks' gestation when considering the general population.

This finding has been validated in a recent study by Clark and colleagues,[14] who performed a retrospective cohort study to review quality-improvement initiatives that were aimed at reducing the rate of elective late preterm and near term birth. A total of 27 hospitals from a large health corporation were included in the study, involving 17,000 deliveries over a 3-month period. The following findings are noteworthy:

- Elective delivery at less than 39 weeks' gestation decreased from 9.6% to 4.3% of deliveries.
- There was a 16% reduction in admissions to the neonatal intensive care unit during the study period.
- There was no increase in the rate of stillbirth during this time.[14]

In brief, it is apparent that some late preterm and early term deliveries can be avoided without increasing the stillbirth rate. Moreover, elective (not medically indicated) late preterm and early term deliveries likely cause more harm than good with respect to the general population.

It also is important to consider the avoidance of morbidity other than stillbirth when considering late preterm or early term birth. Pregnancies at risk for stillbirth are also at risk for other adverse obstetric outcomes such as preeclampsia, neonatal encephalopathy, and neonatal death. Most of the conditions that predispose fetuses to stillbirth are associated with placental insufficiency, which in severe cases leads to stillbirth. However, milder cases may result in live births complicated by problems caused by decreased blood flow to the fetus. Hence, iatrogenic preterm birth before the fetus suffers from profound hypoxia may decrease adverse obstetric and neonatal outcomes other than stillbirth.

These data address the competing risks of preterm birth and stillbirth in the general population. However, there are several maternal and fetal conditions that substantially increase the risk of stillbirth. In such cases, the risk may be so high as to justify the downside of iatrogenic preterm birth.

PREGNANCIES AT INCREASED RISK FOR STILLBIRTH
Hypertension

Hypertensive disorders including chronic hypertension, preeclampsia, and pregnancy-induced hypertension are major risk factors for stillbirth. Indeed, these conditions still account for about 10% of stillbirths.[15] Fortunately, in the United States the risk of stillbirth associated with hypertensive disorders has decreased dramatically over the past 50 years, attributable in large part to iatrogenic preterm birth before maternal and/or fetal deterioration and possible stillbirth occur. In addition, antenatal testing and improved control of maternal blood pressure has contributed to a decreased risk of stillbirth associated with maternal hypertension.

It is generally accepted that pregnancies complicated by severe preeclampsia or gestational hypertension should be delivered at no later than 34 weeks' gestation.[16] Also, most authorities advise delivery between 39 and 40 weeks' gestation for women with well-controlled chronic hypertension with no evidence of fetal compromise or superimposed preeclampsia/gestational hypertension. Thus, controversy exists for pregnancies complicated by mild preeclampsia or gestational hypertension between 34 and 39 weeks' gestation.

The management of such patients has been controversial, with authorities recommending delivery between 37 and 40 weeks' gestation in stable cases.[17] Fortunately, the HYPITAT investigators recently conducted a randomized, controlled clinical trial comparing induction of labor with expectant management of pregnancies complicated by preeclampsia or pregnancy-induced hypertension between 36 and 42 weeks' gestation.[18] Women were randomized to induction of labor (n = 377) or expectant management (n = 379), with close surveillance and delivery for worsening status. Women randomized to induction had a lower rate of a composite maternal adverse outcome (31% vs 44%; relative risk 0.71, 95% confidence interval [CI] 0.59–0.86).[18] There was no difference in neonatal outcomes or rates of cesarean delivery between groups.[18] In fact, the cesarean rate was lower in nulliparous women and in women with "unfavorable cervixes" in the induction group.[18] These findings are important because the primary justifications for expectant management of women with hypertension have been potential increases in the rates of cesarean delivery and neonatal morbidity. These data support induction of labor (or cesarean delivery) in all cases of pregnancies complicated by preeclampsia or gestational hypertension at or beyond 37 weeks' gestation.

Diabetes

Pregnancies complicated by diabetes also are at increased risk for stillbirth. Taken together, diabetes confers a 2- to 4-fold increase in stillbirth risk.[19–21] This point is particularly important because rates of obesity and, consequently, diabetes, are increasing.[22,23] As with hypertension, the rate of stillbirth associated with diabetes has decreased substantially in the past 50 years because of improved glycemic control, antepartum testing, and iatrogenic preterm birth in selected cases.

The optimal timing of delivery for women with diabetes remains controversial, and data from randomized clinical trials are lacking. It is also important to distinguish between pregestational (either type 1 or 2) and gestational diabetes. In a population-based study, women with type 1 pregestational diabetes had a 1.5% rate of stillbirth compared with 0.3% in women without diabetes.[24] Others have confirmed an approximately 3-fold increase in the risk for stillbirth in women with pregestational diabetes.[19–21] Moreover, this risk increases with increasing gestational age, beginning at 34 weeks' gestation.[25] In addition, a considerable proportion of stillbirths in diabetic pregnancies occur after 37 weeks' gestation.[26–28] It thus follows that delivery after 37 weeks' gestation may prevent some cases of stillbirth.

Conversely, the vast majority of infants born to women with diabetes are live-born. Accordingly, the optimal gestational age for delivery of women with pregestational diabetes remains uncertain.[29] The American College of Obstetrics and Gynecology (ACOG) practice bulletin states that pregnancies with well-controlled diabetes and normal antenatal testing may be allowed to progress to their estimated due date.[30] However, they advise that "early delivery" may be indicated in some patients with vasculopathy, nephropathy, poor glycemic control, or a prior stillbirth.[30] The ACOG also recommends amniocentesis to assess fetal pulmonary maturity if there is poor glycemic control and at a gestational age of less than 39 weeks.[30] It is noteworthy that the benefit of assessing fetal pulmonary maturity is controversial, and many obstetricians have abandoned the test.

The risk of stillbirth is considerably less in pregnancies complicated by gestational diabetes. In fact, the risk may not be increased in comparison with women without gestational diabetes.[31] However, in many cases it is not possible to distinguish between true gestational diabetes and unrecognized type 2 pregestational diabetes that is first identified during pregnancy. It is reasonable to manage such women as though they have pregestational diabetes, especially if they require insulin to achieve glycemic control. The ACOG recommends against delivery before 40 weeks' gestation in women with gestational diabetes, good glycemic control, and no other complications.[32] It is possible that delivery at 38 weeks' gestation may decrease the risk of macrosomia in pregnancies with gestational diabetes.[33] Nonetheless, this practice has not been shown to reduce the risk of stillbirth, and benefit relative to the risk of early term birth has not been demonstrated.

Intrauterine Growth Restriction

Intrauterine growth restriction (IUGR) is most commonly defined as an estimated fetal weight less than 10% weight for gestational age.[34] IUGR is a major risk factor for stillbirth, increasing the risk by about 6-fold.[19,20,35] It is important to be cognizant of that IUGR is a "sign" or "risk factor," rather than a diagnosis or disease. Using a definition of an estimated fetal weight of less than 10% identifies a substantial number of normal pregnancies as being IUGR. It is estimated that 70% of such infants less than 10% weight are constitutionally small (smaller than average but entirely normal).[36] In addition, some fetuses may be greater than 10% weight but still be growth impaired relative to their growth potential. The use of "customized" or "individual" growth curves can account for such genetic potential, and may be superior to population-based growth curves in identifying fetuses at risk for stillbirth and other adverse obstetric outcomes.[35,37]

When considering the optimal timing of delivery for IUGR fetuses, it is necessary to consider the reason(s) that the fetus is IUGR. In cases of placental insufficiency (or possible placental insufficiency), iatrogenic preterm birth may prevent stillbirth or other adverse neonatal sequelae. By contrast, if the IUGR is associated with a constitutionally small fetus, genetic abnormalities, birth defects, or in utero viral infection, preterm birth may worsen the outcome.

Galan[38] outlined factors associated with placental insufficiency in pregnancies complicated by IUGR (**Box 1**). First, IUGR can be classified as either symmetric or asymmetric, depending on whether the fetus is uniformly small or if the abdomen is small relative to the size of the head. In general, asymmetric IUGR is more likely to be associated with placental insufficiency than symmetric IUGR, because in cases of decreased blood flow to the fetus, blood is preferentially shunted to the fetal brain, allowing for normal growth of the fetal head. Of note, however, this is not always the case and placental insufficiency may be associated with symmetric IUGR. Second, there is usually an absence of associated fetal malformations. Third, in severe cases, fetal testing may show abnormality, which may include decreased amniotic fluid volume, abnormal fetal heart rate tracings, abnormal biophysical profiles, and abnormal Doppler velocimetry.

Serial fetal/antenatal testing is advised for all fetuses with IUGR. Such tests may consist of nonstress tests, amniotic fluid assessment, biophysical profiles, Doppler studies, or some combination of these tests. It is generally accepted that fetuses with substantially abnormal fetal testing (eg, repetitive late decelerations, abnormal biophysical profile, severe oligohydramnios, reversed end-diastolic velocity on umbilical artery Doppler studies) and IUGR should be delivered after 34 weeks' gestation.[38] Similarly, it is reasonable to deliver a fetus with IUGR but with mildly abnormal fetal testing (eg, increased umbilical artery Doppler index but normal biophysical profile at 36 weeks' gestation).[38] The same is true for fetuses with no or minimal interval growth over a 3-week period.

The optimal timing of delivery for fetuses beyond 34 weeks' gestation with normal antenatal testing is more uncertain. Because most IUGR fetuses with normal antenatal

---

Box 1
Phenotype of the intrauterine growth–restricted fetus with uteroplacental disease

Asymmetric biometric growth

Exclusion of structural abnormalities

Evidence of brain-sparing effect

   Head size maintained

   Reduced MCA Doppler index or CPR

Oligohydramnios

Abnormal umbilical artery Doppler velocimetry

   Elevated Doppler index

   Absent or reserved end-diastolic flow

Abnormal venous Doppler velocimetry

   Increased venous Doppler indexes

   Umbilical venous pulsation

Abnormal biophysical testing

   Spontaneous recurrent late decelerations

   Abnormal biophysical profile score ($\leq$4)

Abbreviations: CPR, cerebral-placental ratio; MCA, middle cerebral artery.

---

testing are constitutionally small, it seems reasonable to deliver them at 38 to 39 weeks' gestation.[38] This approach is supported by good outcomes noted in a small pilot study of IUGR pregnancies with normal Doppler studies.[39] Recently, Boers and colleagues[40] conducted a randomized equivalence trial comparing induction of labor with expectant management in pregnancies with suspected IUGR (DIGITAT trial). Women with suspected IUGR fetuses at or beyond 36 weeks' gestation were randomized to induction (n = 321) or expectant management with close surveillance (n = 329). There were no significant differences among groups with regard to either composite neonatal outcomes or cesarean delivery. The investigators concluded that both expectant management and induction of labor are reasonable options.[40] The same group assessed neurodevelopmental and behavioral outcomes at 2 years of age in the DIGITAT cohort,[41] and also found no differences in developmental or behavioral outcomes in infants in the induction or expectant management groups.[41]

Multiple Gestations

Multiple gestations constitute another condition that often leads to late preterm or early term birth. This fact may account for some of the increase noted in late preterm birth, because the incidence has been steadily increasing alongside increased use of assisted reproductive technologies. First, multiple gestations often are complicated by preterm labor, hypertensive disorders, and IUGR. Second, there is an increased risk of stillbirth in multiple gestations, even in the absence of comorbidities, which is especially true for monochorionic multiple gestations.

The optimal timing of delivery for multiple gestations in the absence of obstetric complications is controversial, and there are no data from randomized clinical trials. Overall, the risk of stillbirth for twins is between 0.2% and 0.4% per week between

32 and 38 weeks' gestation, increasing dramatically after 38 weeks' gestation.[42] Also, the lowest risk for perinatal mortality occurs earlier in gestation for twins than in singleton pregnancies.[42–45] Taken together, these data led authorities to recommend delivery of dichorionic twins with no obstetric complications between 37 and 39 weeks' gestation.[44–46] Newman and Unal[46] advise fetal testing if dichorionic twins are allowed to go past 38 weeks' gestation, and strongly advise delivery at no later than 39 weeks' gestation.

Monochorionic twins are at considerably higher risk of stillbirth than are dichorionic twins, owing in large part to the risks of twin-twin transfusion syndrome. Precise data regarding risks are lacking because most database studies of monochorionic twins do not distinguish between pregnancies with and without complications. A small study noted a risk of unexpected stillbirth after 32 weeks' gestation in monochorionic twins of 4.3% (95% CI 1.9%–9.9%).[47] However, a larger study that included weekly fetal testing noted a smaller risk of stillbirth after 32 weeks' gestation (1.2%; 95% CI 0.3%–4.2%).[48] However, over one-half of their monochorionic twins were delivered preterm because of abnormal fetal testing.[48] Another cohort compared outcomes of almost 200 monochorionic twins with those of more than 800 dichorionic twins.[49] The stillbirth rate was much higher in monochorionic than in dichorionic twins (3.6% vs 1.1%), even when patients with obstetric complications were excluded.[49] Based on these data, authorities recommend delivery of otherwise uncomplicated monochorionic twins between 34 and 37 weeks' gestation.[46] Close surveillance with ultrasonography and fetal testing also is advised. Decisions regarding the precise gestational age for delivery between 34 and 37 weeks' gestation should be made in consultation with the patient with respect to the relative risks of stillbirth and prematurity, given the lack of clear evidence to guide management.[46]

The risk of stillbirth is considerably higher for monoamniotic twins than for diamniotic twins, regardless of chorionicity. Indeed, the mortality rates are 10% to 20%. The mechanism of fetal death is uncertain, but is thought to be due to cord entanglement and fetal asphyxia. Therefore the only way to ensure prevention is with iatrogenic preterm birth (by cesarean). Improved outcomes have been reported with intensive surveillance (often inpatient management and prolonged fetal monitoring) and early delivery.[50–52] Based on poor-quality data, it is estimated that the risk of sudden, unexplained stillbirth after 32 weeks' gestation in monoamniotic twins is 5% to 10%[50,53]; thus, expert recommendations are for delivery between 32 and 34 weeks' gestation.[46] Earlier delivery is advised if there is abnormal fetal testing.

It is common to have IUGR in cases of multiple gestations. There are no randomized clinical trials assessing the management of such pregnancies. Authorities recommend delivery of dichorionic twins with IUGR at 36 weeks' gestation and monochorionic twins with IUGR at 34 to 35 weeks' gestation, in the absence of other indications for delivery.[38]

Placental Abnormalities

The placental abnormality most strongly associated with stillbirth is placental abruption, occurring in 0.4% to 1.0% of pregnancies.[53] Although proof of efficacy is lacking, it is generally accepted that delivery after 34 weeks' gestation is indicated to prevent stillbirth in cases of abruption to prevent stillbirth.[53]

Placenta previa affects about 0.3% to 0.5% of deliveries.[54] This condition can lead to bleeding that can threaten the health of the infant and mother, often prompting preterm birth. Although rare, stillbirth can occur in the setting of maternal hemorrhage. Substantial vaginal bleeding or preterm labor is considered to be an indication for preterm birth after 34 weeks' gestation.[55] In patients with no bleeding or contractions, the optimal timing for delivery is 36 weeks' gestation.[55,56] The placenta accreta spectrum occurs when the placenta is abnormally attached to the myometrium, usually in the setting of placenta previa with a prior cesarean delivery. Perinatal mortality (and maternal morbidity) is much higher than with placenta previa.[57] Delivery is advised at 34 weeks' gestation in stable patients,[57] and earlier in the setting of hemorrhage or labor.[57]

Fetal Abnormalities

Rarely, iatrogenic preterm birth may decrease the risk of stillbirth owing to fetal malformations or genetic abnormalities. These conditions account for approximately 10% to 20% of cases of stillbirth.[15] Indications for preterm birth because of fetal abnormalities have recently been reviewed by Craigo.[58] One of the most common is gastroschisis, which has a substantial risk of stillbirth in the late third trimester. Although controversial, delivery between 37 and 38 weeks' gestation is considered to be a reasonable option.[58] Other anomalies associated with stillbirth include chest masses leading to hydrops, cardiac anomalies leading to hydrops or arrhythmia, tumors leading to cardiovascular compromise, and bowel obstruction.[58]

Prior Stillbirth

Previous stillbirth increases the risk for recurrent stillbirth in future pregnancies over the baseline risk of approximately 1 in 160. Indeed, the risk of recurrent stillbirth is increased 2- to 10-fold for those with previous stillbirth.[3] The risk appears to be somewhat higher for non-Hispanic black women, and lower in cases of unexplained stillbirth.[3] Moreover, there are known medical and genetic conditions for which the risk of recurrence of stillbirth can be precisely determined. For example, α thalassemia is an autosomal recessive condition that carries risk of stillbirth. Medical conditions associated with stillbirth include diabetes and antiphospholipid syndrome, among others.[59,60] However, disease severity and treatment will influence the rate of recurrent stillbirth.

There is no evidence supporting elective preterm birth to lower the rate of recurrent stillbirth. Hence, authorities recommend that delivery occur at 39 weeks' gestation or after fetal lung maturity is established in women with prior stillbirth, if there is no additional indication for induction or delivery.[3,61] Despite this recommendation the risk of preterm birth, induction of labor, or elective cesarean delivery is increased 2- to 3-fold in those with prior stillbirth. It is unclear as to how many of these deliveries are medically indicated rather than patient- and/or physician-driven.

An anonymous survey of Australian obstetricians regarding management of subsequent pregnancies after stillbirth has been completed. The survey had a 69% response rate to a hypothetical question about delivery. Of the respondents, 72% replied that early delivery was appropriate after an unexplained 37-week stillbirth in a prior pregnancy.[62] Specifically, the breakdown included:

- 12% recommending delivery at 36 weeks
- 22% recommending delivery at 37 weeks
- 38% recommending delivery at 38 weeks[62]

Desire for early delivery and extra precautions is even more prominent among patients. A separate Australian study reached out to patients with previous stillbirth through advocacy organizations, and requested that the patients perform an Internet-based survey regarding subsequent pregnancy expectations, which showed the following[63]:

- 81% desired "early delivery"

- 93% desired "testing beyond usual obstetric care"
- 26% requested cesarean regardless of circumstances[63]

Current data suggest that patients should be advised to deliver at 39 weeks' gestation or beyond if there is no medical indication to suggest otherwise. Counseling should include explanation of the risks of early birth and the lack of evidence that early delivery will reduce the risk of stillbirth. Nonetheless, this will be a difficult conversation, as extreme anxiety and emotions surrounding previous stillbirth will weigh heavily on the patient. These patients often blame themselves and feel significant guilt for prior outcomes. It is suggested that physicians work with the families closely in counseling and educating them. Professional counseling may also be considered. Ultimately, delivery at 37 to 38 weeks could still be a reasonable option if extreme anxiety and fear still constitute a major driving force for the patient despite adequate education and counseling.

Abnormal Fetal Testing

Abnormal fetal testing is an indication for late preterm or early term birth, regardless of the underlying condition prompting the fetal testing. Methodologies include fetal movement counting, nonstress tests, contraction stress tests, assessment of amniotic fluid volume, biophysical profile, modified biophysical profile, and Doppler velocimetry of the umbilical, uterine, and middle cerebral arteries. Indications for testing include any disorder associated with an increased risk for stillbirth. Such indications include all of the previously discussed conditions such as hypertension, IUGR, and diabetes, as well as numerous others (eg, systemic lupus erythematosus). A complete discussion of antenatal or fetal testing is beyond the scope of this article, although the subject has been recently reviewed.[64,65]

KNOWLEDGE GAPS

There are numerous unanswered questions that, if answered, could improve our understanding of optimal timing of delivery in women at risk for stillbirth. Clinicians might benefit from further data regarding the burden of early delivery resulting from attempts to reduce stillbirth. In addition, better data are needed regarding the competing risks of stillbirth and preterm birth for all women, as well as those affected by the conditions outlined in this article. Too many of the current generally accepted practices are guided by expert opinion rather than data from appropriately designed clinical trials. The optimal timing of delivery is likely not a "one-size-fits-all" proposition, and further studies allowing risk stratification would be beneficial. Risk stratification inherently would be easier if better predictive models were available to assess which pregnancies are at highest risk of stillbirth.

SUMMARY

Much of the increase in late preterm and early term birth has been due to iatrogenic or medically indicated preterm birth. In large part, this has been intended to reduce the rate of stillbirth. Although stillbirth rates have decrease as late preterm birth rates have increased, most assessments of the practice have not accounted for competing risks with stillbirth, such as neonatal death and neonatal morbidity due to complications of prematurity. Among the general population, there is no evidence that delivery before 39 weeks' gestation causes more good than harm. However, late preterm and early term birth is indicated for many conditions associated with an increased risk of stillbirth, such as preeclampsia, IUGR, and abnormal fetal testing. There is a need for additional studies to identify fetuses at highest risk for stillbirth and to assess the competing risks of delivery (prematurity) in comparisons with expectant management (stillbirth) in appropriately designed clinical trials. Spong and colleagues[66] have proposed guidelines for late preterm and early term birth for a variety of conditions that increase the risk of stillbirth, and these are presented in **Table 1**.

Table 1
Guidance regarding timing of delivery when conditions complicate pregnancy at or after 34 weeks of gestation

Condition	Gestational Age[a] at Delivery	Grade of Recommendation[b]
Placental and Uterine Issues		
Placenta previa[c]	36–37 wk	B
Suspected placenta accreta, increta, or percreta with placenta previa[c]	34–35 wk	B
Prior classic cesarean (upper segment uterine incision)[c]	36–37 wk	B
Prior myomectomy necessitating cesarean delivery[c]	37–38 wk (may require earlier delivery, similar to prior classic cesarean, in situations with more extensive or complicated myomectomy)	B
Fetal Issues		
Fetal growth restriction, singleton	38–39 wk: Otherwise uncomplicated, no concurrent findings	B
	34–37 wk: Concurrent conditions (oligohydramnios, abnormal Doppler studies, maternal risk factors, comorbidity)	B
	Expeditious delivery regardless of gestational age: Persistent abnormal fetal surveillance suggesting imminent fetal jeopardy	—
Fetal growth restriction, twin gestation	36–37 wk: Dichorionic-diamniotic twins with isolated fetal growth restriction	B
	32–34 wk: Monochorionic-diamniotic twins with isolated fetal growth restriction Concurrent conditions (oligohydramnios, abnormal Doppler studies, maternal risk factors, comorbidity)	B
	Expeditious delivery regardless of gestational age: Persistent abnormal fetal surveillance suggesting imminent fetal jeopardy	—

(*continued on next page*)

Table 1
(continued)

Condition	Gestational Age[a] at Delivery	Grade of Recommendation[b]
Fetal congenital malformations[c]	34–39 wk: Suspected worsening of fetal organ damage Potential for fetal intracranial hemorrhage (eg, vein of Galen aneurysm, neonatal alloimmune thrombocytopenia) When delivery before labor is preferred (eg, EXIT procedure) Previous fetal intervention Concurrent maternal disease (eg, preeclampsia, chronic hypertension) Potential for adverse maternal effect from fetal condition	B
	Expeditious delivery regardless of gestational age: When intervention is expected to be beneficial Fetal complications develop (abnormal fetal surveillance, new-onset hydrops fetalis, progressive or new-onset organ injury) Maternal complications develop (mirror syndrome)	B
Multiple gestations: dichorionic-diamniotic[c]	38 wk	B
Multiple gestations: monochorionic-diamniotic[c]	34–37 wk	B
Multiple gestations: dichorionic-diamniotic or monochorionic-diamniotic with single fetal death[c]	If occurs at or after 34 wk, consider delivery (recommendation limited to pregnancies at or after 34 wk; if occurs before 34 wk, individualize based on concurrent maternal or fetal conditions)	B
Multiple gestations: monochorionic-monoamniotic[c]	32–34 wk	B
Multiple gestations: monochorionic-monoamniotic with single fetal death[c]	Consider delivery; individualized according to gestational age and concurrent complications	B
Oligohydramnios, isolated and persistent[c]	36–37 wk	B
Maternal Issues		
Chronic hypertension, no medications[c]	38–39 wk	B
Chronic hypertension, controlled on medication[c]	37–39 wk	B

(continued on next page)

Table 1
(continued)

Condition	Gestational Age[a] at Delivery	Grade of Recommendation[b]
Chronic hypertension, difficult to control (requiring frequent medication adjustments)[c]	36–37 wk	B
Gestational hypertension[d]	37–38 wk	B
Preeclampsia, severe[c]	At diagnosis (recommendation limited to pregnancies at or after 34 wk)	C
Preeclampsia, mild[c]	37 wk	B
Diabetes, pregestational well controlled[c]	LPTB or ETB not recommended	B
Diabetes, pregestational with vascular disease[c]	37–39 wk	B
Diabetes, pregestational poorly controlled[c]	34–39 wk (individualized to situation)	B
Diabetes, gestational well controlled on diet[c]	LPTB or ETB not recommended	B
Diabetes, gestational well controlled on medication[c]	LPTB or ETB not recommended	B
Diabetes, gestational poorly controlled on medication[c]	34–39 wk (individualized to situation)	B
Obstetric Issues		
Prior stillbirth, unexplained[c]	LPTB or ETB not recommended	B
	Consider amniocentesis for fetal pulmonary maturity if delivery planned at less than 39 wk	C
Spontaneous preterm birth: preterm premature rupture of membranes[c]	34 wk (recommendation limited to pregnancies at or after 34 wk)	B
Spontaneous preterm birth: active preterm labor[c]	Delivery if progressive labor or additional maternal or fetal indication	B

Abbreviations: ETB, early term birth at 37-0/7 weeks through 38-6/7 weeks; LPTB, late preterm birth at 34-0/7 weeks through 36-6/7 weeks.

[a] Gestational age is in completed weeks; thus, 34 weeks includes 34-0/7 weeks through 34-6/7 weeks.

[b] Grade of recommendations are based on the following: recommendations or conclusions or both are based on good and consistent scientific evidence (A); limited or inconsistent scientific evidence (B); primarily consensus and expert opinion (C). The recommendations regarding expeditious delivery for imminent fetal jeopardy were not given a grade. The recommendation regarding severe preeclampsia is based largely on expert opinion; however, higher-level evidence is not likely to be forthcoming because this condition is believed to carry significant maternal risk with limited potential fetal benefit from expectant management after 34 weeks.

[c] Uncomplicated; thus no fetal growth restriction, superimposed preeclampsia, and so forth. If these are present, the complicating conditions take precedence and earlier delivery may be indicated.

[d] Maintenance antihypertensive therapy should not be used to treat gestational hypertension.

From Spong CY, Mercer BM, D'Alton M, et al. Timing of indicated late-preterm and early-term birth. Obstet Gynecolol 2011;118:326–7; with permission.

REFERENCES

1. MacDorman MF, Kirmeyer S, Wilson EC. National Vital Statistics Reports; no 8. Fetal and perinatal mortality, United States, 2006, vol. 60. Hyattsville (MD): National Center for Health Statistics; 2012.
2. Information and Statistics Division NHS. Scotland: Scottish perinatal and infant mortality report 2000. Edinburgh (United Kingdom): ISD Scotland Publishing Group; 2001.
3. Reddy UM. Prediction and prevention of recurrent stillbirth. Obstet Gynecol 2007;11:1151–64.
4. McIntire DD, Leveno KJ. Neonatal mortality and morbidity rates in late preterm births compared with births at term. Obstet Gynecol 2008;111:35–41.
5. Tomashek KM, Shapiro-Mendoza CK, Davidoff MJ, et al. Differences in mortality between late-preterm and term singleton infants in the United States, 1995-2002. J Pediatr 2007;151:450–6.
6. Khashu M, Narayanan M, Bhargava S, et al. Perinatal outcomes associated with preterm birth at 33 to 36 weeks' gestation: a population-based cohort study. Pediatrics 2009;123:109–13.
7. Petrini JR, Dias T, McCormick MC, et al. Increased risk of adverse neurological development for late preterm infants. J Pediatr 2009;154:169–76.
8. Tita AT, Landon MB, Spong CY, et al. Timing of elective repeat cesarean delivery at term and neonatal outcomes. N Engl J Med 2009;360:111–20.
9. Lisonkova S, Sabr Y, Butler B, et al. International comparisons of preterm birth: higher rates of late preterm birth are associated with lower rates of stillbirth and neonatal death. BJOG 2012;119:1630–9.
10. MacDorman MF, Kirmeyer S. Fetal and perinatal mortality, United States, 2005. Natl Vital Stat Rep 2009;57:1–20.
11. Yudkin PL, Wood L, Redman CW. Risk of unexplained stillbirth at different gestational ages. Lancet 1987;329:1192–4.
12. Reddy UM, Ko CW, Willinger M. Maternal age and the risk of stillbirth throughout pregnancy in the United States. Am J Obstet Gynecol 2001;184:489–96.
13. Smith GC. Life-table analysis of the risk of perinatal death at term and post term in singleton pregnancies. Am J Obstet Gynecol 2001;184:489–96.
14. Clark SL, Frye DR, Meyers JA, et al. Reduction in elective delivery at <39 weeks of gestation: comparative effectiveness of 3 approaches to change and the impact on neonatal intensive care admission and stillbirth. Am J Obstet Gynecol 2010;203:e1–6.
15. Stillbirth Collaborative Research Network Writing Group. Causes of death among stillbirths. JAMA 2011;306:2459–68.
16. Sibai BM, Barton JR. Expectant management of severe preeclampsia remote from term: patient selection treatment and delivery indications. Am J Obstet Gynecol 2007;146:e1–4.
17. Sibai BM. Induction of labor improves maternal outcomes compared with expectant monitoring in women with gestational hypertension or mild preeclampsia. Evid Based Med 2010;15:11–2.
18. Koopmans CM, Bijlenga D, Groen H, et al. Induction of labour versus expectant monitoring for gestational hypertension or mild preeclampsia after 36 weeks gestation (HYPITAT): a multicenter, open label randomized controlled trial. Lancet 2009;374:979–88.
19. Fretts RC. Etiology and prevention of stillbirth. Am J Obstet Gynecol 2005;193:1923–35.

20. Reddy UM, Laughon SK, Sun L, et al. Prepregnancy risk factors for antepartum stillbirth in the United States. Obstet Gynecol 2010;116:1119–26.
21. Stillbirth Collaborative Research Network Writing Group. Association between stillbirth and risk factors known at pregnancy confirmation. JAMA 2011;306: 2469–79.
22. Flegal KM, Carroll MD, Ogden CL, et al. Prevalence and trends in obesity among US adults, 1999-2008. JAMA 2010;303:235–41.
23. Centers for Disease Control and Prevention. National diabetes fact sheet: general information and national estimates on diabetes in the United States. Atlanta (GA): US Department of Health and Human Services, Centers for Disease Control and Prevention; 2008.
24. Persson M, Norman M, Hanson U. Obstetric and perinatal outcomes in type 1 diabetic pregnancies: a large population based study. Diabetes Care 2009; 32:2005–9.
25. Mondestin MA, Ananth CV, Smulian JC, et al. Birth weight and fetal death in the United States. The effect of maternal diabetes during pregnancy. Am J Obstet Gynecol 2002;187:922–6.
26. Cundy T, Gamble G, Townsend K, et al. Perinatal morbidity in type 2 diabetes mellitus. Diabet Med 1999;17:33–9.
27. Lauenborg J, Mathiesen E, Oveson P, et al. Audit on stillbirths in women with pregestational type 1 diabetes. Diabetes Care 2003;26:1385–9.
28. Macintosh MC, Fleming KM, Baily JA, et al. Perinatal mortality and congenital anomalies in babies of women with type 1 or type 2 diabetes in England, Wales and Northern Ireland: population based study. BMJ 2006;333:177–82.
29. Catalano PM, Sacks DA. Timing of indicated late preterm and early term birth in chronic medical complications: diabetes. Semin Perinatol 2011;35: 297–301.
30. American College of Obstetricians and Gynecologists. Pregestational diabetes mellitus. Practice bulletin number 60. Washington, DC: American College of Obstetricians and Gynecologists; 2005.
31. Fadl HE, Ostlund IK, Magnuson AF, et al. Maternal and neonatal outcomes and time trends of gestational diabetes mellitus in Sweden from 1991 to 2003. Diabet Med 2010;27:436–41.
32. American College of Obstetricians and Gynecologists. Gestational diabetes: practice bulletin number 30. Washington, DC: American College of Obstetricians and Gynecologists; 2001.
33. American Diabetes Association. Gestational diabetes mellitus. Diabetes Care 2004;27(Suppl 1):588–90.
34. ACOG Practice Bulletin no. 134: Fetal growth restriction. Obstet Gynecol 2013; 121:1122–33.
35. Gardosi J, Madurasinghe V, Williams M, et al. Maternal and fetal risk factors for stillbirth: population based study. BMJ 2013;346:f108. http://dx.doi.org/10.1136/bmj.f108.
36. Ott WJ. The diagnosis of altered fetal growth. Obstet Gynecol Clin North Am 1988;15:237.
37. Seeds JW, Peng T. Impaired fetal growth and risk of fetal death. Is the tenth percentile the appropriate standard? Am J Obstet Gynecol 1998;178:658.
38. Galan HL. Timing delivery of the growth-restricted fetus. Semin Perinatol 2011; 35:262–9.
39. McCowan LM, Harding JE, Roberts AB, et al. A pilot randomized controlled trial of two regimens of fetal surveillance for small for gestational age fetuses with

normal results of umbilical artery Doppler velocimetry. Am J Obstet Gynecol 2000;182:81–6.

40. Boers KE, Vijgen SM, Bijlenga D, et al. Induction versus expectant monitoring for intrauterine growth restriction at term: randomizes equivalence trial (DIGITAT). BMJ 2010;341:c7087. http://dx.doi.org/10.1136/bmj.c7087.

41. Van Wyk L, Boers KE, van der Post JA, et al. Effects on (neuro)developmental and behavioral outcome at 2 years of age of induced labor compared with expectant management in intrauterine growth-restricted infants: long term outcomes of the DIGITAT trial. Am J Obstet Gynecol 2012;206:406.e1–7.

42. Sairam S, Costeloe K, Thilaganathan B. Prospective risk of stillbirth in multiple gestation pregnancies: a population-based analysis. Obstet Gynecol 2002;100:638–41.

43. Luke B. Reducing fetal deaths in multiple births: optimal birth weights and gestational ages for infants of twin and triplet births. Acta Genet Med Gemellol (Roma) 1996;45:333–48.

44. Hartley RS, Emanuel I, Hitti J. Perinatal mortality and neonatal morbidity rates among twin pairs at different gestational ages: optimal delivery timing at 37 to 38 weeks gestation. Am J Obstet Gynecol 2001;184:451–8.

45. Kahn B, Lumey LH, Zybert PA, et al. Prospective risk of fetal death in singleton, twin and triplet gestations: implications for practice. Obstet Gynecol 2003;102:685–92.

46. Newman RB, Unal ER. Multiple gestations: timing of indicated late preterm and early term births in uncomplicated dichorionic, monochorionic, and monoamniotic twins. Semin Perinatol 2011;35:277–85.

47. Barigye O, Pasquini L, Gakea P, et al. High risk of unexpected late fetal death in monochorionic twins despite intensive ultrasound surveillance: a cohort study. PloS Med 2005;2:e172.

48. Simoes T, Amaral N, Lerman R, et al. Prospective risk of intrauterine death of monochorionic-diamniotic twins. Am J Obstet Gynecol 2006;195:134–9.

49. Lee YM, Wylie BJ, Simpson LL, et al. Twin chorionicity and the risks of stillbirth. Obstet Gynecol 2008;111:301–8.

50. Rodis JF, McIlveen PF, Egan JF, et al. Monoamniotic twins: Improved perinatal survival with accurate prenatal diagnosis and antenatal fetal surveillance. Am J Obstet Gynecol 1997;177:1046–9.

51. Heyborne KD, Porreco RP, Garite TJ, et al. Improved perinatal survival of monoamniotic twins with intensive inpatient monitoring. Am J Obstet Gynecol 2005;192:96–101.

52. Hack KE, Derks JB, Schaap AH, et al. Perinatal outcome of monoamniotic twin pregnancies. Obstet Gynecol 2009;113:353–60.

53. Tikkanen M. Placental abruption: epidemiology, risk factors and consequences. Acta Obstet Gynecol Scand 2011;90:140–9.

54. Oyelese Y, Smulian JC. Placenta previa, placenta accreta, and vasa previa. Obstet Gynecol 2006;107:927–41.

55. Zlatnik MG, Little SE, Kohli P, et al. When should women with placenta previa be delivered? A decision analysis. J Reprod Med 2010;55:373–81.

56. Blackwell SC. Timing of delivery for women with stable placenta previa. Semin Perinatol 2011;35:249–51.

57. SMFM Clinical Opinion. Placenta accreta. Am J Obstet Gynecol 2010;203:430–9.

58. Craigo SD. Indicated preterm birth for fetal anomalies. Semin Perinatol 2011;35:270–6.

59. Branch DW, Khamashta MA. Antiphospholipid syndrome: obstetric diagnosis, management, and controversies. Obstet Gynecol 2003;101:1333–44.
60. Coletta J, Simpson LL. Maternal medical disease and stillbirth. Clin Obstet Gynecol 2010;53:507–616.
61. ACOG practice bulletin No. 102: management of stillbirth. Obstet Gynecol 2009; 113:748–61.
62. Robson S, Thompson J, Ellwood D. Obstetric management of the next pregnancy after an unexplained stillbirth: an anonymous postal survey of Australian obstetricians. Aust N Z J Obstet Gynaecol 2006;46:278–81.
63. Robson SJ, Leader LR, Dear KB, et al. Women's expectations of management in their next pregnancy after an unexplained stillbirth: an internet-based empirical study. Aust N Z J Obstet Gynaecol 2009;49:642–6.
64. Signore C, Freeman RK, Spong CY. Antenatal testing—a reevaluation: executive summary of a Eunice Kennedy Shriver National Institute of Child Health and Human Development workshop. Obstet Gynecol 2009;113:687–701.
65. Moore TR. The role of amniotic fluid assessment in indicated preterm delivery. Semin Perinatol 2011;35:286–91.
66. Spong CY, Mercer BM, D'Alton M, et al. Timing of indicated late-preterm and early-term birth. Obstet Gynecol 2011;118:323–33.

Early Births and Congenital Birth Defects: A Complex Interaction

Jonathan R. Swanson, MD, Robert A. Sinkin, MD, MPH*

KEYWORDS

• Prematurity • Birth defects • Neonate • Maternal health • Early birth

KEY POINTS

- Neither premature/early birth nor congenital anomalies are caused by a single, simple "one-hit" factor.
- Interactions between genetic coding, the environment (both maternal and uterine), and family history all play a role in fetal and infant well-being.
- There are several interconnected risk factors for both birth defects and early birth; perhaps ongoing or future investigations, including epidemiologic evaluations and animal modeling, will further elucidate these complex interactions.
- In many cases, infants are at risk for not only birth defects or preterm birth, but for both.
- Reduction or elimination of many of the risk factors discussed in this article may prevent both birth defects and premature birth.

INTRODUCTION AND HISTORICAL PERSPECTIVE

In the United States, more than 120,000 babies are born annually with a lethal birth defect, which, according to the March of Dimes, is the leading cause of infant mortality.[1] There are thousands of different birth defects affecting the structure or function of every part of the human body. At present, about 70% of the causes of birth defects are unknown.[2] Not all babies with a birth defect will be delivered prematurely (before 37 completed weeks of gestation). Previous articles have discussed the epidemiology and treatment of preterm and early term neonates. A subset of these babies is born with congenital anomalies that may be responsible for the preterm birth, either electively because of medical compromise to the mother or fetus, or as a specific cause triggering early onset of labor, such as polyhydramnios in a fetus with a gastrointestinal anomaly leading to premature rupture of membranes and premature delivery.

The authors have nothing to disclose.
Department of Pediatrics, University of Virginia Children's Hospital, University of Virginia, Box 800386, Charlottesville, VA 22908, USA
* Corresponding author.
E-mail address: ras9q@virginia.edu

Clin Perinatol 40 (2013) 629–644
http://dx.doi.org/10.1016/j.clp.2013.07.009   **perinatology.theclinics.com**
0095-5108/13/$ – see front matter © 2013 Elsevier Inc. All rights reserved.

Although there are several definitions of birth defects in the literature, they all share a common theme of a genetic or structural defect that is present at birth. The March of Dimes has defined birth defect as "an abnormality of structure, function, or body metabolism (inborn error of body chemistry) presenting at birth or early childhood that results in physical or mental disability, or is fatal."[3]

This article attempts to discriminate those specific factors known to associate premature delivery with congenital birth defects. Beginning with a historical perspective, an attempt is made to classify these complex interactions of early birth and congenital birth defects as neonatal factors of causation and association, after which maternal conditions that may also be both causative and associative with these early deliveries are discussed.

As described in previous articles, there are several identifiable conditions and associations blamed for a premature birth, including early and advanced maternal age, multiple gestations, illicit drug use and smoking, and uterine anomalies. The appreciation that certain medications and ingestions can be harmful to the developing fetus is underscored by the teratogenic effects of alcohol. Fetal alcohol syndrome, a consequence of excessive alcohol consumption during pregnancy, is characterized by growth deficiency and permanent central nervous system damage, specifically mental retardation, and other well-described findings.[4,5] Thalidomide is an example of an unanticipated but devastating teratogen. Thalidomide was prescribed in the late 1950s as an antinausea and sedative drug, initially used as a sleeping pill. It was discovered to help pregnant women with the effects of morning sickness. It was withdrawn in 1962 after being found to be a teratogen, having caused many different forms of birth defects.[6] However, prematurity was not associated with either of these two teratogens.

Diethylstilbestrol (DES) is the most cited example demonstrating an association of prematurity with pharmacopeia. DES, a synthetic form of estrogen, was prescribed to pregnant women between 1940 and 1971 to prevent miscarriage, premature labor, and related complications of pregnancy. The use of DES declined after studies in the 1950s showed that it was not effective in preventing these problems. In 1971, a case series was published revealing a link with prenatal DES exposure and cervical and vaginal clear-cell adenocarcinoma.[7] Soon after, the Food and Drug Administration notified physicians that DES should not be prescribed to pregnant women. It was classified as an endocrine disruptor and is now known to cause cancer, birth defects, and other developmental abnormalities.[8] In addition to the cervical and vaginal neoplasia, several studies found increased risks of premature birth, miscarriage, and ectopic pregnancy associated with DES exposure.[6]

BIRTH DEFECTS CAUSING EARLY BIRTH

Birth defects in the fetus are believed to play a role in the development of preterm labor in several instances. As such, major birth defects have been shown in multiple population studies to be associated with preterm delivery. In one population-based cohort study in metropolitan Atlanta involving 264,000 infants between 1989 and 1995, infants born before 37 weeks' gestation had a greater than 2-fold risk of a birth defect compared with those infants born between 37 and 41 weeks' gestation (relative risk 2.43, 95% confidence interval [CI] 2.30–2.56).[9] Several studies have since confirmed this finding.[10–12]

In the First and Second Trimester Evaluation of Risk (FASTER) trial,[10] singleton live born infants with birth defects were significantly more likely to be delivered prematurely than those without defects. The investigators also found that the risk of birth defects increased as the gestational age decreased. Those with birth defects were 2.7 times more likely to be delivered before 37 weeks, 7 times more likely to be delivered before 34 weeks, and 11.5 times more likely to be delivered before 32 weeks. Infants with birth defects were more likely to have a low birth weight and very low birth weight compared with those without defects.[10] This relationship is not limited to the United States. In a case-control study of nearly 25,000 infants in Brazil, Grandi and colleagues[12] found that newborns with birth defects had a higher adjusted risk for preterm birth than those without birth defects (odds ratio [OR] 2.16, 95% CI 1.92–2.40).

Although no study has shown that birth defects directly cause premature labor and subsequent birth, there are many defects that have a plausible biological cause of early birth. Aneuploidies, polyhydramnios (secondary to both neurologic and gastrointestinal causes), and congenital infections have all been associated with premature labor and subsequent delivery.

Chromosomal Defects

Aneuploidies and other chromosomal anomalies have been well established as major causes of spontaneous early deliveries and spontaneous abortions. The most commonly diagnosed autosomal trisomies are trisomy 21 (T21; Down syndrome), trisomy 18 (T18; Edwards syndrome), and trisomy 13 (T13; Patau syndrome).[13] Parker and colleagues[13] estimated that the rates for live born infants with trisomies per 10,000 live births in the United States population were 13.5 (T21), 2.5 (T18), and 1.2 (T13). In a descriptive study from the Vermont Oxford Network, the prevalence of these defects was much higher in a very low birth weight (<1500 g) population. Rates per 10,000 live births in this population were 31.2 (T21), 26.2 (T18), and 8.1 (T13).[14] The mean gestational age at delivery was 29.4 weeks, 31.8 weeks, and 29.6 weeks for T21, T18, and T13, respectively.

The mechanism behind autosomal aneuploidy and spontaneous early delivery (including spontaneous abortion/miscarriage) is not entirely known but is well established. More than half of all spontaneous abortions before 16 weeks are due to chromosomal abnormalities while 6% to 12% after 20 weeks and 5% to 7% of stillbirths are also due to these defects.[15–17] The lethality of the aneuploidy (miscarriage) has been correlated with the gene content on the involved chromosome.[18] Fetuses with T21, T18, and T13 can survive to term; compared with the more lethal aneuploidies, these three specific chromosomes contain decreased gene content.[19] Certainly the impact and range of neurodevelopmental impairment in infants with T21 and T18 are significant. When coupled to any prematurity-related risk of neurodevelopmental impairment (especially in infants <28 weeks' gestation), the necessity of close follow-up and early intervention is further underscored.

Polyhydramnios

Several defects can lead to excess amniotic fluid within the uterine cavity (ie, polyhydramnios). Fetal congenital anomalies are a significant cause of polyhydramnios, with defects of gastrointestinal or neurologic origins accounting for many of these (**Box 1**).[20] Gastrointestinal causes of polyhydramnios include defects that prevent reabsorption of the amniotic fluid such as atresias of the esophagus, duodenum, or intestines, and defects that interfere with fetal swallowing such as a pharyngeal teratoma.[21] Neurologic conditions such as anencephaly or myotonic dystrophy may also cause swallowing dysfunction, and lead to increased amniotic fluid accumulation.

Some investigators have suggested that polyhydramnios overdistends the uterus, which then leads to spontaneous labor and an increase in the rate of preterm delivery.[22,23] A higher amniotic fluid index, which indicates polyhydramnios, has

---

Box 1
Causes of polyhydramnios

Gastrointestinal Origin

- Tracheoesophageal fistula
- Esophageal atresia
- Congenital diaphragmatic hernia
- Gastroschisis
- Intestinal atresia/stenosis/malrotation

Neurologic Origin

- Anencephaly
- Hydrocephaly
- Spina bifida

Other Origin

- Multiple gestation
- Diabetes mellitus
- Rhesus isoimmunization
- TORCH infections
- Skeletal dysplasias
- Pharyngeal teratoma

Idiopathic

---

been shown to be a risk factor in the frequency of adverse pregnancy outcomes including preterm delivery and perinatal mortality.[24] However, not all causes of polyhydramnios have been associated with premature delivery. In a study examining the role of polyhydramnios and preterm delivery, Many and colleagues[25] showed that polyhydramnios associated with insulin-dependent diabetes mellitus and congenital anomalies had a significantly higher rate of preterm delivery, whereas polyhydramnios with gestational diabetes did not. Of interest, in another observation by this group the rate of premature delivery in mothers with idiopathic polyhydramnios was no higher than in the overall population rate.[26] Thus the interaction between polyhydramnios and premature labor and delivery is not so straightforward.

Congenital Infections

Several congenital infections have been associated with premature delivery. Syphilis, one of the more common sexually transmitted diseases both in the United States and globally, is caused by *Treponema pallidum*. Between 2006 and 2008 there was an 18% increase in the rate of congenital syphilis, which corresponded with an increase in the rate of syphilis among women of childbearing age.[27] Although there has been a subsequent decline in the case rate of syphilis, it remains a significant public health concern. Although 50% of infants with congenital syphilis are asymptomatic, early manifestations including metaphyseal dystrophy, hepatosplenomegaly, anemia, jaundice, snuffles, and periostitis present in the neonatal period.[28]

In a small prospective study on antenatal diagnosis of syphilis and gonorrhea in an African community, Donders and colleagues[29] found that 60% of mothers with syphilis delivered prematurely while 100% of those with syphilis and gonorrhea delivered early. Infection with *Neisseria gonorrhoeae* alone was also a predictor of premature delivery, with 42% of mothers having premature infants. Infection with either syphilis or gonorrhea was also associated with a greater incidence of low birth weight.

The pathogenesis for premature delivery in infants of mothers with syphilis is not widely understood. Along with the physical manifestations of congenital syphilis, it is thought that the fetal immune response to *T pallidum* may be responsible for the premature delivery.[28] This idea is not new. Since 1950, when Knox and Hoerner[30] stated that "infection in the female reproductive tract can cause premature rupture of the membranes and induce premature labor," the role of maternal infection with premature birth has been studied. Other studies have suggested that bacteria invading fetal membranes leading to chorioamnionitis as well as unrecognized amnionitis can cause premature uterine contractions.[31,32]

Other bacteria and viruses that have been shown to cause birth defects such as varicella zoster, rubella, and coxsackie viruses (congenital heart disease) have not been demonstrated to cause premature labor. However, vertical parvovirus infection may be a cause of both anomalies and early birth. There are case reports of fetal anomalies with maternal parvovirus infections including those in the central nervous and cardiovascular systems, and congenital hypoplasia of the abdominal wall and pleural effusions have also been described.[33–36] Parvovirus infection may also lead to fetal nonimmune hydrops, which can cause fetal death or premature delivery, secondary to either the hydrops or early elective delivery because of fetal distress.

EARLY ELECTIVE DELIVERY SECONDARY TO BIRTH DEFECTS

One of the more important quality-improvement initiatives in obstetric medicine in the last 10 years has been the reduction in elective inductions of labor before 39 weeks' gestation. This initiative has certainly reduced infant morbidity and admissions to neonatal intensive care units (NICUs), and has saved billions of health care dollars.[37] There are still several fetal indications (in addition to maternal indications) for the elective induction of labor before 39 weeks' gestation (**Box 2**)[38]; however, the vast majority of these have limited or inconsistent scientific evidence.

Multiple Gestation

In the current era of increased use of fertility-enhancing medications and therapies, twin and other multiple-gestation pregnancies are not an uncommon event. The twin birth rate increased by 76% from 1980 to 2009, rising approximately 3% each year.[39] In 2010, the twin birth rate was 33.2 per 100,000 live births. Infants born in multi-gestational pregnancies tend to be smaller and born earlier than those in singleton pregnancies, leading to a greater risk of early death as well.[39] Of note, twin gestations are also associated with an increased risk of congenital anomalies (**Box 3**). In a birth registry study across several countries in Europe and Central America consisting of more than 12 million deliveries, twins were at significantly higher risk of having a congenital anomaly.[40] Thirty-nine of the 92 malformations studied were more common in twins and affected the central nervous, cardiovascular, gastrointestinal, genitourinary, and musculoskeletal systems. There is some evidence suggesting that the process of "twinning" may lead to the increased risk of congenital anomalies, especially in midline defects.[41] It is thought that this process favors the discordant expression of defects, owing to the multiple opportunities for asymmetry. When these defects are present in one fetus, the normal fetus may be at risk for low birth weight, preterm delivery, and increased rates of morbidity and mortality.[42]

Box 2
Early delivery indicated by placental, fetal, and maternal conditions

Placental Issues

- Placenta previa
- Placenta accreta, increta, or percreta
- Prior classic cesarean

Fetal Issues

- Growth restriction
- Congenital malformations
- Multiple gestation
- Oligohydramnios
- Fetal distress

Maternal Issues

- Chronic and gestational hypertension
- Preeclampsia
- Preexisting and gestational diabetes
- Acute or chronic lung disease
- Cardiac disease
- Renal disease

Obstetric Issues

- Prior stillbirth
- Preterm premature rupture of membranes

Adapted from Spong CY, Mercer BM, D'Alton M, et al. Timing of indicated late-preterm and early-term birth. Obstet Gynecol 2011;118:323; with permission.

Another complex issue with regard to twin gestation is twin-to-twin transfusion syndrome (TTTS) in monozygotic monochorionic twins. Newborns following TTTS have been shown to be at high risk for neurodevelopmental impairment.[43] In addition, monochorionic-diamniotic twins are also at high risk for growth restriction or discordance as well as intrauterine fetal demise (IUFD).[44] There is wide variability in the recommendations of when to deliver these infants. Some have advocated elective preterm delivery because of concerns that the risk of IUFD may actually increase over gestation, and may be more likely after 34 weeks' gestation.[45] However, prospective studies, though not randomized, have suggested that the majority of fetal losses occur earlier than 24 weeks and that TTTS is typically the cause.[46,47] These investigators have questioned the policy of elective preterm delivery; as selective laser photocoagulation continues to evolve and improve, this concern may be substantiated. Stirnemann and colleagues,[48] in the largest cohort of TTTS cases to date, studied postnatal outcome of pregnancies after laser surgery for TTTS. The risk of an unexpected adverse event decreased from 16.8% to 0% between 26 and 36 weeks, and the rate of death or severe brain lesions decreased from 35% in infants delivered at 26 to 28 weeks to 3% at 34 to 36 weeks. The investigators concluded that morbidity after laser therapy for TTTS appears low after 32 weeks, and "the decision for elective delivery should be based on medical history, parental demand, and expert assessment."[48]

Box 3
Malformations more common in twin gestations

Nervous System

- Encephalocele
- Reduction deformities of the brain

Cardiovascular System

- Ventricular septal defect
- Single ventricle
- Hypoplastic left heart syndrome
- Anomalies of pulmonary artery
- Single umbilical artery

Digestive system

- Cleft lip with and without cleft palate
- Tracheoesophageal fistula/esophageal atresia
- Intestinal atresia and stenosis

Genitourinary system

- Hypospadias
- Indeterminate sex
- Renal agenesis
- Cystic kidney disease
- Obstructive defect of the ureter

Musculoskeletal system

- Valgus defect of foot
- Limb reduction defects
- Anomalies of the spine or bones
- Anomalies of the diaphragm
- Anomalies of the abdominal wall

Adapted from Mastroiacovo P, Castilla EE, Arpino C, et al. Congenital malformations in twins: an international study. Am J Med Genet 1999;83:117–24; with permission.

Gastrointestinal Defects

Congenital diaphragmatic hernia (CDH) and gastroschisis are not uncommon congenital anomalies found in NICUs throughout the developed world. Timing of delivery for both of these anomalies has been controversial and is still under debate. Although the morbidity and mortality of these gastrointestinal defects are different, early term delivery has been suggested for both.

Historically, infants with CDH were allowed to remain in utero until spontaneous delivery, in the hopes of increased pulmonary development. However, in a large (628 infants) retrospective cohort study from the CDH Study Group Registry, Stevens and colleagues[49] found that infants born at early term ages (37–38 weeks' gestation) had increased survival when compared with infants born at later term ages (39–41 weeks' gestation). The investigators suggested the reason for the protective advantage of early term delivery may be due to increasing severity of pulmonary hypoplasia and pulmonary vascular abnormalities as the pregnancy progresses. At the time, this study was the best available evidence for the timing of delivery. Further studies, however, have not supported these results. Safavi and colleagues[50] evaluated the Canadian Pediatric Surgery Network (214 infants with CDH) and found no difference between route of delivery or the gestational age at delivery. Most recently, in the largest study to date of infants with CDH (928 infants) evaluating the United States Period Linked Birth-Infant Death database, mortality was found to be higher in infants born at 37 weeks compared with those born at 40 weeks.[51] The adjusted relative risk of infant mortality for early term births versus late term births was 1.56 (95% CI 1.21–2.01). Although there are several differences among all these studies, there does not seem to be a clear benefit for early or late term delivery for infants with CDH, and clinical equipoise remains regarding the optimal timing of delivery.

Two recent studies from Europe have suggested that early delivery of infants with gastroschisis may be of benefit. Although both studies were small retrospective reviews of changes in clinical practice, both found that early elective cesarean section at 35 to 36 weeks' gestation had improved outcomes in comparison with late vaginal or cesarean deliveries.[52,53] The mean time to start feeds and achieve full enteral feeds was shorter in the elective early delivery and the length of stay was decreased, although none of these outcomes were statistically significant. The hypothesis was that early delivery of the fetus might limit the injury to the exposed fetal intestine and thereby promote earlier return of intestinal function. However, early delivery remains controversial. The one randomized controlled trial on elective early delivery found no significant benefit (but also no harm) in early delivery of infants with gastroschisis.[54] However, this study was limited, as the control group had a mean age at delivery of 36.7 weeks, compared with 35.8 weeks in the elective group. Although the hypothesis of reducing intestinal injury is intriguing and physiologically plausible, evidence to suggest that early delivery is of benefit for infants with gastroschisis is limited.

Congenital Heart Disease

Premature or early delivery (<39 weeks) of infants with congenital heart disease is associated with poorer outcomes compared with delivery at 39 to 40 weeks' gestation.[55] In a recent study, Goff and colleagues[55] demonstrated that after cardiac surgery, infants who were born at older gestational ages had improved performance in cognition, visual-motor, and fine-motor skills. In addition, performance of language, executive function, and social skills were also statistically significantly improved in infants born at 39 to 40 weeks' gestation in comparison with those born before 39 weeks. Although early delivery of these infants might be indicated for maternal or fetal health reasons, infants with congenital heart disease should not be delivered before 39 weeks, if possible, to optimize neurodevelopmental outcomes.

Growth Issues

One of the many comorbidities associated with the varying constellations of congenital anomalies is intrauterine growth restriction (IUGR). A significant number of fetuses with IUGR are at risk for complications, including IUFD. The timing of delivery of the late preterm infant with IUGR to prevent IUFD is under debate. Several factors must be evaluated when determining when to deliver the IUGR fetus, including cause of the growth restriction, behavioral responses (nonstress test, biophysical profile), amniotic fluid volume, Doppler studies, current gestational age, interval growth, and maternal comorbidities.[56] Several of these determinants, if abnormal, may warrant urgent delivery if the fetus is beyond 34 weeks' gestation. For example, Doppler studies demonstrating reversed end-diastolic flow in the umbilical artery and a bio-physical profile of less than 4 carry a hypoxemia/acidemia rate as high as 80%.[56] Even without abnormal testing, the small fetus has added risk for morbidity and mortality. There is evidence to suggest that a fetus with IUGR should be delivered at 36 to 37 weeks' gestation even without evidence of fetal lung maturity. McIntire and colleagues[57] demonstrated that infants at or beyond 37 weeks with birth weights below the third percentile have higher rates of acidosis, respiratory failure, seizures, sepsis, and neonatal death.

MATERNAL CONDITIONS ASSOCIATED WITH BIRTH DEFECTS AND EARLY BIRTH

The association between maternal health and fetal well-being is a complex one. There are several maternal medical conditions that can lead to fetal congenital anomalies and several conditions that can lead to premature delivery. Maternal medical problems that may lead to indicated (elective) premature birth are varied and include respiratory, cardiovascular, and immunologic disorders (see **Box 2**). Many of these alter or limit placental blood flow and oxygen delivery to the fetus.

Obesity

Obesity, defined as a body mass index (BMI) of 30 kg/m^2 or higher, is a major health issue in the United States and the rest of the developed world. Obesity not only leads to cardiovascular and renal complications, but is also associated with an increased risk of birth defects. Prepregnancy maternal obesity has been well established as a risk factor for neural tube defects such as spina bifida and anencephaly.[58,59] More recent literature has suggested a modest association between maternal obesity and several other congenital anomalies. In a meta-analysis of 18 observational studies on prepregnancy or early pregnancy weight or BMI, Stothard and colleagues[60] found that obese mothers have increased odds of pregnancies affected by cardiovascular anomalies, cleft lip and palate, anorectal atresia, and limb reduction anomalies, in addition to the aforementioned neural tube defects. Other studies have also found an association between obesity and CDH and omphalocele but, interestingly, an inverse relationship with gastroschisis.[61,62]

The role of maternal weight in prematurity is still under debate. Several studies have shown that low maternal weight and BMI (<20 kg/m^2) are associated with premature delivery after adjusting for confounders. Moutquin[63] noted that women with low BMI were almost 4 times more likely to deliver preterm infants than their heavier counterparts. Additional studies have confirmed these findings. Sebire and colleagues,[64] in a cohort of more than 285,000 singleton pregnancies (70% Caucasian), found that obese women were significantly less likely to deliver before 32 weeks. In addition, Hendler and colleagues[65] found that in a cohort of 2910 women (65% African American), obese women had lower rates of shortened cervical length and lower rates of spontaneous preterm births (OR 0.57, 95% CI 0.39–0.83). However, in a study of more than 350,000 Chinese women, the incidence of preterm birth in obese women, especially nulliparae, was significantly higher (OR 2.94, 95% CI 2.04–4.25).[66] These conflicting studies suggest that there may be other genetic and ethnic factors playing a role. If obesity is protective against premature delivery, it is thought that obesity-related changes in systemic inflammation may be significant.[67]

Diabetes

For decades it has been well known that prepregnancy diabetes mellitus is associated with significant morbidity in the fetus and infant. An increased rate of respiratory distress syndrome resulting from decreased production of surfactant has been well established.[68] Other congenital anomalies associated with poor maternal glycemic control include cardiac malformations and caudal regression syndrome (sacral agenesis). In addition, IUGR (due to maternal vascular disease) and polyhydramnios (see earlier discussion) are also related to maternal diabetes. In a cohort of more than 400,000 pregnancies (1677 with preexisting diabetes), the risk for congenital anomalies in diabetic mothers was approximately 7%, 4 times higher than for the general population.[69] Type and duration of diabetes, age, ethnicity, and BMI were not associated with increased risk for congenital anomalies. Why these anomalies occur is not entirely understood. Certainly, hyperinsulinism in the fetus can lead to organomegaly, but the etiology of sacral agenesis is less well understood. It has been speculated that hyperglycemia leads to release of free radicals; these potent molecules may be directly teratogenic to local cells, or may disrupt signal transduction through enhanced lipid peroxidation and prostaglandin imbalance.[70]

Because of the higher incidence of congenital anomalies, macrosomia, and concern for fetal compromise and IUFD in diabetic mothers, elective early birth is not uncommon. What is less well understood is whether there is an increase in spontaneous preterm birth in diabetic mothers. To answer this question, Kock and colleagues[71] evaluated 187 women with either gestational or preexisting diabetes and compared their perinatal outcomes with those of 192 normoglycemic women. Diabetic women were found to be significantly more likely to deliver prematurely, both electively ($P = .002$) and spontaneously ($P = .047$). These associations were independent of preeclampsia and birth weight. The investigators hypothesized that maternal glucose intolerance impaired pregnancy progression through an unknown mechanism.[71]

Depression

Depression among women of childbearing age is not uncommon, and perhaps underreported and underappreciated, with as many as 3% to 6% of pregnant women receiving medication therapy directed at this problem.[72] Because of this significant incidence of depression, there has been great interest in studying fetal effects of the relatively new selective serotonin reuptake inhibitors (SSRIs) typically prescribed for depression. Although it is difficult to ascertain whether there is a significant association between SSRIs and congenital anomalies, because of the small numbers of exposed infants in the studies and the multiple formulations of SSRIs, it appears that at least 2 SSRIs, fluoxetine and paroxetine, are associated with anomalies (isolated ventricular septal defects and right ventricular outflow tract defects, respectively).[73–76] Of note, Malm and colleagues[73] also found that fetal alcohol spectrum disorders were 10 times more common in the SSRI-exposed offspring than in unexposed infants.

In addition to the birth defects associated with SSRIs, more evidence is emerging that they may be associated with preterm birth. Wisner and colleagues[77] conducted a prospective observational investigation over the course of pregnancy in 238 women with and without depression and SSRI use. Women who were treated with SSRIs throughout pregnancy were found to be more likely to deliver infants prematurely. In addition, women with untreated major depression had similar rates (>20%) of premature delivery. Only 4% of infants partially exposed to SSRIs during gestation and 6% of infants not exposed at all to SSRIs or depression were delivered preterm.[77] More research is needed to determine the best therapy for depression in pregnant women and to identify the differing effects within the SSRI class of drugs.

Behavioral Factors

Behavioral factors such as smoking and alcohol ingestion have been reported to both cause birth defects and be risk factors for preterm birth. Regarding birth defects, the hallmarks of fetal alcohol syndrome, poor growth, decreased tone and coordination, and typical facies may also be accompanied by structural heart defects, including ventricular septal defects and atrial septal defects. The proportion of cases in the literature reported to have a congenital heart defect ranges from 33% to 100%, with septal defects comprising the vast majority.[78] Smoking has also been known to contribute to certain birth defects. Both heavy maternal smoking ($\geq$25 cigarettes per day) and periconceptional smoking have been associated with bilateral cleft lip and cleft palate, as well as atrioventricular septal defects.[79,80]

Regarding prematurity, several studies have demonstrated smoking as a risk factor for premature labor, including the development of preterm premature rupture of membranes. Compared with nonsmokers, adjusted ORs of preterm birth before 32 weeks were 1.4 (95% CI 0.8–2.4) and 2.9 (95% CI 1.5–5.7) for moderate (1–9 cigarettes per day) and heavy ($\geq$10 cigarettes per day) smokers, respectively.[81] A similar dose-response effect can be seen in alcohol consumption. Heavy alcohol consumption (>1.5 drinks per day) during pregnancy increases the risk of fetal growth restriction and preterm birth, whereas moderate to light consumption has not been shown to have a significant effect.[82] The existence of these behavioral risk factors for both birth defects and preterm birth supports close and timely antenatal consultations for high-risk mothers.

SUMMARY

Neither premature/early birth nor congenital anomalies are caused by a single, simple, "one-hit" factor. Interactions between genetic coding, the environment (both maternal and uterine), and family history all play a role in fetal and infant well-being. This article outlines several interconnected risk factors for both birth defects and early birth; perhaps ongoing or future investigations, including epidemiologic evaluations and

---

Box 4
Steps to reduce the risk of birth defects and preterm birth

1. Use a preconception visit to plan for pregnancy and initiate risk factor reduction.

2. Begin a prenatal vitamin including at least 400 µg of folate before conception and continue throughout pregnancy.

3. Screen for and control medical conditions that may lead to adverse events during pregnancy (ie, diabetes, hypertension).

4. Review all medications including prescribed, over-the-counter, and alternative therapies, and review potential side effects (both fetal and maternal).

5. Measure body mass index before pregnancy and review healthy and adequate weight gain during pregnancy.

6. Stop smoking, illicit drug use, and alcohol consumption before conception.

7. Review family history for adverse birth outcomes including history of birth defects and preterm birth. If positive, refer to genetic counselor.

Adapted from Dolan SM, Callaghan WM, Rasmussen SA. Birth defects and preterm birth: overlapping outcomes with a shared strategy for research and prevention. Birth Defects Res A Clin Mol Teratol 2009;85:874–8; with permission.

animal modeling, will further elucidate these complex interactions. The overlapping risk factors and associations provide a common ground for work aimed at reducing the incidence of both birth defects and preterm birth.[3] In many cases, infants are at risk for not one but both of these outcomes. Reduction or elimination of many of the risk factors discussed in this article may prevent both birth defects and premature birth. There are several steps that health care providers and women can take to reduce these risks (**Box 4**). Additional resources are available through several agencies including the American Congress of Obstetricians and Gynecologists, the American Academy of Pediatrics, the March of Dimes, and the World Health Organization.[83–86]

REFERENCES

1. March of Dimes. Birth defects. Available at: www.marchofdimes.com/baby/birthdefects.html. Accessed March 8, 2013.
2. Nelson K, Holmes LB. Malformations due to presumed spontaneous mutations in newborn infants. N Engl J Med 1989;320:19–23.
3. Dolan SM, Callaghan WM, Rasmussen SA. Birth defects and preterm birth: overlapping outcomes with a shared strategy for research and prevention. Birth Defects Res A Clin Mol Teratol 2009;85:874–8.
4. Streissguth AP, Bookstein FL, Barr HM, et al. Risk factors for adverse life outcomes in fetal alcohol syndrome and fetal alcohol effects. J Dev Behav Pediatr 2004;5:228–38.
5. Streissguth AP, Barr HM, Kogan J, et al. Understanding the occurrence of secondary disabilities in clients with fetal alcohol syndrome (FAS) and fetal alcohol effects (FAE). Final report to the Centers for Disease Control and Prevention (CDC). Seattle (WA): University of Washington; 1996. Fetal Alcohol & Drug Unit; August. Tech Rep No 96–06.
6. Franks ME, Macpherson GR, Figg WD. Thalidomide. Lancet 2004;363:1802–11.
7. Herbst AL, Ulfelder H, Poskanzer DC. Adenocarcinoma of the vagina—association of maternal stilbestrol therapy with tumor appearance in young women. N Engl J Med 1971;284:878–81.
8. United States Food and Drug Administration (FDA). Certain estrogens for oral or parenteral use. Drugs for human use; drug efficacy study implementation. Fed Regist 1971;36(217):21537–8.
9. Rasmussen SA, Moore CA, Paulozzi LJ, et al. Risk for birth defects among premature infants: a population-based study. J Pediatr 2001;138:668–73.
10. Dolan SM, Gross SJ, Merkatz IR, et al. The contribution of birth defects to preterm birth and low birth weight. Obstet Gynecol 2007;110:318–24.
11. Honein MA, Kirby RS, Meyer RE, et al. The association between major birth defects and preterm birth. Matern Child Health J 2009;13:164–75.
12. Grandi C, Luchtenberg G, Rittler M. The contribution of birth defects to spontaneous preterm birth. Am J Perinatol 2007;24:487–92.
13. Parker SE, Mai CT, Canfield MA, et al. Updated national birth prevalence estimates for selected birth defects in the United States, 2004-2006. Birth Defects Res A Clin Mol Teratol 2010;88:1008–16.
14. Boghossian NS, Horbar JD, Carpenter JH, et al, Vermont Oxford Network. Major chromosomal anomalies among very low birth weight infants in the Vermont Oxford Network. J Pediatr 2012;160:774–80.e11.
15. Byrne J, Warburton D, Kline J, et al. Morphology of early fetal deaths and their chromosomal characteristics. Teratology 1985;32:297–315.

16. Creasy MR, Alberman ER. A cytogenetic study of human spontaneous abortions using banding techniques. Hum Genet 1976;31:977–96.

17. Angell RR, Sanidson A, Bain AD. Chromosome variation in perinatal mortality: a survey of 500 cases. J Med Genet 1984;21:39–44.

18. Kuhn EM, Sarto GE, Bates BG, et al. Gene-rich chromosome regions and autosomal trisomy. Hum Genet 1987;77:214–20.

19. Wang JC. Autosomal aneuploidies. In: Keagle MB, Gersen SL, editors. The principles of clinical cytogenetics. 2nd edition. Totowa (NJ): Humana Press; 2005. p. 133–64.

20. Guin G, Punekar S, Lele A, et al. A prospective clinical study of feto-maternal outcome in pregnancies with abnormal liquor volume. J Obstet Gynaecol India 2011;61:652–5.

21. Stoll CG, Alembik Y, Dott B. Study of 156 cases of polyhydramnios and congenital malformations in a series of 118,265 consecutive births. Am J Obstet Gynecol 1991;165:586.

22. Peled Y, Hod M, Friedman S, et al. Prenatal diagnosis of familial congenital pyloric atresia. Prenat Diagn 1992;12:151–4.

23. Rudnik-Schoneborn S, Nicholson GA, Morgan G, et al. Different patterns of obstetric complications in myotonic dystrophy in relation to the disease status of the fetus. Am J Med Genet 1998;80:314–21.

24. Pri-Paz S, Khalek N, Fuchs KM, et al. Maximal amniotic fluid index as a prognostic factor in pregnancies complicated by polyhydramnios. Ultrasound Obstet Gynecol 2012;39:648–53.

25. Many A, Lazebnik N, Hill LM. The underlying cause of polyhydramnios determines prematurity. Prenat Diagn 1996;16:55–7.

26. Many A, Hill LM, Lazebnik N, et al. The association between polyhydramnios and preterm delivery. Obstet Gynecol 1995;86:389–91.

27. Centers for Disease Control and Prevention. Syphilis. Available at: www.cdc. gov. Accessed March 11, 2013.

28. LaFond RE, Lukehart SA. Biological basis for syphilis. Clin Microbiol Rev 2006; 19:29.

29. Donders GG, Desmyter J, De Wet DH, et al. The association of gonorrhea and syphilis with premature birth and low birthweight. Genitourin Med 1993;69: 98–101.

30. Knox IC Jr, Hoerner JK. The role of infection in premature rupture of the membranes. Am J Obstet Gynecol 1950;59:190–4.

31. Bobitt JR, Ledger WJ. Unrecognized amnionitis and prematurity: a preliminary report. J Reprod Med 1977;19:8–12.

32. Goldenberg RL, Culhane JF, Johnson DC. Maternal infection and adverse fetal and neonatal outcomes. Clin Perinatol 2005;32:523–59.

33. Pistorius LR, Smal J, de Haan TR, et al. Disturbance of cerebral neuronal migration following congenital parvovirus B19 infection. Fetal Diagn Ther 2008;24: 491–4.

34. Kishore J, Misra R, Paisal A, et al. Adverse reproductive outcome induced by parvovirus B19 and TORCH infections in women with high-risk pregnancy. J Infect Dev Ctries 2011;5:868–73.

35. Mace G, Audry G, Cortey A, et al. Congenital hypoplasia of the abdominal wall muscles following fetal ascites due to parvovirus B19 infection. Ultrasound Obstet Gynecol 2011;37:497–8.

36. Savarese I, De Carolis MP, Costa S, et al. Atypical manifestations of congenital parvovirus B19 infection. Eur J Pediatr 2008;167:1463–6.

37. James BC, Savitz LA. How intermountain trimmed health care costs through robust quality improvement efforts. Health Aff (Millwood) 2011;30:1185–91.
38. Spong CY, Mercer BM, D'Alton M, et al. Timing of indicated late-preterm and early-term birth. Obstet Gynecol 2011;118:323.
39. Martin JA, Hamilton BE, Ventura SJ, et al. Births: final data for 2010. Natl Vital Stat Rep 2012;61:1–65.
40. Mastroiacovo P, Castilla EE, Arpino C, et al. Congenital malformations in twins: an international study. Am J Med Genet 1999;83:117–24.
41. Nance WE. Malformations unique to the twinning process. Prog Clin Biol Res 1981;69A:123.
42. Gul A, Cebecia A, Aslan H, et al. Perinatal outcomes of twin pregnancies discordant for major fetal anomalies. Fetal Diagn Ther 2005;20:244.
43. Rossi AC, Vanderbilt D, Chmait RH. Neurodevelopmental outcomes after laser therapy for twin-twin transfusion syndrome. Obstet Gynecol 2011;118:1145–50.
44. Mahony R, Mulcahy C, McAuliffe F, et al. Fetal death in twins. Acta Obstet Gynecol Scand 2011;90:1274–80.
45. Farah N, Hogan J, Johnson S, et al. Prospective risk of fetal death in uncomplicated monochorionic twins. Acta Obstet Gynecol Scand 2012;91:382–5.
46. Lewi L, Jani J, Blickstein I, et al. The outcome of monochorionic diamniotic twin gestations in the era of invasive fetal therapy: a prospective cohort study. Am J Obstet Gynecol 2008;199:514.e1–8.
47. Simoes T, Amaral N, Lerman R, et al. Prospective risk of intrauterine death of monochorionic-diamniotic twins. Am J Obstet Gynecol 2006;195:134–9.
48. Stirnemann JJ, Quibel T, Essaoui M, et al. Timing of delivery following selective laser photocoagulation for twin-to-twin transfusion syndrome. Am J Obstet Gynecol 2012;207:127.e1–6.
49. Stevens TP, van Wijngaarden E, Ackerman KG, et al, Congenital Diaphragmatic Hernia Study Group. Timing of delivery and survival rates for infants with prenatal diagnoses of congenital diaphragmatic hernia. Pediatrics 2009;123:494–502.
50. Safavi A, Lin Y, Skarsgard ED. Perinatal management of congenital diaphragmatic hernia: when and how should babies be delivered? Results from the Canadian Pediatric Surgery Network. J Pediatr Surg 2010;45:2334–9.
51. Hutcheon JA, Butler B, Lisonkova S, et al. Timing of delivery for pregnancies with congenital diaphragmatic hernia. BJOG 2010;117:1658–62.
52. Hadidi A, Subotic U, Goeppl M, et al. Early elective cesarean delivery before 36 weeks vs late spontaneous delivery in infants with gastroschisis. J Pediatr Surg 2008;43:1342–6.
53. Reigstad I, Reigstad H, Kiserud T, et al. Preterm elective caesarean section and early enteral feeding in gastroschisis. Acta Paediatr 2011;100:71–4.
54. Logghe HL, Mason GC, Thornton JG, et al. A randomized controlled trial of elective preterm delivery of fetuses with gastroschisis. J Pediatr Surg 2005;40:1726–31.
55. Goff DA, Luan X, Gerdes M, et al. Younger gestational age is associated with worse neurodevelopmental outcomes after cardiac surgery in infancy. J Thorac Cardiovasc Surg 2012;143:535–42.
56. Galan HL. Timing delivery of the growth-restricted fetus. Semin Perinatol 2011;35:262–9.
57. McIntire DD, Bloom SL, Casey BM, et al. Birth weight in relation to morbidity and mortality among newborn infants. N Engl J Med 1999;340:1234–8.
58. Shaw GM, Velie EM, Schaffer D. Risk of neural tube defect-affected pregnancies among obese women. JAMA 1996;275:1093–6.

59. Werler MM, Louik C, Shapiro S, et al. Prepregnant weight in relation to risk of neural tube defects. JAMA 1996;275:1089–92.
60. Stothard KJ, Tennant PW, Bell R, et al. Maternal overweight and obesity and the risk of congenital anomalies: a systematic review and meta-analysis. JAMA 2009;301:636–50.
61. Waller DK, Shaw GM, Rasmussen SA, et al. Prepregnancy obesity as a risk factor for structural birth defects. Arch Pediatr Adolesc Med 2007;161: 745–50.
62. Watkins ML, Rasmussen SA, Honein MA, et al. Maternal obesity and risk for birth defects. Pediatrics 2003;111:1152–8.
63. Moutquin JM. Socio-economic and psychosocial factors in the management and prevention of preterm labour. BJOG 2003;110:56–60.
64. Sebire NJ, Jolly M, Harris JP, et al. Maternal obesity and pregnancy outcome: a study of 287,213 pregnancies in London. Int J Obes Relat Metab Disord 2001; 25:1175–82.
65. Hendler I, Goldenberg RL, Mercer BM, et al. The preterm prediction study: association between maternal body mass index and spontaneous and indicated preterm birth. Am J Obstet Gynecol 2005;192:882–6.
66. Wang T, Zhang J, Lu X, et al. Maternal early pregnancy body mass index and risk of preterm birth. Arch Gynecol Obstet 2011;284:813–9.
67. Committee on Understanding Premature Birth and Assuring Healthy Outcomes. Medical and pregnancy conditions associated with preterm birth. In: Behrman RE, Butler AS, editors. Preterm birth: causes, consequences, and prevention. Washington (DC): National Academies Press; 2006. p. 148–68.
68. Wirbelauer J, Speer CP. The role of surfactant treatment in preterm infants and term newborns with acute respiratory distress syndrome. J Perinatol 2009; 29(Supp 2):S18–22.
69. Bell R, Glinianaia SV, Tennant PW, et al. Peri-conception hyperglycaemia and nephropathy are associated with risk of congenital anomaly in women with pre-existing diabetes: a population-based cohort study. Diabetologia 2012. [Epub ahead of print].
70. Reece EA, Homko CJ. Why do diabetic women deliver malformed infants? Clin Obstet Gynecol 2000;43:32–45.
71. Kock K, Kock F, Klein K, et al. Diabetes mellitus and the risk of preterm birth with regard to the risk of spontaneous preterm birth. J Matern Fetal Neonatal Med 2010;23:1004–8.
72. Andrade SE, Raebel MA, Brown J, et al. Use of antidepressant medications during pregnancy: a multisite study. Am J Obstet Gynecol 2008;198:194.e1–5.
73. Malm H, Artama M, Gissler M, et al. Selective serotonin reuptake inhibitors and risk for major congenital anomalies. Obstet Gynecol 2011;118:111–20.
74. Louik C, Lin AE, Werler MM, et al. First-trimester use of selective serotonin-reuptake inhibitors and the risk of birth defects. N Engl J Med 2007;356: 2675–83.
75. Alwan S, Reefhuis J, Rasmussen SA, et al. Use of selective serotonin-reuptake inhibitors in pregnancy and the risk of birth defects. N Engl J Med 2007;356: 2684–92.
76. Greene MF. Teratogenicity of SSRIs—serious concern or much ado about little? N Engl J Med 2007;356:2732–3.
77. Wisner KL, Sit DK, Hanusa BH, et al. Major depression and antidepressant treatment: impact on pregnancy and neonatal outcomes. Am J Psychiatry 2009;166:557–66.

78. Burd L, Deal E, Rios R, et al. Congenital heart defects and fetal alcohol spectrum disorders. Congenit Heart Dis 2007;2:250–5.
79. Patel SS, Burns TL, Botto LD, et al. Analysis of selected maternal exposures and non-syndromic atrioventricular septal defects in the National Birth Defects Prevention Study, 1997-2005. Am J Med Genet A 2012;158:2447–55.
80. Honein MA, Rasmussen SA, Reefhuis J, et al. Maternal smoking and environmental tobacco smoke exposure and the risk of orofacial clefts. Epidemiology 2007;18:226–33.
81. Kyrklund-Blomberg NB, Granath F, Cnattingius S. Maternal smoking and causes of very preterm birth. Acta Obstet Gynecol Scand 2005;84:572–7.
82. Patra J, Bakker R, Irving H, et al. Dose-response relationship between alcohol consumption before and during pregnancy and the risks of low birthweight, preterm birth and small for gestational age (SGA)-a systematic review and meta-analyses. BJOG 2011;118:1411–21.
83. American Congress of Obstetricians and Gynecologists. Available at: www.acog.org. Accessed March 30, 2013.
84. American Academy of Pediatrics. Available at: www.aap.org. Accessed March 30, 2013.
85. March of Dimes. Available at: www.marchofdimes.org. Accessed March 30, 2013.
86. World Health Organization. Available at: www.who.int. Accessed March 30, 2013.

Physiologic Underpinnings for Clinical Problems in Moderately Preterm and Late Preterm Infants

Rakesh Sahni, MD, Richard A. Polin, MD*

KEYWORDS

- Thermoregulation • Respiratory morbidities • Immunologic immaturity
- Glucose homeostasis • Gastrointestinal immaturity • Hepatic immaturity
- Brain dysmaturity

KEY POINTS

- Preterm birth, even a few weeks before term, is associated with a high prevalence of clinical problems.
- Issues arise from functional immaturities of a wide variety of organ systems, acquired problems, and problems associated with inadequate monitoring and/or follow-up plans.
- Different organ systems mature at rates and trajectories that are specific to their functions, whereas maturation rates vary amongst infants. A better understanding of these principles can help guide optimal treatment strategies.

INTRODUCTION

In the United States approximately 1 in 8 infants is born prematurely (<37 weeks).[1] Eighty-four percent of all preterm births are either late preterm infants ($34^{0/7}$–$36^{6/7}$ weeks) or moderately preterm infants ($32^{0/7}$–$33^{6/7}$ weeks) and those groups represent 14% of infant deaths.[2] The causes of preterm birth are heterogeneous, but approximately one-third are medically indicated to protect the well-being of the mother or fetus.[3] Between 10% and 20% of late preterm births may be avoidable by a change in obstetric practices.[4] Late preterm infants experience morbidities 7 times more frequently than term infants (22% vs 3%)[5,6] and add billions of dollars to societal costs of health care.[7] Several major morbidities are associated with late preterm or moderately preterm births:

- Temperature instability
- Respiratory distress

Department of Pediatrics, Columbia University College of Physicians and Surgeons, 3959 Broadway, MSCHN-1201, New York, NY 10032, USA
* Corresponding author.
E-mail address: rap32@columbia.edu

Clin Perinatol 40 (2013) 645–663
http://dx.doi.org/10.1016/j.clp.2013.07.012   perinatology.theclinics.com

- Apnea
- Sepsis
- Hypoglycemia
- Feeding difficulties
- Hyperbilirubinemia

This article discusses the physiologic basis for several of the major morbidities occurring in moderate and late preterm infants.

THERMOREGULATION

Thermoregulation, an important component of physiologic homeostasis, is the ability to maintain body temperature within specific parameters, even when the surrounding temperature is different from that of the subject. It is well established that newborns are predisposed to cold stress at birth unless preventative measures are undertaken.[8] Following birth, the newborn has to mount a variety of physiologic responses to conserve heat loss, increase heat production, and maintain core temperature with the least amount of oxygen consumption in the process.[9–12] For term newborns experiencing cold stress, this is accomplished through nonshivering thermogenesis, increased involuntary activity, and vasoconstriction.[13] Unlike their term counterparts, moderate and late preterm infants are more likely to experience disruptions in thermoregulation. These disruptions are the result of specific challenges to heat production and regulation that are caused by a combination of factors in the context of prematurity, including insufficient brown fat for nonshivering thermogenesis, large surface area compared with body mass, deficient subcutaneous fat and nonkeratinized thin skin, less ability to maintain flexion of extremities, and underdeveloped response of the temperature sensors in the posterior hypothalamus to release thermogenic hormones such as thyroxine and norepinephrine.[9–12,14,15] These hormones peak at term gestation and the moderate or late preterm infant misses those last few weeks of in utero development.[16] In addition, more frequent delivery-room interventions in this group of infants further increase the risk of hypothermia and impede strategies to prevent heat loss. The ineffective thermoregulation in the moderate or late preterm infant predisposes the infant to significant complications. For example, an infant who becomes hypothermic is at risk of developing hypoglycemia.[14] Hypoglycemia and hypothermia are also linked to deteriorating respiratory distress and are often the first signs of sepsis.[17,18] In addition, in moderate and late preterm infants the immature nervous system is unable to respond appropriately to thermal stress, thereby worsening the respiratory and metabolic complications.[19]

RESPIRATORY MORBIDITIES

Pulmonary disorders such as respiratory distress syndrome (RDS), transient tachypnea of the newborn (TTN), pneumonia, and apnea of prematurity are more common, and incur a greater risk of respiratory failure, in moderate and late preterm than in full-term infants.[20] This increased respiratory morbidity is thought to be related to functional immaturity of the lung structure at 34 to 37 weeks of gestation, which predisposes to delayed intrapulmonary fluid absorption, surfactant insufficiency, and ultimately to inefficient gas exchange.[21] Many more moderate and late preterm infants develop respiratory distress soon after birth, compared with those born at term (28.9% vs 4.2%).[22] In addition, for each gestational week of age, infants delivered by elective cesarean section tend to do worse.[23] The risk of ongoing respiratory morbidity after the early neonatal period remains unclear. Some studies suggest that preterm birth may have adverse effects on lung growth and development, with subsequent reduced pulmonary function, even when there has been no significant respiratory disease in the neonatal period.[24]

RDS

The incidence of RDS in late preterm infants is 13-fold higher compared with infants born at 37 to 40 weeks' gestation (5.2% vs 0.4%).[20] RDS thus remains the most common cause of significant respiratory morbidity in moderate and late preterm infants. RDS results from quantitative and/or qualitative deficiency of pulmonary surfactant superimposed on cardiorespiratory immaturity. Surfactant is composed primarily of phospholipids, which represent approximately 80% to 90% of its mass. In mature fetuses, phosphatidylcholine represents 80% of total phospholipids, phosphatidylglycerol is 5% to 10%, and other minor lipids make up the remainder. The phospholipid composition of alveolar lavage fluid changes during perinatal development; there is an increased phosphatidylcholine content during the last one-third of gestation. Around 35 weeks' gestation, there is a significant surge in surfactant pool size, reaching a peak at term. However, preterm infants lack phosphatidylglycerol, which results in deficient surfactant function and predisposes them to RDS. In addition, uterine contractions preceding labor, hormonal surges and cellular factors, and initiation of ventilation enhances secretion of pulmonary surfactant from type-II pneumocytes into the alveoli. All these processes are either deficient or nonexistent in moderate and late preterm infants, thus setting the stage for RDS.[24–26] In affected infants the incidence of respiratory distress requiring mechanical ventilation corresponds with the degree of prematurity: 3.3% of late preterm infants born at 34 weeks' gestation, 1.7% at 35 weeks' gestation, and 0.8% at 36 weeks' gestation need mechanical ventilation.[27]

TTN

The incidence of TTN is about 4% in late preterm infants, making it the second most common respiratory morbidity.[28–30] TTN results from a lack of timely clearance of the pulmonary fluid from the alveolar airspaces. The risk of developing TTN is greater in infants born precipitously without active labor, and in those delivered by elective cesarean section. Although Starling forces and squeeze during vaginal delivery may play some role in the clearing of this lung fluid, amiloride-sensitive sodium transport by lung epithelial cells through epithelial sodium channels (ENaCs) has emerged as the principal event in facilitating transepithelial movement of alveolar fluid.[31,32] Disruption of ENaC function has been implicated in the respiratory distress associated with TTN. Moderate and late preterm infants are more susceptible to this problem, in part because ENaC expression is developmentally regulated and the peak expression in the alveolar epithelium is achieved only at term gestation. Lower expression of these channels in moderate and late preterm infants reduces their ability to clear lung fluid after birth.[33]

Hypoxic Respiratory Failure

Although respiratory disorders are usually transient in most moderate and late preterm infants, some develop severe hypoxic respiratory failure or persistent pulmonary hypertension of the newborn (PPHN) requiring additional therapies such as high-frequency ventilation, inhaled nitric oxide, and extracorporeal membrane oxygenation.[30,34] Many of these infants initially receive high concentrations of oxygen through noninvasive devices, leading to pulmonary nitrogen washout and alveolar atelectasis. Studies have shown that PPHN is more likely to occur in infants born at 34 to 37 weeks' gestation who develop RDS compared with infants born at 32 weeks' gestation.[30]

Such predisposition is attributed to a developmental increase in smooth muscle in the walls of pulmonary blood vessels and the resultant increase in the pulmonary vascular resistance that eventually leads to pulmonary-to-systemic shunting and ventilation-perfusion mismatching.[21]

Pneumonia

Fetal infection as an underlying cause for preterm delivery predisposes moderate and late preterm infants to sepsis and pulmonary infections. In addition, mechanical ventilation can injure the immature lung further and increase the risk for pulmonary infections.[35] The incidence of pneumonia in infants born at 34 weeks' gestation is almost 15-fold higher compared with infants born at 39 weeks' gestation (1.5% vs 0.1%).[20]

Autonomic Regulation, Control of Breathing, and Apnea of Prematurity

The control of breathing and maturation of brainstem regions in moderate and late preterm infants are less mature than those of a full-term infant, making them prone to develop apnea of prematurity. During late gestation, there are dramatic and nonlinear developmental changes in the brainstem with respect to neuronal origin and proliferation, migration pathways, morphologic and neurochemical differentiation, neurotransmitter receptors, transporters, and enzymes, dendritic arborization, spine formation, synaptogenesis, axonal outgrowth, and myelination.[36] These changes translate into immaturity of upper airway and lung volume control, laryngeal reflexes, chemical control of breathing, and sleep mechanisms. The ventilatory response to hypoxia in preterm infants is unique; there is an initial transient hyperventilation followed by a return to baseline and then a decrease to less than baseline.[37] In infants born at 32 to 37 weeks, the parasympathetic nervous system is significantly less mature than in full-term infants, as shown by diminished increases in high-frequency heart rate variability in quiet sleep. This difference suggests that moderate and late preterm infants are more susceptible to bradycardia than full-term infants.[38] Ten percent of late preterm infants have significant apnea of prematurity and they frequently have delays in establishing coordination of feeding and breathing. Obstructive and mixed apnea also occur at greater frequency and severity compared with infants born at term. Developmental features such as highly compliant chest wall and upper airways that tend to collapse when the diaphragm contracts (and generates negative intrathoracic pressure) contribute significantly to these events. Both the presence and severity of apnea of prematurity progressively decrease with advancing postmenstrual age. The incidence of apparent life-threatening events (ALTE) is also more common in preterm infants (8%–10%) than in full-term infants (1% or less). In the Collaborative Home Infant Monitoring Evaluation study, 86% of infants experiencing an ALTE were born between 34 and 37 weeks' gestation.[39] The rate for sudden infant death syndrome in preterm infants born at 33 to 36 weeks is 1.37/1000 live births compared with 0.69/1000 live births in infants born full-term.[40] Affected late preterm infants die at an older mean postmenstrual age compared with less mature infants (48 and 46 weeks, respectively), but die at a younger postmenstrual age than full-term infants (53 weeks).[41]

IMMUNOLOGIC IMMATURITY AND INFECTIONS

Preterm infants have a higher rate of early-onset sepsis and health care–associated infections.[42,43] Although some of these infections are the result of invasive monitoring, host defense impairments contribute to the increased susceptibility to both categories of infections as well as to necrotizing enterocolitis. Moreover, chorioamnionitis is thought to be responsible for a significant proportion of infants delivered to women with preterm labor or preterm premature rupture of membranes.

Unlike older children and adults, neonates are highly dependent on the innate immune system to defend against an infectious challenge, especially in the first several days of life.[44] Innate responses are defined as those present at the time of birth before exposure to a bacterial or fungal pathogen. The innate immune system consists of skin and mucosal barriers, sentinel cell (phagocytic cells and antigen-presenting cells) pathogen recognition systems, inflammatory response proteins, host defense proteins and peptides, and passively acquired maternal immunoglobulin. Although most studies have not focused on late preterm or moderate preterm infants, several generalizations about host susceptibility are possible.

At the time of birth, the skin of the newborn infant is covered by vernix caseosa.[45] Vernix is a complex proteolipid cellular cream and is reduced in infants born prematurely. The vernix not only reduces insensible water losses but also serves as a shield against antioxidants and promotes colonization with commensal organisms rather than pathogens.[46] The stratum corneum of the skin is the major mechanical barrier against bacterial infection[47]; however, it may take weeks to become fully functional.[48] The variables affecting colonization of the skin include development of the acid mantle, local environmental factors such as occlusion and humidity, and skin care practices.[49] At birth the skin has a neutral pH, which decreases over the ensuing weeks. Acid mantle development is delayed in very low birth weight infants and likely develops more slowly in late preterm and moderate preterm infants.[50] The acid mantle is thought to be important in antimicrobial defense; however, there are a variety of antimicrobial agents produced by the epidermis, including complement components, defensins, cathelicidins, cytokines, chemokines, and reactive oxygen species.[47] Other epidermal cells have an important role in host defense. For example, keratinocytes have been shown to internalize and kill bacteria, and Langerhans cells in the mid to lower epidermis are critical for immune surveillance. The density and function of Langerhans cells in the preterm population has not been investigated.

Pattern recognition receptors (PRRs) sit on the cell surface, within intracellular vesicles, and in the cytoplasm of immune cells (macrophages, dendritic cells, and neutrophils) and on the surface of nonimmune cells (eg, epithelial cells of the gastrointestinal tract). They are the critical link between pathogen recognition and the innate immune response. In humans, the major PRRs are Toll-like receptors (TLRs), 10 of which have been described. Activation of TLRs results in downstream production of cytokines, chemokines, complement, and coagulation proteins, and enhances phagocytic function (**Fig. 1**).[51] TLR4 is the major PRR for gram-negative bacteria and its expression has been shown to increase with advancing gestational age.[52] Another important PRR is beta 2 integrin complement receptor type 3 (CR3). CR3 functions as a pathogen sensor on the surface of phagocytes. Engagement of the CR3 receptor on the surface of phagocytes leads to production of reactive oxygen intermediates and enhances phagocytosis. There is decreased expression of CR3 on neonatal phagocytes, which may impair their accumulation at sites of inflammation.[53] CR3 expression is further reduced in preterm neonates.[54]

TLR-mediated cytokine production differs in newborn infants and adults.[55] Monocytes derived from infants produce less T helper cell (T_H1)-polarizing cytokines (interleukin [IL]-1β, tumor necrosis factor alpha [TNF-α], interferon alfa [IFN-α], and interferon gamma [IFN-γ]), but more T_H2/T_H17-polarizing cytokines (IL-6, IL-10, IL-17, and IL-23). T_H1 cells develop from naive CD4+ T cells following exposure to IFN-γ and IL-12 and promote cell-mediated immunity against intracellular pathogens. T_H2 cells develop in the presence of IL-2 and IL-4. T_H2 responses support humoral

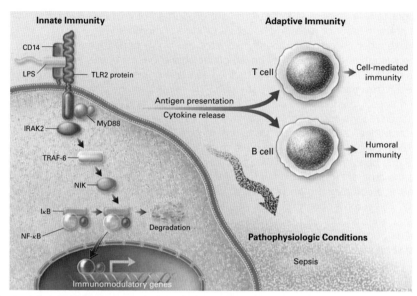

Fig. 1. Role of Toll-like receptor 2 (TLR2) in the regulation of the response of macrophages to bacterial lipopolysaccharide (LPS). (*From* Modlin RL, Brightbill HD, Godowski PJ. The toll of innate immunity on microbial pathogens. N Engl J Med 1999;340(23):1834–5; with permission.)

immunity but also downregulate T_H1 responses. T_H17 cells are produced in the presence of IL-6, IL-21, and IL-23 and are important in the defense against extracellular bacteria and fungi (**Fig. 2**). The decrease in T_H1-polarizing cytokines likely decreases the ability of neonates to respond to microorganisms that are intracellular pathogens

Th Group	Cell Products	Cell Target	Infectious Agents
Th1	Interferon-γ Interleukin-2 Interleukin-12R	Macrophages Dendritic cells	Intracellular bacteria Fungi Viruses
Th17	Interleukin-17A Interleukin-17F Interleukin-21 Interleukin-22 Interleukin-23R	Neutrophils	Extracellular bacteria Fungi
Th2	Interleukin-4 Interleukin-13 Interleukin-5 Interleukin-4R	Eosinophils Basophils	Parasites

Fig. 2. Helper T-cell (Th) subgroups and effector functions. (*From* Miossec P, Korn T, Kuchroo VK. Interleukin-17 and type 17 helper T cells. N Engl J Med 2009;361(9):888–98; with permission.)

(eg, *Listeria monocytogenes*) and limits the response to vaccines.[56] The imbalance in T_H1 and T_H2 responses may also have positive effects including (1) avoidance of harmful alloimmune reactions between fetus and mother, (2) decreased inflammation when neonates become colonized, and (3) enhanced production of antimicrobial proteins and peptides to avoid microbial penetration and infection.[57] Cells derived from newborn infants are less able than cells from adults to produce multiple cytokines simultaneously in response to TLR agonists. In addition, adenosine levels are increased in newborn blood and inhibit production of TNF-α and T_H1-polarizing cytokines by monocytes.[55,58] Stress and hypoxia, common events in preterm infants, further increase adenosine levels.

Antigen-presenting cells (monocytes, macrophages, and dendritic cells) promote cellular recruitment (by production of cytokines and chemokines), ingest and kill pathogens, and present antigens to cells of the adaptive immune system. The presentation of foreign antigens to cells of the adaptive immune system is less efficient in the newborn infant.[59,60] Monocytes and dendritic cells derived from newborn infants have impaired expression of class II histocompatibility antigens and costimulatory molecules, resulting in reduced antigen presentation to CD4+ T cells. Neonatal dendritic cells require increased stimulation for activation and show impaired stimulation of T-cell proliferation.[61] Monocyte phagocytosis and chemotaxis are reduced in infants with sepsis[62,63]; however, the ability to produce oxygen radicals is normal.[64] Macrophages derived from neonates are poorly responsive to TLR agonists and IFN-γ.[65]

A wide variety of abnormalities in neutrophil (polymorphonuclear cell [PMN]) numbers and function have been described in newborn infants. Neutropenia is commonly observed during gram-negative sepsis and bone marrow reserves are quickly depleted in infants with sepsis.[66] PMN chemotaxis and random migration are diminished in the newborn infant,[67] and this abnormality is accentuated in neonates with sepsis. Diminished upregulation of adhesion molecules limits diapedesis and migration to sites of inflammation.[68] PMNs derived from neonates contain reduced amounts of several antimicrobial proteins and peptides (lactoferrin, elastase, and bactericidal permeability increasing protein).[69,70] Oxygen-dependent and oxygen-independent microbicidal activity are comparable with those seen in adults.[71] However, at high ratios of bacteria to phagocytes or in PMNs derived from premature infants or neonates with sepsis, killing may be impaired. Phagocytosis of PMNs derived from late preterm and term infants is equivalent to that of adult controls.[71] The use of granulocyte and granulocyte-macrophage colony-stimulating factors improves PMN function and numbers, but does not decrease the risk of nosocomial infections.[72]

Abnormalities in the complement system have also been shown in newborn infants. Neonates show gestational age–related decreases in complement levels (**Fig. 3**).[73] Decreased levels of the ninth component of complement may increase the susceptibility to gonococcal ophthalmia in the neonate.[74] In contrast with adults, neonates are particularly dependent on the alternative complement pathway during bacterial sepsis. However, mannose-binding lectin (MBL) levels are decreased in the neonate and MBL is an important activator of the alternative pathway.[75] Some bacteria (eg, group B streptococci) have cell wall components that can also inhibit the alternative pathway.[76]

In addition, preterm neonates have reduced levels of immunoglobulin (Ig) G compared with term infants and adults (**Fig. 4**).[77] The physiologic nadir in IgG levels in some preterm infants can be low and this has been associated with an increased risk of bacteremia. Use of intravenous immunoglobulin has not been efficacious in decreasing the risk of infection.

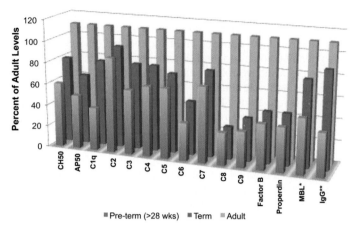

Fig. 3. Comparison of neonatal and adult levels of opsonins and antimicrobial proteins and peptides (APPs). Complement functional assays and complement proteins, mannose-binding lectin (MBL), and immunoglobulin (Ig) G concentrations in preterm neonates, term neonates, and adults. (*From* Wynn JL, Levy O. Role of innate host defenses in susceptibility to early-onset neonatal sepsis. Clin Perinatol 2010;37(2):307–37; with permission.)

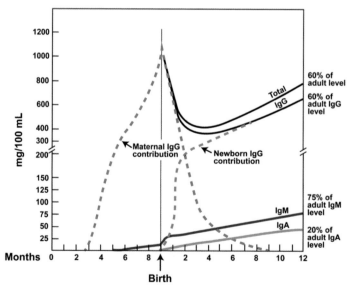

Fig. 4. Immunoglobulin (Ig)G, IgM, and IgA levels in the fetus and in the infant in the first year of life. IgG of the fetus and newborn infant is solely of maternal origin. Maternal IgG disappears by age 9 months, by which time endogenous synthesis of IgG by the infant is well established. IgM and IgA of the neonate are entirely endogenously synthesized because maternal IgM and IgA do not cross the placenta. (*From* Insel RA, Looney RJ. The B-lymphocyte system. In: Stiehm ER, Ochs HD, Winkelstein JA, editors. Immunologic disorders in infants and children. 5th edition. Philadelphia: Elsevier Saunders; 2004. p. 53–84; with permission.)

GLUCOSE HOMEOSTASIS

All preterm infants are at high risk of hypoglycemia and it is estimated that 10% to 15% of late preterm infants experience an episode of hypoglycemia during the neonatal period. The pathophysiology of hypoglycemia in the preterm infant is complex and multifactorial. During fetal life, 80% of energy needs are met by glucose, which is transported across the placenta by facilitative diffusion.[78] The gradient between maternal and fetal glucose concentrations increases with advancing gestational age (**Fig. 5**) and is greater in growth-restricted infants. Glucose is transported via specific membrane transporter proteins (glucose transporter [GLUT] proteins). GLUT-1 is the primary placental transporter during fetal life. Studies in a variety of animal species and humans estimate net uptake by the fetus to be 4 to 7 mg/kg/min. The major storage form of glucose in the fetus is glycogen, which peaks in liver and muscle at term gestation.[79,80]

During the transition to postnatal life, glucose concentrations decrease, accompanied by a surge in regulatory hormones (epinephrine, norepinephrine, and glucagon) and decrease in insulin concentrations, which increase mobilization of glycogen and fatty acids.[81] The plasma glucose concentration reaches its lowest point at 1 hour of age and recovers by 2 to 4 hours of postnatal life. Glucose production rates have been estimated to be 4 to 6 mg/kg/min.[82] Those values are higher than are observed in the human adult and reflect the higher brain/body weight ratio in the newborn.[82] In the human newborn, oxidation of glucose is thought to supply 70% of the energy needs of the brain; therefore the energy needs of the brain are partially met by alternative fuels. Low birth weight infants can produce glucose at an appropriate weight-specific rate to meet metabolic demands. The major contributors to glucose production in the newborn infant are glycogenolysis, and various substrates including alanine and glycerol.[78] Gluconeogenesis is active in preterm infants, even when they receive parenteral nutrition. Premature infants are at increased risk for hypoglycemia because of reduced glycogen stores and low activity of key gluconeogenic and glycolytic enzymes. The risk of hypoglycemia is increased when there are increased energy demands (eg, sepsis, hypoxia, and cold stress) and when enteral intake is inadequate (eg, abnormal suck and swallow or feeding intolerance).

During the metabolic adaptation to postnatal life, blood glucose concentrations as low as 30 mg/dL are commonly observed.[83] When these low values occur in

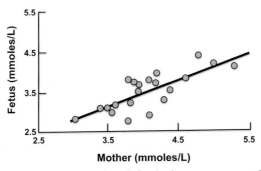

Fig. 5. Relationship between maternal and fetal glucose concentrations. Simultaneous maternal venous and umbilical venous blood samples (via percutaneous umbilical blood sample) were obtained in the third trimester of pregnancy. (*From* Ashmead GG, Kalhan SC, Lazebnik N, et al. Maternal-fetal substrate relationships in the third trimester in human pregnancy. Gynecol Obstet Invest 1993;35(1):18–22; with permission.)

healthy-appearing infants, they are considered physiologic and likely represent the presence of alternative fuels to meet metabolic demands. Symptomatic hypoglycemia occurs when there is an imbalance in the supply and demand of glucose and alternative fuels. Therefore, the plasma glucose concentration at which infants develop clinical signs is highly variable.[84] Late preterm infants are considered to be a high-risk group for neonatal hypoglycemia and screening of asymptomatic newborns after an initial feeding is recommended (**Fig. 6**). The response to a low plasma glucose value depends on whether the infant is showing abnormal clinical signs or is asymptomatic. Symptomatic hypoglycemia must always be treated with intravenous glucose because of the risk of neurologic injury. A proposed cutoff value for treating symptomatic infants is 40 mg/dL. Symptomatic infants should receive a minibolus of 200 mg/kg followed by a constant infusion of glucose supplying 4 to 6 mg/kg/min to maintain a plasma glucose concentration between 40 and 50 mg/dL. Asymptomatic infants with low plasma glucose values can be treated with enteral feedings with a target glucose value of greater than or equal to 45 mg/dL before each feeding (see **Fig. 6**). If that value cannot be maintained, treatment with intravenous glucose is indicated. Late preterm infants should be screened for hypoglycemia for at least the first 24 hours of life. Any infant with documented hypoglycemia must be monitored for at least 3 feed-fast cycles to be certain that the hypoglycemia does not recur.

GASTROINTESTINAL IMMATURITY AND FEEDING

The gastrointestinal tract continues to develop throughout gestation, but moderate and late preterm infants adapt quickly to enteral feedings, including the digestion

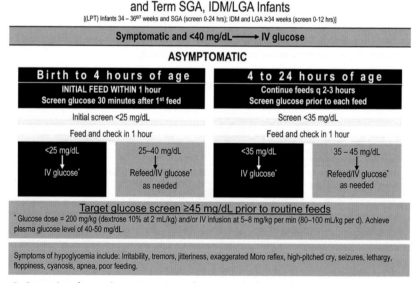

Screening and Management of Postnatal Glucose Homeostasis in Late Preterm and Term SGA, IDM/LGA Infants

[(LPT) Infants 34 – 36^6/7 weeks and SGA (screen 0-24 hrs); IDM and LGA ≥34 weeks (screen 0-12 hrs)]

Symptomatic and <40 mg/dL ⟶ IV glucose

ASYMPTOMATIC

Birth to 4 hours of age	4 to 24 hours of age
INITIAL FEED WITHIN 1 hour Screen glucose 30 minutes after 1st feed	Continue feeds q 2-3 hours Screen glucose prior to each feed
Initial screen <25 mg/dL	Screen <35 mg/dL
Feed and check in 1 hour	Feed and check in 1 hour

| <25 mg/dL
↓
IV glucose* | 25–40 mg/dL
↓
Refeed/IV glucose*
as needed | <35 mg/dL
↓
IV glucose* | 35 – 45 mg/dL
↓
Refeed/IV glucose*
as needed |

Target glucose screen ≥45 mg/dL prior to routine feeds

* Glucose dose = 200 mg/kg (dextrose 10% at 2 mL/kg) and/or IV infusion at 5–8 mg/kg per min (80–100 mL/kg per d). Achieve plasma glucose level of 40-50 mg/dL.

Symptoms of hypoglycemia include: Irritability, tremors, jitteriness, exaggerated Moro reflex, high-pitched cry, seizures, lethargy, floppiness, cyanosis, apnea, poor feeding.

Fig. 6. Screening for and management of postnatal glucose homeostasis in late preterm (LPT 34–36 6/7 weeks) and term small for gestational age (SGA) infants and infants who are born to mothers with diabetes (IDM)/large for gestational age (LGA) infants. IV, intravenous. (*From* Committee on Fetus and Newborn, Adamkin DH. Postnatal glucose homeostasis in late-preterm and term infants. Pediatrics 2011;127(3):575–9; with permission.)

and absorption of lactose, proteins, and lipids.[85–87] However, orobuccal coordination, deglutination mechanisms, peristaltic functions, and the sphincter controls in the esophagus, stomach, and intestines are immature in moderate and late preterm infants compared with term infants.[87] This immaturity may lead to difficulty in coordinating suck and swallowing, difficulty in establishing successful breastfeeding, poor weight gain, and dehydration during early postnatal weeks.[88–90] In addition, mild oromotor hypotonia, rapid fatigue, cold stress, and general lack of strength add to the difficulty that moderate and late preterm infants have in establishing and maintaining adequate breastfeeding. All preterm infants have a higher frequency of gastroesophageal reflux, further reducing food intake and affecting weight gain. Changes in the ecology of gastrointestinal bacteria in the immature gut of the late preterm infant, and their potential impact on growth and later health (allergy, diabetes), remain to be studied.[91,92] There is limited evidence of ongoing feeding problems in moderate and late preterm infants. In a prospective cohort study using parental questionnaires to collect information about feeding behavior during the first year of life in infants born between 25 and 36 weeks of gestation, DeMauro and colleagues[93] reported similar rates of feeding dysfunction in late preterm infants. Feeding difficulties improved during the first 12 months of life in both groups and episodes of hospitalization for feeding problems did not differ between the two groups. A Brazilian population-based study found significantly increased risks of poor weight and height attainment in late preterm infants at 12 and 24 months of age compared with those born at term.[94] Data from the Millennium Cohort Study showed lower height attainment at both 3 and 5 years in late preterm infants compared with infants born at 39 to 41 weeks'.[95]

HEPATIC IMMATURITY AND HYPERBILIRUBINEMIA

Jaundice and hyperbilirubinemia occur more commonly in late preterm infants than in term infants because of developmental immaturity in the liver and feeding difficulties.[96,97] Furthermore, late preterm infants are overly represented in hospital readmissions for hyperbilirubinemia and in the Kernicterus Registry.[51] Bilirubin neurotoxicity may occur at an earlier postnatal age and the margin of safety for late preterm infants may be narrower.[97,98]

Compared with infants born at term gestation, preterm infants have higher rates of bilirubin production, a shortened red blood cell life span, decreased hepatic uptake and conjugation, and an increased enterohepatic circulation (especially in sick preterm infants who are not fed).[97] The recommendations for management of late preterm infants have been summarized in 2 separate management guidelines. In 2004, the Subcommittee on Hyperbilirubinemia of the AAP published a clinical practice guideline for infants greater than or equal to 35 weeks' gestation.[99] The AAP recommended 2 alternatives for the assessment of bilirubin risk: (1) predischarge measurement of bilirubin (serum bilirubin or transcutaneous bilirubin), or (2) assessment of clinical risk factors. The discriminating ability using the clinical risk factor approach may be lower than that of predischarge bilirubin assessment. The recommendations for the timing of evaluations following discharge were based on the presence or absence of risk factors, age at discharge, and risk of other neonatal problems. Infants born at 35 to 36 weeks were considered to have a major risk factor for jaundice. In 2009, these recommendations were updated and new algorithms were published for infants of 35 to 37[6/7] weeks with or without other risk factors for hyperbilirubinemia (**Figs. 7** and **8**).[100] Maisels and colleagues[101] subsequently published management guidelines for infants of less than 35 weeks' gestation that were consensus based, but not evidence based. These guidelines made new recommendations for the timing of

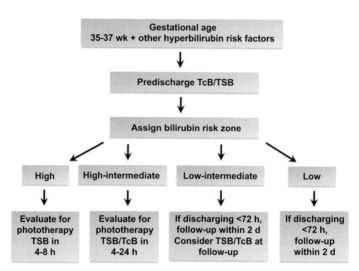

Fig. 7. Algorithm providing recommendations for management and follow-up according to predischarge bilirubin measurements, gestation, and risk factors for subsequent hyperbilirubinemia. TcB, transcutaneous bilirubin; TSB, total serum bilirubin. (*From* Maisels MJ, Bhutani VK, Bogen D, et al. Hyperbilirubinemia in the newborn infant > or =35 weeks' gestation: an update with clarifications. Pediatrics 2009;124(4):1193–8; with permission.)

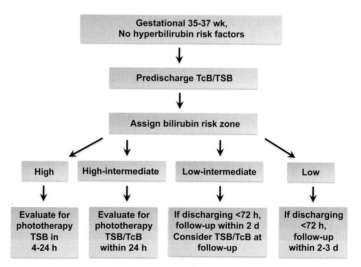

Fig. 8. Algorithm providing recommendations for management and follow-up according to predischarge bilirubin measurements, gestation, and risk factors for subsequent hyperbilirubinemia. TcB, transcutaneous bilirubin; TSB, total serum bilirubin. (*From* Maisels MJ, Bhutani VK, Bogen D, et al. Hyperbilirubinemia in the newborn infant > or =35 weeks' gestation: an update with clarifications. Pediatrics 2009;124(4):1193–8; with permission.)

phototherapy and exchange transfusion. Several recent studies have established new normograms for transcutaneous bilirubin values in late preterm infants.[102,103]

BRAIN DYSMATURITY AND RISK FOR PERIVENTRICULAR LEUKOMALACIA

Periventricular leukomalacia (PVL) is the most common neurologic disorder responsible for neurologic disabilities in infants born very prematurely.[104] This disorder affects the immature white matter of the cerebral hemispheres, and is most common in infants born at 24 to 32 gestational weeks.[104] Nevertheless, it is not restricted to the very prematurely born infant but also occurs in the moderate or late preterm (and term) infant.[105–108] The last half of gestation is a critical period in the growth and development of the human brain. The brain volume increases at a rate of approximately 15 mL (1.4%) per week between 29 and 41 weeks of gestation. At 28 weeks of gestation, brain volume is about 13% of that observed at term, and by about 34 weeks of gestation the brain weighs only 65% of the term infant's brain.[109] Thus, more than one-third of brain size increase takes place during final 6 to 8 weeks of gestation (**Fig. 9**). The white matter increases greatly as term approaches, with a 5-fold increase in white matter volume between 35 and 41 weeks of gestation.[110] Furthermore, in the last several weeks of pregnancy, there are important structural changes that occur in the brains of moderate and late preterm infants, including increases in neuronal connectivity, dendritic arborization, and connectivity; increasing synaptic junctions; and maturation of neurochemical and enzymatic processes augmenting growth and maturation of the brain.[111,112] The precise incidence of PVL in moderate and late preterm infants is unknown, because systematic ultrasound scanning of the newborn head is not done in this group. Further, with early discharge and limited follow-up, the prevalence of other brain disorders in this population remains unknown. An autopsy study of term infants dying after surgery for congenital heart diseases revealed an incidence of PVL of 61%,[108] which implies that, although they are more mature than very preterm infants, the brains of moderate and late preterm infants are still immature and vulnerable for white matter injury under adverse conditions.

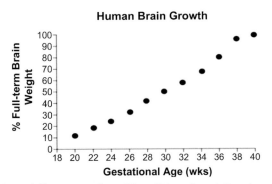

Human Brain Growth

% Full-term Brain Weight vs Gestational Age (wks)

Fig. 9. Brain weight at different ages from 20 to 40 (term) gestational weeks is expressed at each age as a percentage of term brain weight. Late preterm, at 34 gestational weeks, the overall brain weight is 65% of term weight. (*From* Guihard-Costa AM, Larroche JC. Differential growth between the fetal brain and its infratentorial part. Early Hum Dev 1990;23:27–40; and Kinney HC. The near-term (late preterm) human brain and risk for periventricular leukomalacia: a review. Semin Perinatol 2006;30(2):81–8, with permission.)

SUMMARY

This article highlights some of the important developmental characteristics that function as underpinnings for common problems seen in moderate and late preterm infants. Preterm birth, even a few weeks before term, is associated with a high prevalence of clinical problems caused by immaturity of a wide variety of organ systems (eg, the lungs, brain, gastrointestinal system), acquired problems (eg, infections, hypothermia), and problems associated with inadequate monitoring and/or follow-up plans (eg, hypoxic respiratory failure, hypoglycemia, kernicterus). There are variations in the degree of maturation among infants of similar gestational ages because the developmental process is nonlinear. Therefore, different organ systems mature at rates and trajectories that are specific to their functions. A better understanding of these principles can help guide optimal treatment strategies.

REFERENCES

1. Shapiro-Mendoza CK, Lackritz EM. Epidemiology of late and moderate preterm birth. Semin Fetal Neonatal Med 2012;17(3):120–5.
2. Mathews TJ, MacDorman MF. Infant mortality statistics from the 2007 period linked birth/infant death data set. Natl Vital Stat Rep 2011;59(6):1–30.
3. Mohan SS, Jain L. Late preterm birth: preventable prematurity? Clin Perinatol 2011;38(3):547–55.
4. Holland MG, Refuerzo JS, Ramin SM, et al. Late preterm birth: how often is it avoidable? Am J Obstet Gynecol 2009;201(4):404.e1–4.
5. Shapiro-Mendoza CK, Tomashek KM, Kotelchuck M, et al. Effect of late-preterm birth and maternal medical conditions on newborn morbidity risk. Pediatrics 2008;121(2):e223–32.
6. Kamath BD, Marcotte MP, DeFranco EA. Neonatal morbidity after documented fetal lung maturity in late preterm and early term infants. Am J Obstet Gynecol 2011;204(6):518.
7. Petrou S, Khan K. Economic costs associated with moderate and late preterm birth: primary and secondary evidence. Semin Fetal Neonatal Med 2012; 17(3):170–8.
8. Johanson RB, Spencer SA, Rolfe P, et al. Effect of post-delivery care on neonatal body temperature. Acta Paediatr 1992;81:859–63.
9. Schroder HJ, Power GG. Engine and radiator: fetal and placental interactions for heat dissipation. Exp Physiol 1997;82:403–14.
10. Cummings KJ, Li A, Nattie EE. Brainstem serotonin deficiency in the neonatal period: autonomic dysregulation during mild cold stress. J Physiol 2011;589: 2055–64.
11. Sahni R, Schulze KF. Temperature Control in Newborn Infants. In: Polin R, Fox WW, Abman SH, editors. Fetal and Neonatal Physiology. 4th edition. Philadelphia: Elsevier; 2011. p. 624–48.
12. Tews D, Wabitsch M. Renaissance of brown adipose tissue. Horm Res Paediatr 2011;75:231–9.
13. Gardner S, Carter B, Enzman-Hines M, et al. Merenstein & Gardner's handbook of neonatal intensive care. 7th edition. St Louis (MO): Mosby; 2011.
14. Laptook A, Jackson GL. Cold stress and hypoglycemia in late preterm ("near term") infant: impact on nursery admission. Semin Perinatol 2006;30:24–7.
15. Fairchild KD, Sun CC, Gross GC, et al. NICU admission hypothermia, chorioamnionitis, and cytokines. J Perinat Med 2011;39:731–6.

16. Engle WA, Tomashek KM, Wallman C, Committee on Fetus and Newborn, American Academy of Pediatrics. "Late-preterm" infants: a population at risk. Pediatrics 2007;120(6):1390–401.
17. Darcy A. Complications of the late preterm infant. J Perinat Neonatal Nurs 2009; 23(1):78–86.
18. Raju T, Higgins R, Stark A, et al. Optimizing care an outcome for late-preterm (near-term) infants: a summary of the workshop sponsored by the national institutional of child health and human development. Pediatrics 2006;118(3): 1207–14.
19. Cinar N, Filiz T. Neonatal thermoregulation. J Neonatal Nurs 2006;12:69–74.
20. Consortium on Safe Labor, Hibbard JU, Wilkins I, et al. Respiratory morbidity in late preterm births. JAMA 2010;304:419–25.
21. Dudell GG, Jain L. Hypoxic respiratory failure in the late preterm infant. Clin Perinatol 2006;33:803–30.
22. Wang ML, Dorer DJ, Fleming MP, et al. Clinical outcomes of near-term infants. Pediatrics 2004;114(2):372–6.
23. De Luca R, Boulvain M, Irion O, et al. Incidence of early neonatal mortality and morbidity after late-preterm and term cesarean delivery. Pediatrics 2009;123(6): e1064–71.
24. Colin AA, McEvoy C, Castile RG. Respiratory morbidity and lung function in preterm infants of 32 to 36 weeks' gestational age. Pediatrics 2010;126:115–28.
25. Smith LJ, McKay KO, van Asperen PP, et al. Normal development of the lung and premature birth. Paediatr Respir Rev 2010;11:135–42.
26. Ramachandrappa A, Rosenberg ES, Wagoner S, et al. Morbidity and mortality in late preterm infants with severe hypoxic respiratory failure on extracorporeal membrane oxygenation. J Pediatr 2011;159:192–8.
27. McIntire DD, Leveno KJ. Neonatal mortality and morbidity rates in late preterm births compared with births at term. Obstet Gynecol 2008;111(1):35–41.
28. Jain L, Eaton DC. Physiology of fetal lung fluid clearance and the effect of labor. Semin Perinatol 2006;30:34–43.
29. Eaton DC, Helms MN, Koval M, et al. The contribution of epithelial sodium channels to alveolar function in health and disease. Annu Rev Physiol 2009;71: 403–23.
30. Keszler M, Carbone MT, Cox C, et al. Severe respiratory failure after elective repeat cesarean delivery: a potentially preventable condition leading to extracorporeal membrane oxygenation. Pediatrics 1992;89:670–2.
31. Jain L. Alveolar fluid clearance in developing lungs and its role in neonatal transition. Clin Perinatol 1999;26(3):585–99.
32. Bland RD. Loss of liquid from the lung lumen in labor: more than a simple "squeeze". Am J Physiol Lung Cell Mol Physiol 2001;280(4):L602–5.
33. Smith DE, Otulakowski G, Yeger H, et al. Epithelial Na(+) channel (ENaC) expression in the developing normal and abnormal human perinatal lung. Am J Respir Crit Care Med 2000;161(4 Pt 1):1322–31.
34. Heritage CK, Cunningham MD. Association of elective repeat cesarean delivery and persistent pulmonary hypertension of the newborn. Am J Obstet Gynecol 1985;152(6 Pt 1):627–9.
35. Raju TN. Developmental physiology of late and moderate prematurity. Semin Fetal Neonatal Med 2012;17(3):126–31.
36. Darnall RA, Ariagno RL, Kinney HC. The late preterm infant and the control of breathing, sleep, and brainstem development: a review. Clin Perinatol 2006; 33(4):883–914.

37. Rigatto H. Control of breathing in fetal life and onset and control of breathing in the neonate. In: Polin RA, Fox WW, editors. Fetal and neonatal physiology. Philadelphia: WB Saunders; 1992. p. 790–801.
38. Patural H, Barthelemy JC, Pichot V, et al. Birth prematurity determines prolonged autonomic nervous system immaturity. Clin Auton Res 2004;14:391–5.
39. Ramanathan R, Corwin MJ, Hunt CE, et al. Cardiorespiratory events recorded on home monitors: comparison of healthy infants with those at increased risk for SIDS. JAMA 2001;285(17):2199–207.
40. Malloy DH, Freeman DH Jr. Birth weight- and gestational age-specific sudden infant death syndrome mortality United States, 1991 versus 1995. Pediatrics 2000;6:1227–31.
41. Malloy MH, Hoffman HJ. Prematurity, sudden infant death syndrome, and age of death. Pediatrics 1995;3:464–71.
42. Polin RA, Committee on Fetus and Newborn. Management of neonates with suspected or proven early-onset bacterial sepsis. Pediatrics 2012;129(5):1006–15.
43. Polin RA, Denson S, Brady MT, Committee on Fetus and Newborn, Committee on Infectious Diseases. Epidemiology and diagnosis of health care-associated infections in the NICU. Pediatrics 2012;129(4):e1104–9.
44. Wynn JL, Levy O. Role of innate host defenses in susceptibility to early-onset neonatal sepsis. Clin Perinatol 2010;37(2):307–37.
45. Visscher MO, Narendran V, Pickens WL, et al. Vernix caseosa in neonatal adaptation. J Perinatol 2005;25(7):440–6.
46. Ushijima T, Takahashi M, Ozaki Y. Acetic, propionic, and oleic acid as the possible factors influencing the predominant residence of some species of *Propionibacterium* and coagulase-negative *Staphylococcus* on normal human skin. Can J Microbiol 1984;30(5):647–52.
47. Chuong CM, Nickoloff BJ, Elias PM, et al. What is the 'true' function of skin? Exp Dermatol 2002;11(2):159–87.
48. Rutter N. The immature skin. Eur J Pediatr 1996;155(Suppl 2):S18–20.
49. Sidbury R, Darmstadt GL. Microbiology. In: Hoath SB, Maibach H, editors. Neonatal Skin. 2nd edition. New York (NY): Marcel Dekker; 2002. p. 21–46.
50. Fox C, Nelson D, Wareham J. The timing of skin acidification in very low birth weight infants. J Perinatol 1998;18(4):272–5.
51. Kawai T, Akira S. The role of pattern-recognition receptors in innate immunity: update on Toll-like receptors. Nat Immunol 2010;11(5):373–84.
52. Förster-Waldl E, Sadeghi K, Tamandl D, et al. Monocyte toll-like receptor 4 expression and LPS-induced cytokine production increase during gestational aging. Pediatr Res 2005;58(1):121–4.
53. Kim SK, Keeney SE, Alpard SK, et al. Comparison of L-selectin and CD11b on neutrophils of adults and neonates during the first month of life. Pediatr Res 2003;53(1):132–6.
54. Nupponen I, Pesonen E, Andersson S, et al. Neutrophil activation in preterm infants who have respiratory distress syndrome. Pediatrics 2002;110(1 Pt 1):36–41.
55. Cuenca AG, Wynn JL, Moldawer LL, et al. Role of innate immunity in neonatal infection. Am J Perinatol 2013;30(2):105–12.
56. PrabhuDas M, Adkins B, Gans H, et al. Challenges in infant immunity: implications for responses to infection and vaccines. Nat Immunol 2011;12(3):189–94.
57. Levy O. Innate immunity of the newborn: basic mechanisms and clinical correlates. Nat Rev Immunol 2007;7(5):379–90.

58. Power Coombs MR, Belderbos ME, Gallington LC, et al. Adenosine modulates Toll-like receptor function: basic mechanisms and translational opportunities. Expert Rev Anti Infect Ther 2011;9(2):261–9.
59. Hunt DW, Huppertz HI, Jiang HJ, et al. Studies of human cord blood dendritic cells: evidence for functional immaturity. Blood 1994;84(12):4333–43.
60. Velilla PA, Rugeles MT, Chougnet CA. Defective antigen-presenting cell function in human neonates. Clin Immunol 2006;121(3):251–9.
61. Wong OH, Huang FP, Chiang AK. Differential responses of cord and adult blood-derived dendritic cells to dying cells. Immunology 2005;116(1):13–20.
62. Hallwirth U, Pomberger G, Zaknun D, et al. Monocyte phagocytosis as a reliable parameter for predicting early-onset sepsis in very low birthweight infants. Early Hum Dev 2002;67(1–2):1–9.
63. Klein RB, Fischer TJ, Gard SE, et al. Decreased mononuclear and polymorpho-nuclear chemotaxis in human newborns, infants, and young children. Pediatrics 1977;60(4):467–72.
64. Spear GT, June RA, Landay AL. Oxidative burst capability of human monocyte subsets defined by high and low HLA-DR expression. Immunol Invest 1989; 18(8):993–1005.
65. Maródi L. Innate cellular immune responses in newborns. Clin Immunol 2006; 118(2–3):137–44.
66. Christenesen RD, Rothsetin G. Exhaustion of mature marrow neutrophils in neonates with sepsis. J Pediatr 1980;96(2):316–8.
67. Türkmen M, Satar M, Atici A. Neutrophil chemotaxis and random migration in preterm and term infants with sepsis. Am J Perinatol 2000;17(2):107–12.
68. Bührer C, Graulich J, Stibenz D, et al. L-selectin is down-regulated in umbilical cord blood granulocytes and monocytes of newborn infants with acute bacterial infection. Pediatr Res 1994;36(6):799–804.
69. Kjeldsen L, Sengeløv H, Lollike K, et al. Granules and secretory vesicles in human neonatal neutrophils. Pediatr Res 1996;40(1):120–9.
70. Levy O, Martin S, Eichenwald E, et al. Impaired innate immunity in the newborn: newborn neutrophils are deficient in bactericidal/permeability-increasing protein. Pediatrics 1999;104(6):1327–33.
71. Urlichs F, Speer CP. Neutrophil function in preterm and term infants. Neoreviews 2004;5:e417.
72. Suri M, Harrison L, Van de Ven C, et al. Immunotherapy in the prophylaxis and treatment of neonatal sepsis. Curr Opin Pediatr 2003;15(2):155–60.
73. Strunk T, Doherty D, Richmond P, et al. Reduced levels of antimicrobial proteins and peptides in human cord blood plasma. Arch Dis Child Fetal Neonatal Ed 2009;94(3):F230–1.
74. Lassiter HA, Watson SW, Seifring ML, et al. Complement factor 9 deficiency in serum of human neonates. J Infect Dis 1992;166(1):53–7.
75. Dzwonek AB, Neth OW, Thiébaut R, et al. The role of mannose-binding lectin in susceptibility to infection in preterm neonates. Pediatr Res 2008;63(6):680–5.
76. Edwards MS, Nicholson-Weller A, Baker CJ, et al. The role of specific antibody in alternative complement pathway-mediated opsonophagocytosis of type III, group B *Streptococcus*. J Exp Med 1980;151(5):1275–87.
77. Malek A, Sager R, Schneider H. Maternal-fetal transport of immunoglobulin G and its subclasses during the third trimester of human pregnancy. Am J Reprod Immunol 1994;32(1):8–14.
78. Garg M, Devaskar SU. Glucose metabolism in the late preterm infant. Clin Perinatol 2006;33(4):853–70.

79. Shelley HJ. Carbohydrate metabolism in the foetus and the newly born. Proc Nutr Soc 1969;28(1):42–9.
80. Shelley HJ. Carbohydrate reserves in the newborn infant. Br Med J 1964; 1(5378):273–5.
81. Mayor F, Cuezva JM. Hormonal and metabolic changes in the perinatal period. Biol Neonate 1985;48(4):185–96.
82. Bier DM, Leake RD, Hamond MW, et al. Measurement of "true" glucose production rates in infancy and childhood with 6,6-dideuteroglucose. Diabetes 1977; 26(11):1016–23.
83. Ward PM, Deshpande S. Metabolic adaptation at birth. Semin Fetal Neonatal Med 2005;10(4):341–50.
84. Adamkin DH, Committee on Fetus and Newborn. Postnatal glucose homeostasis in late-preterm and term infants. Pediatrics 2011;127(3):575–9.
85. Kien CL. Digestion, absorption, and fermentation of carbohydrates in the newborn. Clin Perinatol 1996;23:211–28.
86. Kien CL, McClead RE, Cordero L Jr. Effects of lactose intake on lactose digestion and colonic fermentation in preterm infants. J Pediatr 1998;133:401–5.
87. Neu J. Gastrointestinal maturation and feeding. Semin Perinatol 2006;30:77–80.
88. Escobar GJ, Gonzales VM, Armstrong MA, et al. Rehospitalization for neonatal dehydration: a nested case-control study. Arch Pediatr Adolesc Med 2002;156: 155–61.
89. Tomashek KM, Shapiro-Mendoza CK, Weiss J, et al. Early discharge among late preterm and term newborns and risk of neonatal morbidity. Semin Perinatol 2006;30:61–8.
90. Shapiro-Mendoza CK, Tomashek KM, Kotelchuck M, et al. Risk factors for neonatal morbidity and mortality among "healthy," late preterm newborns. Semin Perinatol 2006;30:54–60.
91. Martinez-Tallo E, Claure N, Bancalari E. Necrotizing enterocolitis in full-term or near-term infants: risk factors. Biol Neonate 1997;71:292–8.
92. Hooper LV, Stappenbeck TS, Hong CV, et al. Angiogenins: a new class of microbicidal proteins involved in innate immunity. Nat Immunol 2003;4:269–73.
93. DeMauro SB, Patel PR, Medoff-Cooper B, et al. Postdischarge feeding patterns in early- and late-preterm infants. Clin Pediatr 2011;50:957–62.
94. Santos IS, Matijasevich A, Domingues MR, et al. Late preterm birth is a risk factor for growth faltering in early childhood: a cohort study. BMC Pediatr 2009;9:71.
95. Boyle EM, Poulsen G, Field DJ, et al. Population-based cohort study of the effects of gestational age at birth on health outcomes at three and five years. BMJ 2012;344:e896.
96. Watchko JF, Maisels MJ. Jaundice in low birthweight infants: pathobiology and outcome. Arch Dis Child Fetal Neonatal Ed 2003;88(6):F455–8.
97. Bhutani VK. Late preterm births major cause of prematurity and adverse outcomes of neonatal hyperbilirubinemia. Indian Pediatr 2012;49(9):704–5.
98. Bhutani VK, Johnson L. Kernicterus in late preterm infants cared for as term healthy infants. Semin Perinatol 2006;30(2):89–97.
99. American Academy of Pediatrics Subcommittee on Hyperbilirubinemia. Management of hyperbilirubinemia in the newborn infant 35 or more weeks of gestation. Pediatrics 2004;114(1):297–316.
100. Maisels MJ, Bhutani VK, Bogen D, et al. Hyperbilirubinemia in the newborn infant > or =35 weeks' gestation: an update with clarifications. Pediatrics 2009; 124(4):1193–8.

101. Maisels MJ, Watchko JF, Bhutani VK, et al. An approach to the management of hyperbilirubinemia in the preterm infant less than 35 weeks of gestation. J Perinatol 2012;32(9):660–4.
102. Fouzas S, Karatza AA, Skylogianni E, et al. Transcutaneous bilirubin levels in late preterm neonates. J Pediatr 2010;157(5):762–6.e1.
103. Kaur S, Chawla D, Pathak U, et al. Predischarge non-invasive risk assessment for prediction of significant hyperbilirubinemia in term and late preterm neonates. J Perinatol 2012;32(9):716–21.
104. Kinney HC, Haynes RL, Folkerth RD. White matter lesions in the perinatal period. In: Golden JA, Harding B, editors. Pathology and genetics: acquired and inherited diseases of the developing nervous system. Basel (Switzerland): ISN Neuropathology Press; 2004. p. 156–70.
105. Mahle WT, Tavani F, Zimmerman RA, et al. An MRI study of neurological injury before and after congenital heart surgery. Circulation 2002;106(Suppl 12): I109–14.
106. Galli KK, Zimmerman RA, Jarvik GP, et al. Periventricular leukomalacia is common after neonatal cardiac surgery. J Thorac Cardiovasc Surg 2004;127: 692–704.
107. Pierson CR, Folkerth RD, Haynes RL, et al. Gray matter injury in premature infants with or without periventricular leukomalacia (PVL). J Neuropathol Exp Neurol 2004;62:5.
108. Kinney HC, Panigrahy A, Newburger JW. Hypoxic ischemic brain injury in infants with congenital heart disease dying after cardiac surgery. Acta Neuropathol 2005;110:563–78.
109. Guihard-Costa AM, Larroche JC. Differential growth between the fetal brain and its infratentorial part. Early Hum Dev 1990;23:27–40.
110. Huppi PS, Warfield S, Kikinis R, et al. Quantitative magnetic resonance imaging of brain development in premature and mature newborns. Ann Neurol 1998;43: 224–35.
111. Kinney HC. The near-term (late preterm) human brain and risk for periventricular leukomalacia: a review. Semin Perinatol 2006;30(2):81–8.
112. Kinney HC, Armstrong DL. Perinatal neuropathology. In: Graham DI, Lantos PE, editors. Greenfield's neuropathology. 7th edition. London: Arnold; 2002. p. 557–9.

Respiratory Disorders in Moderately Preterm, Late Preterm, and Early Term Infants

Ashley Darcy Mahoney, PhD, NNP-BC[a,b,]*, Lucky Jain, MD, MBA[c]

KEYWORDS

- Moderately preterm • Late preterm • Early term • Respiratory distress
- Transient tachypnea of the newborn • Respiratory distress syndrome

KEY POINTS

- Even when it is just a few weeks before term gestation, early birth has consequences, resulting in higher morbidity and mortality.
- Respiratory issues related to moderate prematurity include delayed neonatal transition to air breathing, respiratory distress resulting from delayed fluid clearance (transient tachypnea of the newborn), surfactant deficiency (respiratory distress syndrome), and pulmonary hypertension.
- Management approaches emphasize appropriate respiratory support to facilitate respiratory transition and minimize iatrogenic injury.
- Studies are needed to determine the impact of respiratory distress coupled with mild-moderate prematurity on long-term outcome.

EPIDEMIOLOGY

Evidence accumulated in recent years shows that moderately preterm, late preterm, and early term births lead to significant acuity and expense. Twenty-four studies published between 2000 and 2009 have documented a consistently higher risk of respiratory morbidity in infants born at less than 37 weeks (**Fig. 1**).[1] Overall morbidities in late preterm infants have been noted to increase 20-fold with each week lost before 38 weeks' gestation.[2] The rate of respiratory compromise in 19 US hospitals was 10.5% of 19,334 late preterm and 1.13% of 165,993 term infants.[3] Often beginning as delayed respiratory transition and transient tachypnea, the course of respiratory distress in late preterm infants can be unpredictable. The scope and causes of

Disclosure: Ashley Darcy Mahoney is on the speaker's bureau for Ikaria Therapeutics.
[a] Nell Hodgson Woodruff School of Nursing, Emory University School of Nursing, 1520 Clifton Road, Atlanta, GA 30322, USA; [b] South Dade Neonatology, Miami, FL, USA; [c] Department of Pediatrics, Emory University School of Medicine, 2015 Uppergate Drive, Atlanta, GA 30322, USA
* Corresponding author. 1520 Clifton Road #317, Atlanta, GA 30309.
E-mail address: ashley.darcy@emory.edu

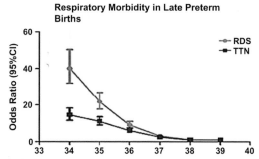

Fig. 1. Respiratory morbidity in late preterm births (infants born <37 weeks). CI, confidence interval; RDS, respiratory distress syndrome; TTN, transient tachypnea of the newborn. (*From* Kotecha S. Long term respiratory outcomes of late preterm-born infants. Semin Fetal Neonatal Med 2012;17(2):78; with permission; and *Data from* Hibbard JU, Wilkins I, Sun L, et al, Consortium on Safe Labor. Respiratory morbidity in late preterm births. JAMA 2010;304(4):419–25.)

respiratory disorders in this population can be varied and often overlap with transient tachypnea of the newborn (TTN), respiratory distress syndrome (RDS), persistent pulmonary hypertension (PPHN), and apnea.[4–17] Of the affected babies, the incidence of respiratory distress requiring mechanical ventilation corresponded with the degree of prematurity: 3.3% of late preterm infants born at 34 weeks' gestation, 1.7% at 35 weeks, and 0.8% at 36 weeks' gestation (**Fig. 2**).[10] Further, 29% of late preterm infants required intensive care, with 13% of those infants presenting with respiratory failure. Higher morbidity persists in early childhood; in one study, 30% of children less than the age of 2 years admitted to the pediatric intensive care unit for respiratory diseases were born prematurely (17% of these infants were classified as early preterm; 12% were classified as late preterm).[18]

Many late preterm infants develop respiratory distress soon after birth (sustained distress for more than 2 hours after birth accompanied by grunting, flaring, tachypnea, retractions, or supplemental oxygen requirement). Studies indicate that such

Neonatal Morbidity in Live Births Delivered Late Preterm (34, 35, 36 wk) and at 37 Weeks Compared With 39 Weeks as Referent

	Weeks of Gestation				
Morbidity	34 (n=3,498)	35 (n=6,571)	36 (n=11,702)	37 (n=26,504)	39 (n=84,747)
Respiratory distress					
Ventilator	116 (3.3)*	109 (1.7)*	89 (0.8)*	130 (0.5)*	275 (0.3)
Transient tachypnea	85 (2.4)*	103 (1.6)*	130 (1.1)*	187 (0.7)*	34 (0.4)
Intraventricular hemorrhage					
Grades 1, 2	16 (0.5)*	13 (0.2)*	7 (0.06)†	9 (0.03)	13 (0.01)
Grades 3, 4	0	1 (0.02)*	1 (0.01)	1 (0.004)	3 (0.004)
Sepsis					
Work-up	1,073 (31)*	1,443 (22)*	1,792 (15)*	3,274 (12)	10,588 (12)
Culture proven	18 (0.5)*	23 (0.4)*	26 (0.2)†	60 (0.2)*	97 (0.1)
Phototherapy	213 (6.1)*	227 (3.5)*	36 (2.0)*	418 (1.6)*	857 (1)
Necrotizing enterocolitis	3 (0.09)*	1 (0.02)†	1 (0.01)	3 (0.01)*	1 (0.001)
Apgar 3 or less at 5 min	5 (0.1)*	12 (0.2)*	10 (0.9)	21 (0.08)	54 (0.06)
Intubation in delivery room	49 (1.4)*	55 (0.8)†	36 (0.6)	154 (0.6)	477 (0.6)
One or more of the above	1,175 (34)*	1,565 (24)*	1,993 (17)*	3,652 (14)	11,513 (14)

Data are expressed as n (%).
* P<.001 compared with the 39 weeks referent.
† P<.05 compared with the 39 weeks referent.

Fig. 2. Percentage of infants born at late preterm gestations who require mechanical ventilation. (*From* McIntire DD, Leveno KJ. Neonatal mortality and morbidity rates in late preterm births compared with births at term. Obstet Gynecol 2008;111:38; with permission.)

conditions occur more often in late preterm infants than in term newborns (28.9% vs 5.3% respectively)[19] and that neonates born at 35 weeks are 9 times more likely to have respiratory distress compared with infants born at 38 to 40 weeks' gestation.[14] For each week before expected term of delivery, infants delivered by elective cesarean section tend to experience greater morbidity.[20] Madar and colleagues[21] found the incidence of respiratory distress to be significantly increased with every week of gestation less than 39 weeks: 30 of 1000 infants born at 34 weeks developed respiratory distress versus 14 of 1000 infants born at 35 weeks and 7.1 of 1000 infants born at 36 weeks' gestation. More recently, Ghartey and coleagues[22] replicated this result, describing a decreasing trend in the incidence of adverse respiratory outcomes with additional weeks of gestation (37 weeks, 8.2%; 38 weeks, 5.5%; 39 weeks, 3.4%). Recognizing the importance of morbidity in late preterm and early elective births, quality programs have begun targeting births in these groups that are not medically indicated. In one multistate collaborative undertaken over 12 months, elective scheduled early term deliveries decreased from 27.8% in the first month to 4.8% in the 12th month; in addition, rates of elective, scheduled, singleton, early term inductions and cesarean deliveries decreased significantly.[23]

FETAL LUNG DEVELOPMENT AND NEONATAL RESPIRATORY TRANSITION

The causes of respiratory distress stem from the inability of a neonate's lungs to adapt to the new environment. The last few weeks of gestation prepare the fetus for success in the transition from intrauterine life. Late preterm infants are born in the late saccular stage of development when surfactant and antioxidant systems are still immature.[24] For effective gas exchange to occur, alveolar spaces must be cleared of excess fluid and ventilated, and pulmonary blood flow must be increased to match ventilation and perfusion.[25] From 34 to 36 weeks' gestation, terminal respiratory units of the lung evolve from alveolar saccules lined with both cuboidal type II and flat type I epithelial cells (terminal sac period) to mature alveoli lined primarily with extremely thin type I epithelial cells (alveolar period). During the alveolar period, pulmonary capillaries also begin to bulge into the space of each terminal sac, and adult pool sizes of surfactant are attained. The immature lung structure present before term may be associated functionally with delayed intrapulmonary fluid absorption, surfactant insufficiency, and inefficient gas exchange.[11] In addition, during the last 6 weeks of gestation, the fetus begins to develop synchrony and control over breathing; delivery before this maturation increases the risk of apnea of prematurity.[26]

Fetal lung maturity is often used as the sole criterion to show that late preterm infants are at low risk for RDS and are ready for postnatal life. Fetal lung maturity tests may aid clinicians in determining when delivery can occur. The American College of Obstetricians and Gynecologists (ACOG) currently recommends the delay of elective delivery until 39 weeks' gestation and that a fetal lung maturity test should be performed to avoid iatrogenic prematurity if the scheduled delivery is planned at less than 39 weeks' gestation.[27,28]

Although most fetal lung maturity tests perform well in predicting maturity, they are poor at predicting respiratory morbidity including, RDS and TTN.[27–30] If an initial test shows immature or indeterminate lung maturity, reflex tests are performed; if they, in turn, show fetal lung maturity, the likelihood of RDS is presumed to be low, even though the initial test did not predict maturity. The ACOG Practice Bulletin on fetal lung maturity notes that, "The negative predictive value for mature neonatal lung function is high, and if one of these test results for fetal lung maturity is positive, RDS is unlikely. The main value for fetal lung maturity testing is predicting the absence of

RDS. An immature test result for fetal lung maturity is less reliable in predicting the presence of RDS."[27]

The most popular initial test for assessing fetal lung maturity is the TDx-FLM II (Fetal Lung Maturity II) surfactant/albumin ratio assay. If this test is indeterminate or negative, other studies such as lecithin/sphingomyelin (L/S) ratio or phosphatidylglycerol (PG) presence may then be performed. Tennant and colleagues[29] found that L/S ratios may provide false reassurance when used after immature or indeterminate TDx-FLM II testing. Using PG or L/S ratios as a reflex test to confirm lung maturity was associated with a high risk for respiratory morbidity, particularly when PG was not present. Another study found that, despite documented fetal lung maturity, infants who were born at less than 39 weeks had significantly higher rates of neonatal morbidities compared with infants who were born at greater than or equal to 39 weeks' gestation.[31] Lamellar body count in the amniotic fluid as a measure of fetal lung maturity has also gained popularity. A recent meta-analysis recommended replacing the L/S ratio with the lamellar body count as the gold standard because the lamellar body count is easy to perform, rapid, inexpensive, and available to all hospitals 24 hours per day.[32]

After birth, rapid clearance of fetal lung fluid is key to a successful neonatal transition. In fetal sheep, fetal lung fluid is actively secreted from alveolar type I and II cells at a rate of up to 50 mL/kg/d at mid-gestation and 120 mL/kg/d at term.[33–35] Increased fetal epinephrine and steroid concentration during labor normally reduces lung fluid production and activates sodium channels, leading to reabsorption. Failure to properly clear lung fluid leads to TTN and/or respiratory distress. This fluid is chloride rich and low in protein, being the product of chloride secretion into the nascent airspaces after the creation of an electrochemical gradient by basolateral channels in epithelial cells.[33,36] In the fetus, sodium follows chloride; water follows the newly developed osmotic gradient, resulting in a net secretion of fluid by the fetal lung. Underlying mechanisms that allow the volume of fluid to be sensed and adjusted are still unknown; however, fluid secretion is inhibited by diuretics such as bumetanide, suggesting a role for Na-K-2Cl cotransport.[33] However, there is evidence that this fluid is essential to normal lung growth and provides a distending volume similar to functional residual capacity. Processes that interfere with normal production and volume of fetal lung fluid, such as oligohydramnios and pulmonary artery ligation, result in pulmonary hypoplasia and respiratory distress.[37,38]

Late preterm infants are sometimes still at risk for developing respiratory distress even when amniotic fluid testing shows a mature surfactant profile.[31] A 2011 study of a cohort of neonates in Cincinnati revealed that, despite documented fetal lung maturity, infants born at 34 to 38 weeks' gestation had significantly higher rates of neonatal morbidities compared with infants who were born at greater than or equal to 39 weeks' gestation (**Fig. 3**).[31] This finding may be attributable to a delay in clearing fetal lung fluid. At the time of delivery, the lung epithelium becomes integral to the process of switching from placental to pulmonary gas exchange.[39,40] For effective gas exchange to occur in the lungs, alveolar spaces must be cleared of excess fluid and pulmonary blood flow must be increased to match ventilation with the perfusion that is taking place. If either the ventilation or perfusion is inadequate, the infant has a difficult time transitioning and develops respiratory distress.[25]

Although a small role in the clearance of this fluid can be attributed to Starling forces and vaginal squeeze,[39,40] amiloride-sensitive sodium transport by lung epithelial cells through epithelial sodium channels (ENaC) has emerged as a key event in the transepithelial movement of alveolar fluid (**Fig. 4**).[39,40] Research has shown that these ENaC channels regulate the clearing of fluid from the fetal lungs, and

Risk of neonatal morbidity in infants with positive fetal lung maturity

Neonatal outcome	Adjusted odds ratio (95% CI)[a]
Composite adverse neonatal outcome[b]	3.66 (1.48–9.09)
Delivery room interventions: oxygen or more	1.43 (0.77–2.66)
Hypoglycemia	3.95 (1.76–8.85)
Phototherapy	6.67 (1.52–29.18)
Sepsis evaluation	2.72 (0.95–7.81)
Treatment with antibiotics	4.23 (0.55–32.69)
Neonatal intensive care admission	2.68 (0.91–7.89)
Oxygen supplementation	19.14 (1.62–225.88)

The risk of neonatal morbidity in infants born at <39 weeks with documented fetal lung maturity, compared to the reference group born at 39 0/7 to 40 6/7 weeks' gestation is shown.

[a] Adjusted for hypertensive disease, diabetes mellitus, birthweight of the infant, use of antenatal steroids, and presence of labor before delivery.

[b] Consists of neonatal intensive care admission, phototherapy, antibiotic treatment, intravenous fluids for hypoglycemia, or gavage feeding.

CI, confidence interval.

Fig. 3. Risk of adverse outcome in newborns (<39 weeks) with documented lung maturity. (*From* Kamath B, Marcotte M, DeFranco E. Neonatal morbidity after documented fetal lung maturity in late preterm and early term infants. Am J Obstet Gynecol 2011;204(6):518.e6; with permission.)

disruption of their function has been implicated in several disease processes affecting the newborn, including TTN and hyaline membrane disease. The moderately preterm and late preterm infant is more susceptible to these problems in part because ENaC expression is developmentally regulated. Peak expression in the alveolar epithelium is achieved only at term gestation; this leaves preterm infants with lower expression of these channels, thus reducing their ability to clear fetal lung fluid after birth.[41]

It is clear that infants born early (including late preterm and early term) are at increased risk for respiratory distress, which is in part explained by evidence in animal and human studies that ENaC expression is developmentally regulated.[42,43] Nasal potential difference studies in preterm infants with respiratory distress show a smaller decrease in potential difference in response to amiloride than occurs in preterm infants without respiratory distress, indicating a lower level of ENaC activity.[44] Further studies have confirmed lower levels of α-ENaC, β-ENaC, and γ-ENaC in preterm infants with respiratory distress compared with healthy term infants.[45] During the first 30 hours of life, ENaC levels decrease quicker in vaginally delivered term infants as lung fluid is cleared. The decrease in ENaC levels is slower in preterm and cesarean-delivered term infants. Thus low levels of epithelial sodium transport caused by low levels of ENaC production, whether caused by gestational immaturity, lack of spontaneous labor, or both, contribute to the development of TTN.

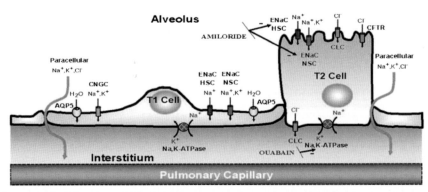

Fig. 4. Epithelial sodium (Na) absorption in the fetal lung near birth. Na enters the cell through the apical surface of both alveolar type I (ATI) and alveolar type II (ATII) cells via amiloride-sensitive ENaC, both highly selective channels (HSC) and nonselective channels (NSC), and via cyclic nucleotide–gated channels (seen only in ATI cells). Electroneutrality is conserved with chloride movement through cystic fibrosis transmembrane conductance regulator (CFTR) or through chloride channels (CLC) in ATI and ATII cells, and/or paracellularly through tight junctions. The increase in cell Na stimulates Na-K-ATPase activity on the basolateral aspect of the cell membrane, which drives out 3 Na ions in exchange for 2 K ions, a process that can be blocked by the cardiac glycoside ouabain. If the net ion movement is from the apical surface to the interstitium, an osmotic gradient is created, which in turn directs water transport in the same direction, either through aquaporins or by diffusion. (*From* Jain L. Respiratory morbidity in late-preterm infants: prevention is better than cure! Am J Perinatol 2008;25:76; with permission.)

How retention of fetal lung fluid leads to such predictable tachypnea, in spite of normal or low arterial CO_2 levels, is a puzzling biological phenomenon. Early studies by Paintal[46] suggested a role for pulmonary C-fibers (J-receptors) in initiating reflex activity leading to tachypnea and bronchoconstriction, among other effects. Paintal[46] postulated that C-fibers respond to excess fluid in the interstitial space as interstitial stretch receptors trigger rapid shallow breathing. A similar role has since been described for bronchial C-fibers.[47,48]

Healthy late preterm infants have significantly lower respiratory compliance and expiratory flow ratio (Ratio of Time to Reach Peak Tidal Expiratory Flow to Total Expiratory Time [TPTEF/TE]) than term infants.[49] The physiologic deficiencies that result from incomplete lung development described earlier are likely to account for the early morbidity and vulnerability to infection. With growth in the first to second years of life, the physiologic instability of the chest wall and the inadequate maintenance of lung volume likely correct themselves and should not account for the long-term deficiencies. It seems that impairment of the potential for full growth is related to early birth; however, one of the consequences of altered lung development in preterm infants is their increased vulnerability to respiratory syncytial virus infection.[1]

Based on some of the information presented earlier, intrapartum interventions, including antenatal corticosteroid (ACS) administration, have recently been investigated to determine the health consequences in infants born late preterm. In a large cohort study (n = 11,783 infants), 8620 infants were exposed to ACS. Results showed a reduced risk of RDS in infants exposed to ACS earlier in fetal life and born after 34 weeks. This finding is similar to the risk reduction in infants born before 34 weeks' gestation. This risk reduction was mainly in infants born at 34 to 36 weeks' gestation.

Further ACS given earlier in pregnancy seem to have prolonged beneficial effects for infants born after 34 weeks' gestation without increased risk of neurologic side effects.[50] The National Institute of Child Health and Human Development (NICHD) is currently conducting a large randomized multicenter trial (Antenatal Late Preterm Steroid [ALPS] trial) to evaluate the efficacy of antenatal betamethasone in late preterm gestation (34–36 weeks) mothers.

RESPIRATORY MORBIDITIES

Several factors may contribute to the overall burden of respiratory morbidity in the late preterm infant.[5,9,51–55] Given the shortcomings clinicians face in accurate estimation of gestational age, elective inductions and cesarean sections may have increased the burden of iatrogenic prematurity. Colin and colleagues[1] postulated that preterm birth, even if there is no significant neonatal respiratory disease, may have adverse effects on lung growth and development, leading to reduced pulmonary function and increased morbidity.

Rates of RDS, transient TTN, pneumonia, surfactant use, and oscillator use were all higher at 37 weeks compared with 39 weeks. Ghartey and colleagues[22] showed a 2-fold increased risk of respiratory morbidity among neonates delivered in the early term period compared with those delivered at 39 weeks. Multiple studies have shown that the risk of all types of respiratory distress, and of TTN specifically, increases with each week less than 39 weeks.[3,9,51] The Consortium on Safe Labor evaluated respiratory outcomes at delivery in 233,844 infants of more than 34 weeks, with a special focus on late preterm infants ($34^{0/7}$ to $36^{6/7}$ weeks' gestation), and the incidence of TTN was highest at 34 weeks (64 of 1000 births) and 35 weeks (46 of 1000 births) and decreased with advancing gestational age.[3]

The severity of respiratory disease often depends on gestational age. In moderate preterm birth, 30% of these infants needed nasal continuous positive airway pressure (nCPAP) alone, another 30% were mechanically ventilated, and 35% were administered surfactant (**Fig. 5**). Up to 45% of infants born late preterm with respiratory failure were given surfactant.

It is widely accepted that RDS is the result of a primary absence or deficiency of this highly surface-active alveolar lining layer (pulmonary surfactant). Surfactant, a

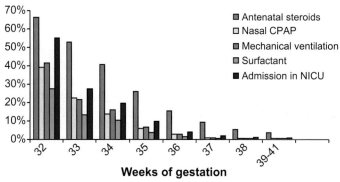

Weeks of gestation

Fig. 5. Gestational age and rates of respiratory treatments and admission in a neonatal intensive care unit (NICU) in a population of 173,058 live-born infants (years 2000–2009). CPAP, continuous positive airway pressure. (*From* Guoyon JB, Iacobelli S, Ferdunus C, et al. Neonatal problems of late and moderate preterm infants. Semin Fetal Neonatal Med 2012;17:147; with permission.)

complex lipoprotein rich in saturated phosphatidylcholine molecules, binds to the internal surface of the lung and markedly lessens the forces of surface tension at the air-water interphase, thereby reducing the pressure tending to collapse the alveolus. The distal respiratory epithelium responsible for gas exchange features 2 distinct cell types in the mature infant lung. Type I pneumocytes cover most of the alveolus, in close proximity to capillary endothelial cells. Type II cells have been identified in the human fetus as early as 22 weeks' gestation, but become prominent at 34 to 36 weeks of gestation.[25,40] These highly metabolically active cells contain the cytoplasmic lamellar bodies that are the source of pulmonary surfactant. Surfactant synthesis is a complex process that requires an abundance of precursor substrates, such as glucose, fatty acid, and choline, and a series of key enzymatic steps that are regulated by various hormones, including corticosteroids. For neonates born at 34 weeks, the odds of RDS were increased 40-fold; that risk decreases with each advancing week of gestation until 38 weeks. Even at 37 weeks, the odds of RDS were still 3-fold greater than that of a 39-week or 40-week birth.[3]

Although respiratory issues tend to be transient in most neonates, some neonates develop persistent pulmonary hypertension of the neonate (PPHN) or severe hypoxic respiratory failure, conditions requiring additional therapies such as nitric oxide, high-frequency ventilation, and extracorporeal membrane oxygenation (ECMO).[15,17] Studies have shown that PPHN is more likely in 34-week to 37-week preterm infants who develop RDS than in similar infants born at 32 weeks' gestation. Such predisposition is attributed to a developmental increase in smooth muscle in the walls of pulmonary blood vessels. In a retrospective study of 228,668 deliveries with 19,334 late preterm births, the incidence of PPHN was 0.38% in late preterm infants compared with 0.08% in term infants, and the incidence of respiratory failure was 0.94% in late preterm infants compared with 0.11% in term infants.[3] Many of these infants are asymptomatic immediately after birth but subsequently show an escalating need for respiratory support with evidence of PPHN.[4,17]

PPHN of the newborn is associated with increased pulmonary vascular resistance, which eventually leads to right-to-left shunting by means of fetal pathways and ventilation-perfusion (V/Q) mismatching.[56] Management of neonates who develop significant pulmonary hypertension can be challenging, given the self-propagated nature of hypoxia-induced pulmonary vasoconstriction. Treatment options include exogenous surfactant (shown to be effective if used early in the disease course),[56] inhaled nitric oxide (selectively lowers pulmonary vascular resistance and decreases extrapulmonary right-to-left shunting),[57,58] high-frequency ventilation, and ECMO.

A review of the Extracorporeal Life Support Organization (ELSO) Neonatal Registry by Dudell and Jain[56] found that, from 1989 to 2006, 14.5% of the patients receiving ECMO were late preterm infants and had a mean gestational age of 35.3 weeks. Affected infants were more likely to require ECMO secondary to hypoxic respiratory failure/RDS instead of aspiration syndromes, which is the primary insult for term babies requiring ECMO.[56] A more recent study[4] from the ELSO Neonatal Registry found that late preterm and early term infants comprised 15% and 21% of the neonatal ECMO population, respectively (for reference, late preterm infants comprise 12.8% of all births and early term infants comprise 17.5% of all births in the United States). Late preterm and early term infants experience higher mortality on ECMO (late preterm, 26.2%; early term, 18%; full term, 11.2%; $P<.001$) and have longer ECMO runs compared with term infants. Late preterm infants with a primary diagnosis of sepsis and PPHN had a 3-fold higher risk of mortality on ECMO than those with meconium aspiration. Nearly 23% of late preterm infants with severe hypoxic respiratory failure were born by elective cesarean section, which is a higher rate than the

16.5% reported by Keszler and colleagues[17] in their 1985 to 1991 data, and almost twice the estimated national rate of ~12% repeat cesarean sections of all live births in the United States. Late preterm infants born by elective repeat cesarean section are over-represented in the ECMO population. In addition, late preterm infants were older at cannulation (likely because most of these infants are asymptomatic at birth but gradually develop an increasing oxygen requirement with subsequent development of PPHN), had a longer duration of ECMO support, and were more likely to have intraventricular hemorrhage and other neurologic complications than term infants.

LONG-TERM RISK OF RESPIRATORY DISORDERS

Moderate, late, and near term infants are born during the third trimester of pregnancy when the rate of lung maturation is greatest.[59] Higher risk of respiratory illnesses and rehospitalizations in infancy and early childhood have been found in the neonatal period in infants born at 32 to 36 weeks' gestation.[1,59] A recent review article noted that, "the respiratory vulnerability of preterm infants born 32–36 weeks gestational age, usually considered low risk for subsequent respiratory problems, is more similar to that of very preterm infants than that of term infants."[60]

Although very preterm infants are at a higher risk of psychomotor, behavioral, cognitive, and other developmental disabilities, late preterm infants have more subtle findings of language delay, attention deficits, lower intelligence, behavioral problems, and academic achievement issues. There are few studies of long-term outcomes in late preterm infants. A large Swedish population-based study including 903,402 children (32,945 late preterm infants) who were born alive without any congenital anomalies from 1967 to 1983 and followed through adulthood until 2003 found a higher incidence of cerebral palsy (relative risk, 2.7; 95% confidence interval [CI], 2.2 to 3.3; $P<.001$), mental retardation (relative risk, 1.6; 95% CI, 1.4 to 1.8; $P<.001$), disorders of psychological development, behavior and emotional disturbances, other major disabilities (blindness, low vision, hearing loss, and epilepsy), and medical disability affecting working capacity.[61] A more recent study by Williams and colleagues[62] evaluated the role of prematurity and maternal factors in first-grade academic failure. After adjusting for maternal and child characteristics, there was an increased chance of failure of each component of the first-grade Criterion-referenced Competency Test (CRCT) for children born late preterm versus term.

Short-term lung function outcomes are compromised in these infants as well. Lung physiologic measurements in children born very preterm (<32 weeks' gestation) have been reported, but there is a paucity of data regarding lung function of infants born late preterm. Friedrich and colleagues[63] compared healthy infants born at 30 to 34 weeks' gestation with term controls, reporting decreased forced expiratory flow between 25% and 75% of forced vial capacity at 4 and 16 months of age. These measurements seemed to continue without showing any catch-up time between these 2 time points.[64] Another study by Hoo and colleagues[65] investigated airway function in healthy premature infants with a mean gestational age of 33.2 weeks who did not have respiratory illness in the neonatal period. This group had significantly diminished maximal expiratory flow at functional residual capacity at 1 year of age.

Data on long-term respiratory outcomes of children born at 32 to 36 weeks is sparse. Todisco and colleagues[66] studied children born late preterm without RDS or mechanical ventilation and compared them with their term siblings. Late preterm children had significantly increased mean values of residual volume compared with their siblings. Using the Avon Longitudinal Study of Parents and Children (ALSPAC), Kotecha and Kotecha[67] recently showed that, at 8 to 9 years of age, measures of forced expiratory spirometry are lower in children born at 33 to 34 weeks' gestation compared with children born at term, and are of similar magnitude to those in the extremely preterm (25–32 weeks' gestation) group, who had received a higher proportion of respiratory intervention during the neonatal period.[67] The association between extremely low birthweight infants and asthma has been established; however, few studies have focused on the impact of late prematurity and asthma. A retrospective cohort study of 7925 infants revealed that, compared with term gestation, late preterm gestation was associated with significant increases in persistent asthma diagnoses (adjusted odds ratio [aOR], 1.68), inhaled corticosteroid use (aOR, 1.66), and numbers of acute respiratory visits (incidence rate ratio, 1.44). Further, infants born at 37 to 38 weeks' gestation also had increases in asthma diagnoses (aOR, 1.34) and inhaled corticosteroid use (aOR, 1.39).[68]

Late preterm infants have been termed The Great Imposters. Their size and shape make them appear deceivingly innocent and much like a full-term infant. Their physiologic complications may or may not manifest until 48 to 72 hours of life, and in many cases these complications do not manifest until they have already been discharged from the hospital. Late preterm infants have rehospitalization rates that are 2-fold to 3-fold higher than the rates for full-term infants.[69]

Late preterm infants are at an increased risk of respiratory morbidity in the neonatal period, with a higher incidence of respiratory interventions, such as mechanical ventilation, and an increased rate of early respiratory infections, all of which may have a negative impact on later lung function. Although data on lung function later in life are lacking, available data suggest that these children may be at risk for respiratory consequences later in life.[67,70]

In 2005, the Association of Women's Health, Obstetric and Neonatal Nurses announced an initiative in collaboration with Johnson & Johnson to improve health care and guidelines for this vulnerable population.[71] These guidelines have now been published and the new protocols and pathways are designed to fit the needs of the late preterm infant in a variety of settings from well-baby nurseries to level III neonatal intensive care units to pediatrician offices. Further research on the long-term respiratory outcomes of these infants is needed and more educational tools will help care providers identify morbidities in these preterm neonates and advocate for appropriate clinical care for this subgroup of premature infants.[72]

ACKNOWLEDGMENTS

We would like to thank Dr Kara del Valle and Dr Ken Hepburn for their editorial comments and critiques in an effort to make this manuscript scientifically accurate and readable.

REFERENCES

1. Colin A, McEvoy C, Castile RG. Respiratory morbidity and lung function in preterm infants of 32 to 36 weeks' gestational age. Pediatrics 2010;126(1):115–28. http://dx.doi.org/10.1542/peds.2009-1381.
2. Shapiro-Mendoza C, Tomashek K, Kotelchuck M, et al. Effect of late-preterm birth and maternal medical conditions on newborn morbidity risk. Pediatrics 2008;121(2):e223–32. http://dx.doi.org/10.1542/peds.2006-3629.
3. Hibbard JU, Wilkins I, Sun L, et al, Consortium on Safe Labor. Respiratory morbidity in late preterm births. JAMA 2010;304(4):419–25. http://dx.doi.org/10.1001/jama.2010.1015.

4. Ramachandrappa A, Rosenberg E, Wagoner S, et al. Morbidity and mortality in late preterm infants with severe hypoxic respiratory failure on ECMO. J Pediatr 2011;159(2):192–8.e3. http://dx.doi.org/10.1016/j.jpeds.2011.02.015.

5. Roth-Kleiner M, Wagner BP, Bachmann D, et al. Respiratory distress syndrome in near-term babies after caesarean section. Swiss Med Wkly 2003;133(19–20): 283–8 [PubMed: 12844271].

6. Hack M, Fanaroff AA, Klaus MH, et al. Neonatal respiratory distress following elective delivery. A preventable disease? Am J Obstet Gynecol 1976;126: 43–7 [PubMed: 961745].

7. Goldenberg RL, Nelson K. Iatrogenic respiratory distress syndrome. An analysis of obstetric events preceding delivery of infants who develop respiratory distress syndrome. Am J Obstet Gynecol 1975;123:617–20 [PubMed: 1242870].

8. Maisels MJ, Rees R, Marks K, et al. Elective delivery of the term fetus. An obstetrical hazard. JAMA 1977;238:2036–9 [PubMed: 410962].

9. Villar J, Carroli G, Zavaleta N, et al. Maternal and neonatal individual risks and benefits associated with caesarean delivery: multicentre prospective study. BMJ 2007;335(7628):1025 [PubMed: 17977819].

10. McIntire DD, Leveno KJ. Neonatal mortality and morbidity rates in late preterm births compared with births at term. Obstet Gynecol 2008;111(1):35–41 [PubMed: 18165390].

11. Engle WA, Tomashek KM, Wallman C. "Late-preterm" infants: a population at risk. Pediatrics 2007;120:1390–401 [PubMed: 18055691].

12. Wang ML, Dorer DJ, Fleming MP, et al. Clinical outcomes of near-term infants. Pediatrics 2004;114:372–6 [PubMed: 15286219].

13. Rubaltelli FF, Bonafe L, Tangucci M, et al. Epidemiology of neonatal acute respiratory disorders. A multicenter study on incidence and fatality rates of neonatal acute respiratory disorders according to gestational age, maternal age, pregnancy complications and type of delivery. Biol Neonate 1998;74:7–15 [PubMed: 9657664].

14. Escobar GJ, Clark RH, Greene JD. Short-term outcomes of infants born at 35 and 36 weeks gestation: we need to ask more questions. Semin Perinatol 2006;30:28–33 [PubMed: 16549211].

15. Heritage CK, Cunningham MD. Association of elective repeat cesarean delivery and persistent pulmonary hypertension of the newborn. Am J Obstet Gynecol 1985;152:627–9 [PubMed: 4025421].

16. Hernandez-Diaz S, Van Marter LJ, Werler MM, et al. Risk factors for persistent pulmonary hypertension of the newborn. Pediatrics 2007;120:e272–82 [PubMed: 17671038].

17. Keszler M, Carbone MT, Cox C, et al. Severe respiratory failure after elective repeat cesarean delivery: a potentially preventable condition leading to extracorporeal membrane oxygenation. Pediatrics 1992;89:670–2 [PubMed: 1557250].

18. Gunville CF, Sontag MK, Stratton KA, et al. Scope and impact of early and late preterm infants admitted to the PICU with respiratory illness. J Pediatr 2010; 157(2):209–14.e1. http://dx.doi.org/10.1016/j.jpeds.2010.02.006.

19. Boyle J, Boyle E. Born just a few weeks early: does it matter? Arch Dis Child Fetal Neonatal Ed 2013;98(1):F85–8. http://dx.doi.org/10.1136/archdischild-2011-300535.

20. De Luca R, Boulvain M, Irion O, et al. Incidence of early neonatal mortality and morbidity after late-preterm and term cesarean delivery. Pediatrics 2009;123(6): e1064–71. http://dx.doi.org/10.1542/peds.2008-2407.

21. Madar J, Richmond S, Hey E. Surfactant-deficient respiratory distress after elective delivery at "term". Acta Paediatr 1999;88:1244.

22. Ghartey K, Coletta J, Lizarraga L, et al. Neonatal respiratory morbidity in the early term delivery. Am J Obstet Gynecol 2012;207(4):292.e1–4. http://dx.doi.org/10.1016/j.ajog.2012.07.022.

23. Oshiro B, Kowalewski L, Sappenfield W, et al. A multistate quality improvement program to decrease elective deliveries before 39 weeks of gestation. Obstet Gynecol 2013;121(5):1025–31. http://dx.doi.org/10.1097/AOG.0b013e31828ca096.

24. Joshi S, Kotecha S. Lung growth and development. Early Hum Dev 2007;83: e789–94.

25. Jain L, Eaton DC. Physiology of fetal lung fluid clearance and the effect of labor. Semin Perinatol 2006;30:34.

26. Zhao J, Gonzalez F, Mu D. Apnea of prematurity: from cause to treatment. Eur J Pediatr 2011;170(9):1097–105. http://dx.doi.org/10.1007/s00431-011-1409-6 PMCID: PMC3158333.

27. American College of Obstetricians and Gynecologists. ACOG practice bulletin no. 97: fetal lung maturity. Obstet Gynecol 2008;112:717–26.

28. Bates E, Rouse DJ, Mann ML, et al. Neonatal outcomes after demonstrated fetal lung maturity before 39 weeks of gestation. Obstet Gynecol 2010;116: 1288–95.

29. Tennant C, Friedman A, Pare E, et al. Performance of lecithin-sphingomyelin ratio as a reflex test for documenting fetal lung maturity in late preterm and term fetuses. J Matern Fetal Neonatal Med 2012;25(8):1460–2.

30. Hallman M, Teramo K. Measurement of the lecithin/sphingomyelin ratio and phosphatidylglycerol in amniotic fluid: an accurate method for the assessment of fetal lung maturity. Br J Obstet Gynaecol 1981;88:806–13.

31. Kamath B, Marcotte M, DeFranco E. Neonatal morbidity after documented fetal lung maturity in late preterm and early term infants. Am J Obstet Gynecol 2011; 204(6):518.e1–8. http://dx.doi.org/10.1016/j.ajog.2011.03.038.

32. Besnard AE, Wirjosoekarto SA, Broeze KA, et al. Lecithin/sphingomyelin ratio and lamellar body count for fetal lung maturity: a meta-analysis. Eur J Obstet Gynecol Reprod Biol 2013. http://dx.doi.org/10.1016/j.ejogrb.2013.02.013. pii:S0301–2115(13)00099-7.

33. Cassin S, Gause G, Perks AM. The effects of bumetanide and furosemide on lung liquid secretion in fetal sheep. Proc Soc Exp Biol Med 1986;181(3): 427–31.

34. Olver R, Ramsden C, Strang L, et al. The role of amiloride-blockable sodium transport in adrenaline-induced lung liquid reabsorption in the fetal lamb. J Physiol 1986;376:321–40.

35. Adamson IY, Bowden DH. Reaction of cultured adult and fetal lung to prednisolone and thyroxine. Arch Pathol 1975;99(2):80–5.

36. McCray PB Jr, Reenstra WW, Louie E, et al. Expression of CFTR and presence of cAMP-mediated fluid secretion in human fetal lung. Am J Physiol 1992;262: L472–81.

37. Wallen LD, Perry SF, Alston JT, et al. Morphometric study of the role of pulmonary arterial flow in fetal lung growth in sheep. Pediatr Res 1990;27(2):122–7.

38. Moessinger AC, Collins MH, Blanc WA, et al. Oligohydramnios-induced lung hypoplasia: the influence of timing and duration in gestation. Pediatr Res 1986;20: 951–4.

39. Bland RD. Loss of liquid from the lung lumen in labor: more than a simple "squeeze". Am J Physiol Lung Cell Mol Physiol 2001;280:L602.

40. Jain L, Chen XJ, Ramosevac S, et al. Expression of highly selective sodium channels in alveolar type II cells is determined by culture conditions. Am J Physiol Lung Cell Mol Physiol 2001;280:L646.
41. Smith DE, Otulakowski G, Yeger H, et al. Epithelial Na(+) channel (ENaC) expression in the developing normal and abnormal human perinatal lung. Am J Respir Crit Care Med 2000;161:1322.
42. Jesse NM, McCartney J, Feng X, et al. Expression of ENaC subunits, chloride channels, and aquaporins in ovine fetal lung: ontogeny of expression and effects of altered fetal cortisol concentrations. Am J Physiol Regul Integr Comp Physiol 2009;297(2):R453–61. http://dx.doi.org/10.1152/ajpregu.00127.
43. O'Brodovich H, Canessa CM, Ueda J, et al. Expression of the epithelial Na1 channel in the developing rat lung. Am J Physiol 1993;265:C491–6.
44. Barker PM, Gowen CW, Lawson EE, et al. Decreased sodium ion absorption across nasal epithelium of very premature infants with respiratory distress syndrome. J Pediatr 1997;130:373–7.
45. Helve O, Andersson S, Kirjavainen T, et al. Expression of epithelial sodium channel (ENAC) in the airways of healthy term infants during the first postnatal days. Pediatr Res 2004;56:482. http://dx.doi.org/10.1203/00006450-200409000-00131.
46. Paintal AS. Mechanism of stimulation of type J pulmonary receptors. J Physiol 1969;203:511–32.
47. Widdicombe JG. Respiratory reflexes from the trachea and bronchi of the cat. J Physiol 1954;123:55–70.
48. Widdicombe J. Reflexes from the lungs and airways: historical perspective. J Appl Physiol 2006;101:628–34.
49. McEvoy C, Venigalla S, Schilling D, et al. Respiratory function in healthy late preterm infants delivered at 33-36 weeks of gestation. J Pediatr 2013;162(3):464–9. http://dx.doi.org/10.1016/j.jpeds.2012.09.042.
50. Eriksson L, Haglund B, Ewald U, et al. Health consequences of prophylactic exposure to antenatal corticosteroids among children born late preterm or term. Acta Obstet Gynecol Scand 2012;91(12):1415–21. http://dx.doi.org/10.1111/aogs.12014.
51. Hansen AK, Wisborg K, Uldbjerg N, et al. Risk of respiratory morbidity in term infants delivered by elective caesarean section: cohort study. BMJ 2008; 336(7635):85–7.
52. Kolas T, Saugstad OD, Daltveit AK, et al. Planned cesarean versus planned vaginal delivery at term: comparison of newborn infant outcomes. Am J Obstet Gynecol 2006;195(6):1538–43.
53. Levine EM, Ghai V, Barton JJ, et al. Mode of delivery and risk of respiratory diseases in newborns. Obstet Gynecol 2001;97(3):439–42.
54. Morrison JJ, Rennie JM, Milton PJ. Neonatal respiratory morbidity and mode of delivery at term: influence of timing of elective caesarean section. Br J Obstet Gynaecol 1995;102(2):101–6.
55. Tita AT, Landon MB, Spong CY, et al. Timing of elective repeat cesarean delivery at term and neonatal outcomes. N Engl J Med 2009;360:111.
56. Dudell GG, Jain L. Hypoxic respiratory failure in the late preterm infant. Clin Perinatol 2006;33(4):803–30.
57. Kinsella JP, Neish SR, Ivy DD, et al. Clinical responses to prolonged treatment of persistent pulmonary hypertension of the newborn with low doses of inhaled nitric oxide. J Pediatr 1993;123:103.
58. Kinsella JP, Neish SR, Shaffer E, et al. Low-dose inhalation nitric oxide in persistent pulmonary hypertension of the newborn. Lancet 1992;340:819.

59. Resch B, Paes B. Are late preterm infants as susceptible to RSV infection as full term infants? Early Hum Dev 2011;87S:S47–9.
60. Raju TN, Higgins RD, Stark AR, et al. Optimizing care and outcome for late-preterm (near-term) infants: a summary of the workshop sponsored by the National Institute of Child Health and Human Development. Pediatrics 2006;118: 1207–14.
61. Moster D, Terje R, Markestad T. Long-term medical and social consequences of preterm birth. N Engl J Med 2008;359:262.
62. Williams B, Dunlop A, Kramer M, et al. Perinatal origins of first-grade academic failure: role of prematurity and maternal factors. Pediatrics 2013;131:693–700.
63. Friedrich L, Pitrez PM, Stein RT, et al. Growth rate of lung function in healthy preterm infants. Am J Respir Crit Care Med 2007;176:1269–73.
64. Kotecha SJ, Watkins WJ, Paranjothy S, et al. Effect of late preterm birth on longitudinal lung spirometry in school age children and adolescents. Thorax 2012; 67:e54–61.
65. Hoo AF, Dezateux C, Henschen M, et al. Development of airway function in infancy after preterm delivery. J Pediatr 2002;141:652–8.
66. Todisco T, de Benedictis FM, Iannacci L, et al. Mild prematurity and respiratory functions. Eur J Pediatr 1993;152:55–8.
67. Kotecha S, Kotecha SJ. Long term respiratory outcomes of perinatal lung disease. Semin Fetal Neonatal Med 2012;17:65–6.
68. Goyal N, Fiks A, Lorch S. Association of late-preterm birth with asthma in young children: practice-based study. Pediatrics 2011;128:e830.
69. Bhutani VK, Johnson L. Kernicterus in late preterm infants cared for as term healthy infants. Semin Perinatol 2006;30:89–97.
70. Kotecha S, Dunstan F, Kotecha S. Long term respiratory outcomes of late preterm-born infants. Semin Fetal Neonatal Med 2012;17(2):77–81.
71. Medoff-Cooper B, Holditch-Davis D, Verklan T, et al. Newborn clinical outcomes of the AWHONN late preterm infant research-based practice project. J Obstet Gynecol Neonatal Nurs 2012;41:774–85.
72. Darcy A. Complications of the late preterm infant. J Perinat Neonatal Nurs 2009; 23(1):78–86.

Jaundice and Kernicterus in the Moderately Preterm Infant

Matthew B. Wallenstein, MD, Vinod K. Bhutani, MD*

KEYWORDS

- Kernicterus • Bilirubin-induced neurologic dysfunction • Jaundice
- Hyperbilirubinemia • Bilirubin encephalopathy • Newborn jaundice
- Moderately preterm

KEY POINTS

- Moderately preterm infants remain at increased risk for adverse outcomes, including acute bilirubin encephalopathy (ABE) relative to term infants. Evidence-based guidelines for the management of hyperbilirubinemia in moderately preterm infants, however, are lacking.
- High concentrations of unconjugated bilirubin can cause permanent neurologic damage in infants, known as chronic bilirubin encephalopathy or kernicterus.
- There is growing concern that exposure to even moderate concentrations of bilirubin may lead to subtle but permanent neurodevelopmental impairment (NDI), known as bilirubin-induced neurologic dysfunction (BIND).
- Clinical manifestations of ABE in preterm infants are similar to, but often more subtle than, those of term infants.
- This article provides clinical strategies to operationalize the thresholds for the management of hyperbilirubinemia in moderately preterm infants, based on recently published consensus-based recommendations.

INTRODUCTION

The American Academy of Pediatrics published guidelines for management of hyperbilirubinemia in infants greater than or equal to 35 weeks' gestational age (GA) in 2004.[1] This management protocol, based on available evidence, has been widely

Funding Source: No external funding was secured for this study.
Financial Disclosure: None of the authors has financial relationships relevant to this article to disclose.
Conflict of Interest: None of the authors has conflicts of interest to disclose.
Division of Neonatal-Developmental Medicine, Department of Pediatrics, Lucile Packard Children's Hospital, Stanford University School of Medicine, 750 Welch Road #315, Stanford, CA 94304, USA
* Corresponding author.
E-mail address: bhutani@stanford.edu

Clin Perinatol 40 (2013) 679–688
http://dx.doi.org/10.1016/j.clp.2013.07.007
0095-5108/13/$ – see front matter © 2013 Elsevier Inc. All rights reserved.

accepted as standard practice and has been successfully implemented for late preterm infants.[2] Similar guidelines in the United States for infants less than 35 weeks' GA have been elusive due to absence of a rigorous standard of evidence and the practical inability to test the hypothesis of bilirubin-induced injury in vulnerable infants. As a result, management of hyperbilirubinemia in moderately preterm infants ($28^{0/7}$ to $34^{6/7}$-wk GA) varies greatly among neonatal intensive care units (NICUs).[3–5] A consensus-based recommendation was recently proposed for use of phototherapy and exchange transfusion in preterm infants less than 35 weeks' GA.[6] These practical recommendations are based on expert consensus because there are insufficient data to establish evidence-based guidelines.

Posticteric complications are infrequent, with liberal and effective use of phototherapy in current clinical practice. The risk is not zero, however, and several recent studies have shown that even moderate or low total serum/plasma bilirubin (TB) levels can lead to development of kernicterus in sick premature infants.[7–10] Furthermore, recent population studies suggest that moderate elevations in TB may be associated with NDI,[10,11] although additional studies failed to identify increased risk of NDI with moderate TB elevation.[12,13] Studies of extremely low birth weight (ELBW) infants have been informative. A recent randomized controlled trial showed that aggressive phototherapy in ELBW infants reduced NDI and hearing loss among surviving infants versus those receiving conservative phototherapy. A post hoc statistical analysis reported, however, a 5% higher mortality among those infants weighing 501 g to 750 g in the aggressive phototherapy group, although the CI included 1.0.[14] This subcohort of the smallest of infants with translucent and fragile skin was exposed to light irradiance that lowered their concentration of plasma bilirubin (a powerful antioxidant).

There is extensive literature on phototherapy guidelines for full-term and ELBW infants; however, management of hyperbilirubinemia in infants less than 35 weeks' GA has not been subject to similar scientific rigor. This review outlines clinical strategies that would operationalize the management of hyperbilirubinemia in moderately preterm infants to meet the recently published consensus-based recommendations[6] and examines the scope of the problem of hyperbilirubinemia in moderately preterm infants, the mechanism of brain injury, clinical manifestations of untreated and progressive hyperbilirubinemia, and the spectrum of BIND.

SCOPE OF THE PROBLEM

Infants 30 to 35 weeks' GA constitute almost one-third of all NICU admissions.[15] This moderately preterm population is more vulnerable to adverse outcomes at lower TB concentrations, including ABE, relative to term infants.[15–17]

The prevalence of hyperbilirubinemia among preterm infants 30 to 34 weeks' GA is difficult to quantify. The thresholds for excessive hyperbilirubinemia in this group are not standardized by GA, and clinicians often utilize lower TB thresholds to intervene with decreasing GA.[18] As a result, the exact prevalence of BIND and kernicterus in preterm infants who survive to discharge is not known.[19]

The consequence of hyperbilirubinemia in premature infants is more severe than in term infants, with mean peak TB levels approaching 10 to 12 mg/dL (171–205 μmol/L).[17] Premature infants face higher bilirubin burdens due to increased bilirubin production, decreased hepatic uptake, decreased uridine-diphosphoglucuronate glucuronosyltransferase (UGT) activity, and increased enterohepatic circulation. Disorders in binding of bilirubin to albumin augment the vulnerability of both sick and healthy preterm infants. Furthermore, preterm infants are at higher risk for ABE due to their immature and developing nervous systems.[20–22]

Given the prevalence of hyperbilirubinemia among preterm infants and the relative proportion of moderately preterm infants among NICU populations, neonatal health care providers are encouraged to review their institutional policies for a systems-based approach to manage hyperbilirubinemia in these preterm infants that includes screening, diagnostic evaluation, frequency and duration of monitoring, TB thresholds for intervention adjusted for GA and presence of hemolysis, risk assessment for neurotoxicity, and effective, but judicious, use of phototherapy. Local implementation of these approaches has been successful in the apparent reduction of exchange transfusion among NICUs in the United States. Continued assessment of best practices would be helpful to minimize overtreatment or unintended consequences of bilirubin reduction strategies.

MECHANISM OF BRAIN INJURY

High concentrations of unconjugated bilirubin can cause permanent neurologic damage in infants, known as chronic bilirubin encephalopathy or kernicterus. This relationship has been well established.[23–26] More than half of term infants with TB greater than 30 mg/dL (513 μmol/L) develop permanent neurologic sequelae.[27] Similar data are not available for moderately preterm infants. Disordered binding of bilirubin to albumin may cause increased vulnerability among preterm infants. The fraction of free bilirubin (unbound bilirubin) increases as bilirubin approaches the binding capacity of albumin. Increased unbound bilirubin levels have been linked to bilirubin neurotoxicity.[28] Current evidence does not provide for precise prediction (sensitivity and/or specificity) for bilirubin neurotoxicity based on either TB or unbound (or free) bilirubin. Use of basic pharmacokinetic models of bilirubin transport and tissue uptake suggests that either unbound bilirubin alone or in combination with TB may better discriminate the risk for an individual infant.[28] Diagnosis of kernicterus is made via microscopic evaluation at autopsy. History of exposure to severe or prolonged duration of hyperbilirubinemia, association of clinical signs characterized by diverse processing disorders, sensorineural hearing abnormalities (auditory brainstem-evoked responses or cochlear microphonics), and MRI in surviving infants assist clinicians in diagnosing posticteric sequelae. Classically, injury is evident in the basal ganglia (globus pallidus), central/peripheral auditory pathways, hippocampus, diencephalon, subthalamic nuclei, or midbrain, among other regions.[24,29] MRI often reveals increased signal intensity in these locations.

The mechanism of bilirubin neurotoxicity has not yet been elucidated. On crossing the blood-brain barrier, bilirubin may damage neurons by interfering with energy metabolism in subcellular organelles, binding to and inhibiting function of specific organelle or cyoplasmic proteins, and/or directly damaging DNA.[30] In vitro studies have found that bilirubin exposure causes neuritic atrophy, cell death, decreased neuronal arborization, arrested neuritic growth, and neuritic hypoplasia.[29]

Acute kernicterus (or ABE) can result from unmonitored or insufficiently treated progressive hyperbilirubinemia. There is growing concern that exposure to even moderate concentrations of bilirubin may also lead to isolated neurodevelopmental injury or subtle but permanent impairment known as BIND.[31] The spectrum of neurologic impairment from BIND may manifest as disturbances of myriad processes, including visual-motor, auditory, speech, cognition, and language. The effect of bilirubin on neuronal differentiation and development in vitro provides biologic plausibility for the spectrum of BIND. Evidence for a causal link between hyperbilirubinemia and subtle NDI, however, is lacking at present. Also, some evidence suggests that infants may benefit from the antioxidant properties of bilirubin, making ideal management less straightforward.[13,21]

CLINICAL MANIFESTATIONS OF HYPERBILIRUBINEMIA IN THE MODERATELY PRETERM INFANT

Clinical manifestations of ABE include changes in mental status, muscle tone, feeding, and pitch of cry, leading to progressive hypotonia, retrocollis, and opisthotonos. Mortality during ABE approaches 10%, usually due to respiratory failure or seizures refractory to antiepileptic administration.[31] Kernicterus, which refers to permanent neurologic damage in infants who survive ABE, is characterized by chronic manifestations of the acute syndrome of ABE, including dystonia, athetoid cerebral palsy, gaze paralysis, and sensorineural hearing loss. Cognitive function may be spared, although some studies suggest otherwise.[32]

Clinical manifestations of ABE in preterm infants are similar to, but often more subtle than, those of term infants. Immature neuronal architecture and masking clinical conditions (eg, ventilatory support), however, often produce subtle clinical changes that make diagnosis of ABE a challenge in preterm infants. In a case series of preterm infants with kernicterus, only one-half displayed evidence of ABE, such as arching, seizures, posturing, abnormal muscle tone, or apnea/periodic breathing.[19] A recent study identified 3 biomarkers (activin A, S100B protein, and adrenomedullin) for brain injury in preterm infants.[33] Further characterization of these biomarkers may eventually aid in the diagnosis of ABE, although brain injury was defined broadly and was not specific to bilirubin-related injury in their study.

The clinical spectrum of BIND, in which moderate elevations of bilirubin affect narrow neural pathways, has yet to be fully characterized in term and preterm populations. There is a persuasive theoretic support, however, for increased vulnerability to BIND among preterm populations. Several studies have found a dose-response relationship between bilirubin concentration and subtle neurodevelopmental outcomes, including minor motor/gait abnormalities, learning disabilities, autism, and developmental delay, among others.[31,32,34–38] Some studies, however, found no relationship after controlling for confounding variables using logistic regression.[39] Another recent study found no increase in minor neurologic dysfunction at 18 months of age among term infants with moderate hyperbilirubinemia, but they did find a significant association among infants with bilirubin concentrations above 330 μmol/L (19.3 mg/dL).[40]

To date, there is no direct causal relationship between moderate hyperbilirubinemia and neurotoxicity, but observational literature and a recent review support the spectrum of BIND and its relationship to subtle neurologic disorders associated with abnormal bilirubin-albumin binding.[31] Future research is needed to confirm these relationships.

CLINICAL MANAGEMENT OF HYPERBILIRUBINEMIA IN THE MODERATELY PRETERM INFANT

Management of hyperbilirubinemia in moderately preterm infants varies greatly among institutions, with little evidentiary support for these differences in management.[3–5] This review outlines clinical strategies to operationalize the management of hyperbilirubinemia in moderately preterm infants to meet the recently published consensus-based recommendations.[6] Technical aspects of effective phototherapy, including irradiance and light source, as well as method and risks of exchange transfusion are not reviewed here and have been the subject of several recent reports.[3,41,42] **Fig. 1** shows the recommended guidelines for initiation of phototherapy and exchange transfusion in preterm infants by postmenstrual age, for infants less than 35 weeks' GA.

Operational total bilirubin thresholds
to manage moderately preterm infants

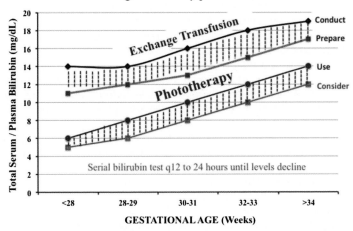

Fig. 1. Suggested use of phototherapy and exchange transfusion in preterm infants less than 35 weeks' GA. The operational thresholds have been demarcated by recommendations of an expert panel. The shaded bands represent the degree of uncertainty. Recommended thresholds to prepare for exchange transfusion assume that these infants are already being managed by effective phototherapy. Increase in exposure of BSA to phototherapy may inform the decision to conduct an exchange transfusion based on patient response to phototherapy. (*Adapted from* Maisels MJ, Watchko JF, Bhutani VK, et al. An approach to the management of hyperbilirubinemia in the preterm infant less than 35 weeks of gestation. J Perinatol 2012;32(9):660–4; with permission.)

Operational strategies
1. TB levels
   a. **Fig. 1** is based on recommendations for operational or therapeutic TB threshold levels at, or above which, treatment is likely to do more good than harm.[6] These TB levels are not based on high-quality evidence but on consensus expert opinion.
   b. Use TB measurements. Do not subtract direct-reacting or conjugated bilirubin from the TB.
   c. These TB thresholds reflect a degree of uncertainty for these recommendations. Clinicians should consider the lower range of the thresholds for infants at greater risk for bilirubin neurotoxicity, for example, (1) lower GA; (2) serum albumin levels <2.5 g/dL; (3) rapidly rising TB levels, suggesting hemolytic disease; and (4) those who are clinically unstable (if they have one or more of the following conditions): (a) blood pH <7.15; (b) blood culture positive sepsis in the prior 24 h; (c) apnea and bradycardia requiring cardiopulmonary resuscitation (bagging and or intubation) during the previous 24 h; (d) hypotension requiring intervention during the previous 24 h; and (e) respiratory support at the time of blood sampling.
   d. Use postmenstrual age; for example, when a $29^{0/7}$-wk infant is 7 days old, use the TB level for $30^{0/7}$-wk GA.
2. Bilirubin-albumin molar ratio (BAMR). Measure the serum albumin level in all infants and calculate the BAMR. Bilirubin that is unbound from albumin has been considered responsible for the neurotoxic effects of hyperbilirubinemia.[28,43] As a result, incorporation of BAMR has been advocated to better define exchange transfusion

criteria. From a clinical perspective, BAMR may be estimated by dividing TB (mg/dL) by serum albumin (g/dL). In term infants, BAMR values >0.8 are considered dangerous because bilirubin/albumin binding is unpredictable at these levels. Using data presented by Ahlfors,[44] the calculated values at which bilirubin is likely to be displaced from albumin in moderately preterm infants are provided (**Fig. 2**).

3. Effective phototherapy. The use of phototherapy, akin to pharmacotherapy, is usually prophylactic with a goal of containing the rate-of-rise of bilirubin. The most effective phototherapy is administered using blue light in the wavelength range of 430 to 490 nm. A recent technical report details further evidence and operational considerations.[41] The effectiveness of irradiance delivered may be modulated by an infant's hematocrit.[45]

   a. Measure irradiance at regular intervals with an appropriate spectroradiometer.

   b. If the TB continues to rise, additional phototherapy devices may be used to increase exposure to the body surface area (BSA).

   c. The irradiance should be increased by using a higher intensity setting on the device or by bringing the overhead light closer to the infant. Fluorescent and light-emitting diode light sources can be brought closer to an infant, but this cannot be done with halogen or tungsten lamps because of the danger of a burn.

   d. Discontinue phototherapy when TB is 1 to 2 mg/dL (17–34 μmol/L) below the initiation level for an infant's postmenstrual age.

   e. Discontinue TB measurements when TB is declining and phototherapy is no longer required.

4. Exchange transfusions

   a. These thresholds assume that infants are already receiving intensive phototherapy to the maximal BSA (approximately 80%), but whose TB levels continue to increase to these thresholds.

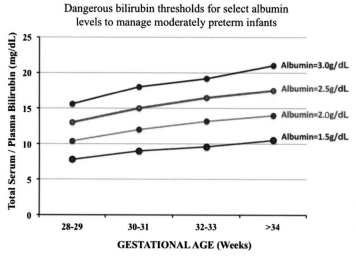

Fig. 2. Recommended use of BAMR for initiation of exchange transfusions. BAMR values have been calculated to bilirubin (mg/dL)/albumin (g/dL). Values above the thresholds for select serum albumin values of 1.5, 2, 2.5, and 3 g/dL are presented as bands above which bilirubin is likely to be displaced and may be neurotoxic. (*Data from* Ahlfors CE. Criteria for exchange transfusion in jaundiced newborns. Pediatrics 1994;93:488–94.)

b. Exchange transfusion is recommended for any infant who shows signs of ABE (hypertonia, arching, retrocollis, opisthotonos, and high-pitched cry) although these signs are often subtle.

These recommendations may assist with the establishment of a systems-based approach to operationalize the management of hyperbilirubinemia in moderately preterm infants. Clinicians also are encouraged to review their institutional policies for screening, diagnostic evaluation, frequency and duration of monitoring, TB thresholds for intervention adjusted for GA and presence of hemolysis, risk assessment for neurotoxicity, and effective, but judicious, use of phototherapy.

FUTURE DIRECTIONS

The recommendations for management of hyperbilirubinemia presented in this article are consensus based. Long-term follow-up data and randomized controlled clinical trials are required to determine if these guidelines produce the best outcomes for moderately preterm infants. Comparing these guidelines with routine care or other established guidelines, or comparing the higher versus lower ranges of TB thresholds in **Fig. 1**, will allow for evidence-based recommendations in the future. There is a delicate balance between risk of BIND and overtreatment in the setting of reducing the potential antioxidant properties of bilirubin. This balance must be the subject of future investigation before true evidence-based management of hyperbilirubinemia in moderately preterm infants can be realized. Continued assessment of best practices would be helpful to minimize overtreatment or unintended consequences of bilirubin reduction strategies.

SUMMARY

Moderately preterm infants remain at increased risk for adverse outcomes, including ABE relative to term infants. Evidence-based guidelines for management of hyperbilirubinemia in preterm infants, however, are not yet optimized. High concentrations of unconjugated bilirubin can cause permanent neurologic damage in infants, known as chronic posticteric sequelae, including kernicterus. There is growing concern that exposure to even moderate concentrations of bilirubin may lead to isolated neurodevelopmental injury or subtle, but permanent, impairment known as BIND. Clinical manifestations of ABE in preterm infants are similar to, but often more subtle than, those of term infants. Clinical strategies to operationalize the management of hyperbilirubinemia in moderately preterm infants to meet the recently published consensus-based recommendations are outlined.

ACKNOWLEDGMENTS

The authors gratefully appreciate the contributions of Ronald J. Wong, Senior Research Scientist, at Stanford University Medical Center.

REFERENCES

1. American Academy of Pediatrics Subcommittee on hyperbilirubinemia. Clinical practice guidelines: management of hyperbilitubinemia in the newborn infant 35 or more weeks of gestation. Pediatrics 2004;114:297–316.
2. Wolff M, Schinasi DA, Lavelle J, et al. Management of neonates with hyperbilirubinemia: improving timeliness of care using a clinical pathway. Pediatrics 2012; 130:e1688–94.

3. Bratlid D, Nakstad B, Hansen TW. National guidelines for treatment of jaundice in the newborn. Acta Paediatr 2011;100:499–505.
4. Rennie JM, Sehgal A, De A, et al. Range of UK practice regarding thresholds for phototherapy and exchange transfusion in neonatal hyperbilirubinaemia. Arch Dis Child Fetal Neonatal Ed 2009;94:F323–7.
5. Hansen TW. Therapuetic approaches to neonatal jaundice: an international survey. Clin Pediatr 1996;35:309–16.
6. Maisels MJ, Watchko JF, Bhutani VK, et al. An approach to the management of hyperbilirubinemia in the preterm infant less than 35 weeks of gestation. J Perinatol 2012;32:660–4.
7. Govaert P, Lequin M, Swarte R, et al. Changes in globus pallidus with (pre) term kernicterus. Pediatrics 2003;112:1256–63.
8. Moll M, Goelz R, Naegele T, et al. Are recommended phototherapy thresholds safe enough for extremely low birth weight (ELBW) infants? A report on 2 ELBW infants with kernicterus despite only moderate hyperbilirubinemia. Neonatology 2011;99:90–4.
9. Sugama S, Soeda A, Eto Y. Magnetic resonance imaging in three children with kernicterus. Pediatr Neurol 2001;25:328–31.
10. Mazeiras G, Roze JC, Ancel PY, et al. Hyperbilirubinemia and neurodevelopmental outcome of very low birth weight infants: results from the LIFT cohort. PLoS One 2012;7:1–8.
11. Oh W, Tyson JE, Fanaroff AA, et al. Association between peak serum bilirubin and neurodevelopmental outcomes in extremely low birth weight infants. Pediatrics 2003;112:773–9.
12. O'Shea TM, Dillard RG, Klinepeter KL, et al. Serum bilirubin levels, intracranial hemorrhage, and the risk of developmental problems in very low birth weight infants. Pediatrics 1992;90:888–92.
13. Yeo KL, Perlman M, Hao Y, et al. Outcomes of extremely premature infants related to their peak serum bilirubin concentrations and exposure to phototherapy. Pediatrics 1998;102:1426–31.
14. Morris BH, Oh W, Tyson JE, et al. Aggressive vs. conservative phototherapy for infants with extremely low birth weight. N Engl J Med 2008;359:1885–96.
15. Escobar GJ, McCOrmick MC, Zupancic JAF, et al. Unstudies infants: outcomes of moderately premature infants in the neonatal intensive care unit. Arch Dis Child 2006;91:F238–44.
16. Matthew T. Infant mortality statistics from 2002 period linked birth/infant death data set: National Vital Statistics Report. Hyattsville (MD): National Center for Health Statistics; 2002.
17. Kaplan M, Wong RJ, Sibley E, et al. Neonatal jaundice and liver disease. In: Martin RJ, Fanaroff AA, Walsh MC, editors. Neonatal-perinatal medicine. St Louis (MO): Elsevier Mosby; 2011. p. 1443–96.
18. Altman M, Vanpee M, Cnattingius S, et al. Neonatal morbidity in moderately preterm infants: a Swedish national population-based study. J Pediatr 2011;158:239–44.
19. Bhutani VK, Johnson LH, Shapiro SM. Kernicterus in sick and preterm infants (1999-2002): a need for an effective preventive approach. Semin Perinatol 2004;28:319–25.
20. Gartner LM, Snyder RN, Chabon RS, et al. Kernicterus: high incidence in premature infants with low serum bilirubin concentrations. Pediatrics 1970;45:906–17.
21. Cashore WJ. Bilirubin metabolism and toxicity in the newborn. In: Polin RA, Fox WW, editors. Fetal and neonatal physiology. 1st edition. Philadelphia: WB Saunders; 1992. p. 1160–4.

22. Watchko JF, Claasen D. Kernicterus in premature infants: current prevalaence and relationship to NICHD phototherapy study exchange criteria. Pediatrics 1994;93:996–9.
23. Perlstein M. Neurologic sequelae of erythroblastosis fetalis. Am J Dis Child 1950; 79:605–6.
24. Volpe JJ. Bilirubin and brain injury. In: Volpe JJ, editor. Neurology of the newborn. 4th edition. Philadelphia: Elsevier; 2001.
25. Van Praagh R. Diagnosis of kernicterus in the neonatal period. Pediatrics 1961; 28:870–4.
26. Johnson L, Brown AK, Bhutani VK. System-based approach to management of neonatal jaundice and prevention of kernicterus. J Pediatr 2002;93:488–94.
27. Mollison PL, Cutbush M. A method of measuring the severity of a series of cases of hemolytic disease of the newborn. Blood 1951;6:777–88.
28. Wennberg RP, Ahlfors CE, Bhutani V, et al. Toward understanding kernicterus: a challenge to improve the mangement of jaundiced newborns. Pediatrics 2006; 117:474–85.
29. Byers RK, Paine RS, Crothers B. Extrapyramidal cerebral palsy with hearing loss following erthroblastosis. Pediatrics 1955;15:248–54.
30. Chuniaud L, Dessante M, Chantoux F, et al. Cytotoxicity of bilirubin for human fibroblasts and rat astrocytes in culture. Effect of the ratio of bilirubin to serum albumin. Clin Chim Acta 1996;256:103–14.
31. Johnson L, Bhutani VK. The clinical syndrome of bilirubin-induced neurologic dysfunction. Semin Perinatol 2011;35:101–13.
32. Newman TB, Klebanof MA. Neonatal hyperbilirubinemia and long-term outcome: another look at the collaborative perinatal project. Pediatrics 1993;92:651–7.
33. Risso FM, Sannia A, Gavilanes DA, et al. Biomarkers of brain damage in preterm infants. J Matern Fetal Neonatal Med 2012;25:101–4.
34. Soorani-Lunsing I, Woltil HA, Hadders-Algra M. Are moderate degrees of hyperbilirubinemia in healthy term neonates really safe for the brain? Pediatr Res 2006; 117:474–85.
35. Jangaard KA, Fell DB, Dodds L, et al. Outcomes in a population of healthy term and near-term infants with serum bilirubin levels of >or= 325 micromol/L who were born in Nova Scotia, Canada, between 1994 and 2000. Pediatrics 2008;122:119–24.
36. Good WV, Hou C. Sweep visual evoked potential grating acuity thresholds paradoxically improve in low-luminance conditions in children with cortical visual impairment. Invest Ophthalmol Vis Sci 2006;47:3220–4.
37. Boggs T, Hardy J, Frazier T. Correlation of neonatal serum total bilirubin concentration and evelopmental status at age eight months. Preliminary report from the collaborative project. J Pediatr 1967;71:553–60.
38. Maimburg RD, Bech BH, Vaeth M. Neonatal jaundice, autism, and other disorders of psychological development. Pediatrics 2010;126:872–8.
39. Croen LA, Yoshida CK, Odouli R. Neonatal hyperbilitubinemia and risk of autism spectrum disorders. Pediatrics 2005;115:e135–8.
40. Lunsing RJ, Pardoen WF, Hadders-Algra M. Neurodevelopment after moderate hyperbiliruinemia at term. Pediatr Res 2013;73:655–60.
41. Bhutani VK, Committee on Fetus and Newborn. Phototherapy to prevent severe neonatal hyperbilirubinemia in the newborn infant 35 or more weeks of gestation. Pediatrics 2011;128:e1046–52.
42. National Institute for Health and Clinical Excellence. Neonatal Jaundice. National Institute for Health and Clinical Excellence. 2010. Available at: www.nice.org.uk/CG98. Accessed May 18, 2013.

43. McDonagh AF, Maisels MJ. Bilirubin unbound: déjà vu all over again? Pediatrics 2006;117:523–5.
44. Ahlfors CE. Criteria for exchange transfusion in jaundiced newborns. Pediatrics 1994;93:488–94.
45. Lamola AA, Bhutani VK, Wong RJ, et al. Effect of hematocrit on efficacy of phototherapy for neonatal jaundice. Pediatr Res 2013;74(1):54–60.

Management of Breastfeeding During and After the Maternity Hospitalization for Late Preterm Infants

Paula Meier, PhD, RN[a,b,*], Aloka L. Patel, MD[a],
Karen Wright, PhD, RN, NNP-BC[b],
Janet L. Engstrom, PhD, RN, CNM, WHNP-BC[b,c]

KEYWORDS

- Late preterm infant • Moderately preterm infant • Early term infant • Lactation
- Breastfeeding • Lactation technologies

KEY POINTS

- Human milk is especially important for infants who are born before the final maturation of body organs and systems, including moderately preterm, late preterm, and early term infants.
- Late preterm infants (LPIs) are at risk for underconsumption of milk during feedings at the breast because of immature suction pressures and sleepy behavior, and their mothers are at risk for delayed onset of lactation.
- In-hospital management strategies should focus on protecting the maternal milk volume and ensuring that the infant is fed appropriately, and may be inconsistent with the Baby Friendly Hospital Initiative's Ten Steps for Successful Breastfeeding, which were intended for healthy term infants.
- During and after the maternity hospitalization, breastfeeding management for the LPI and mother should incorporate evidence-based lactation technologies, including the breast pump, in-home test-weighing, and the nipple shield, until the infant approximates term corrected age, and can remove milk from the breast effectively.
- Many of the management strategies outlined for the LPI can be adapted to moderately preterm and early term infants.

Funding: This work was partially supported by NIH Grant Number NR0100009.
[a] Division of Neonatology, Department of Pediatrics, Rush University Medical Center, 1653 West Congress Parkway, Chicago, IL 60612, USA; [b] Department of Women, Children and Family Nursing, Rush University Medical Center, 600 South Paulina, Chicago, IL 60612, USA; [c] Department of Research, Frontier Nursing University, 195 School Street, Hyden, KY 41749, USA
* Corresponding author. Rush University Medical Center, Room 625 Jones Pavilion, 1653 West Congress Parkway, Chicago, IL 60612.
E-mail address: paula_meier@rush.edu

perinatology.theclinics.com

Human milk reduces the risk of short-term and long-term morbidities in recipient infants through a combination of nutritional, anti-infective, anti-inflammatory, antioxidative, epigenetic, and gut-colonizing substances.[1-6] These substances function synergistically to downregulate inflammatory and oxidative stress processes that manifest in lifelong health problems, including infections, atopic disease, neurocognitive and neurodevelopmental delay, and many chronic diseases.[1,7-9] Late and moderately preterm infants, and even those infants delivered early term, are born before the maturation of many body organs and systems,[10-16] and are especially protected by the bioactive components in human milk. In contrast, several lines of inquiry indicate that the components in commercial formulas may be separately detrimental in that they upregulate inflammatory and oxidative stress processes by a variety of mechanisms, including increased intestinal permeability and toxicity to immature gut epithelial cells.[17-26] Thus, while human milk is important for all infants, it is especially important for infants who are born early and have a compromised immunomodulatory response, and immature organs, including the brain, that are susceptible to inflammatory injury and oxidative stress.

Among the infants born moderately and late preterm or early term, the greatest challenge for breastfeeding management is the late preterm infant (LPI) who is cared for with the mother in the maternity setting.[27] The lack of management strategies is underscored by the fact that exclusive breastfeeding at the time of hospital discharge is a major risk factor for rehospitalization in LPIs because of dehydration, hyperbilirubinemia, and suspected sepsis.[27-31] In less severe situations, LPIs who are exclusively breastfed tend to gain weight slowly and have protracted jaundice. These and other complications can be termed lactation-associated morbidities, in that human milk does not cause the morbidity, but inadequate milk intake during breastfeeding contributes to its severity.[27] It is well documented that LPIs demonstrate ineffective breastfeeding behaviors such as sleepiness and slipping off the mother's nipple during feeding that translate into compromised milk transfer during breastfeeding.[27,32] Whether or not rehospitalization is required, common outcomes in this population include routine formula supplementation and early cessation of breastfeeding.[27,32]

Although breastfeeding for LPIs and their mothers is commonly managed according to practices designed for healthy term infants, LPIs are much more like premature infants being discharged from the neonatal intensive care unit (NICU) with respect to consuming an adequate volume of milk during feedings at the breast.[27] However, unlike mothers of NICU infants who have used a breast pump to establish their milk supply by the time of NICU discharge, mothers of LPIs must rely on the sucking stimulation of the infant to establish the milk supply. Furthermore, delayed onset of lactation is especially common among mothers of LPIs, meaning that despite an effective sucking stimulus from the breast pump or the infant, little milk is available for several days after birth.[27,33-37] As a consequence, breastfeeding failure among LPIs and their mothers is high, and clinicians need evidence-based strategies to protect infant hydration and growth, as well as the maternal milk supply, until complete feeding at the breast can be established. This article reviews the evidence for lactation and breastfeeding risks in LPIs and their mothers, and describes strategies for managing these immaturity-related feeding problems. Application to moderate preterm infants (MPIs) and early term infants (ETIs) is made throughout.

LATE PRETERM INFANTS AND MOTHERS: A POPULATION AT RISK FOR POOR LACTATION OUTCOMES

LPIs and their mothers each bring risk factors to effective breastfeeding that contribute to the high rates of lactation-associated morbidities and shortened duration of breastfeeding in this population.[27] In combination, these risk factors predispose infants to inadequate intake during feedings at the breast and predispose mothers to an inadequate milk supply. LPIs have weak suction pressures and immature sleep-wake regulation that place them at risk for underconsumption of milk during breastfeeding. Mothers of LPIs are at risk for delayed onset of lactation, such that the availability of adequate milk occurs later and less predictably than for healthy term births. These maternal and infant risk factors compromise the intricate interplay in lactation hormones and changes in mammary epithelial cells during the transition to lactogenesis II and the establishment of a full milk supply (**Fig. 1**).[38–40] An understanding of these LPI-mother lactation dynamics is essential for establishing evidence-based practices to prevent, identify, and manage these problems.

Suction Pressures and Milk Removal During Breastfeeding in Late Preterm Infants

Suction (eg, vacuum) occurs during feeding when the infant lowers the mandible, creating negative pressure in the oral cavity.[41–43] In contrast to bottle feedings, strong baseline suction pressures (mean = −64 mm Hg) are essential for breastfeeding because the infant must create the nipple shape by elongating the maternal nipple approximately 3 times its resting length so that the tip is almost at the juncture of the hard and soft palate.[42,44,45] The infant maintains this baseline suction pressure throughout the feeding, even while not actively sucking.[42,44] Furthermore, even stronger suction pressures are used to transfer the bolus of milk from the maternal breast to the infant during the suction phase.[42,44–46] By contrast, suction pressures are not really essential to the removal of milk from a standard bottle and nipple unit.[41–43,47] The bottle nipple shape is already "created" so that baseline suction pressures are not required for the infant to maintain a "latch" on the nipple, and the hydrostatic pressure associated with bottle feeding allows milk transfer with minimal or no suction on the part of the infant.[41,44,46,48] Thus, suction pressures are critical to creating the nipple shape and removing milk from the breast, but not for removing milk from a typical bottle unit.

Suction pressures mature more slowly than expression pressures in premature infants,[43,49] and explain many of the common behaviors associated with breastfeeding

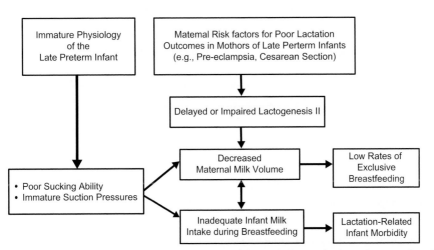

Fig. 1. The interplay of maternal and late preterm infant risk factors for lactation-associated morbidities and poor lactation outcomes. (*Courtesy of* L. Furman, MD, Cleveland, OH; and P. Meier, PhD, RN, FAAN, Chicago, IL.)

problems for MPIs, LPIs, and ETIs, such as the inability to latch onto the breast, slipping off of the breast repeatedly during a feeding, and the ability to consume milk more efficiently from a bottle than from the breast.[27] In combination with immature sleep-wake regulation,[11] these weak suction pressures predispose infants to underconsumption of milk directly from the breast until approximately term corrected age.[27] Several studies of test-weighing, in which milk intake during breastfeeding can be accurately and precisely measured,[50–54] are consistent with the fact that MPIs, LPIs, and ETIs do not consume adequate amounts of milk directly from the breast, even when the milk is available and can be removed with a breast pump.[27,51]

Lactation Risk for Mothers of Late Preterm Infants

Delayed onset of lactation (eg, delayed lactogenesis II) is a temporary problem whereby the availability of milk during the early days after birth is extremely limited.[33] During uncomplicated lactogenesis, milk synthesis is triggered by the withdrawal of progesterone with the birth of the placenta.[39] The dramatic decline in serum progesterone removes its inhibiting effect on prolactin, so that milk synthesis can begin.[39,40,55] These abrupt hormonal changes are catalyzed by a uniquely human infant sucking rate and rhythm that is applied to the breast when milk flow is limited.[46,56–62] The combination of hormonal changes and breast stimulation rapidly transition the breast from producing approximately 15 mL of colostrum during the entire first 24 hours post birth to 500 to 600 mL of milk by days 4 to 7 post birth.[56,63–65]

These early days are conceptualized as a critical period for the mammary gland, which must receive timely and appropriate stimulation from the infant, and during which time the number of secretory cells and the density of prolactin receptors in the mammary epithelial cells increase.[39,40,56,66,67] Central to this transition is the closure of tight junctions in the mammary epithelium, an anatomic change that keeps lactose within the mammary gland rather than allowing it to pass into the maternal serum via open paracellular pathways.[39,40] The osmotic properties of lactose remaining in the mammary gland result in copious milk output.[66,67] The transition from lactogenesis I to lactogenesis II normally occurs between 40 and 72 hours after birth, but in delayed onset of lactation a longer duration of very little available milk is typical.[33,34,37,39,40,68,69] Risk factors for delayed onset of lactogenesis II are listed in **Box 1**.

Delayed onset of lactation is prevalent worldwide, and mothers who deliver LPIs often have 1 or more of the risk factors for delayed onset of lactation.[33,34,37,39,40,68,69]

Box 1
Major maternal risk factors for delayed onset of lactation

- High body mass index
- Diabetes
- Pregnancy-induced hypertension
- Preterm labor
- Prolonged bed rest
- Cesarean delivery
- Intrapartum complications, including excessive blood loss
- Medications, including magnesium sulfate and other antepartum/intrapartum medications, and selective serotonin reuptake inhibitors

These risk factors frequently go unnoticed, especially when infants are considered "healthy" and cared for in the maternity area with their mothers. However, despite little milk being available, the effective sucking stimulus of the infant (or a breast pump substitute) is necessary to catalyze the hormonal, structural, and biochemical processes in the breast.[56] Many LPIs and some ETIs are incapable of providing the stimulation and milk removal necessary to correct delayed onset of lactation, and what should be a temporary problem segues into a permanent low milk volume that is difficult to correct once the early critical period for mammary stimulation has passed.[27]

LATE PRETERM INFANTS CARED FOR IN THE MATERNITY SETTING SHOULD NOT BE CONSIDERED HEALTHY TERM INFANTS

Most LPIs are cared for in the maternity area with their mothers, where lactation care is guided by polices consistent with the Joint Commission Core Perinatal Measure on exclusive breastfeeding and/or the Baby Friendly Hospital Initiative (BFHI).[70-72] Both of these sets of guidelines are intended to establish effective breastfeeding practices in the hospital setting for healthy term infants and their mothers.[73,74] However, it is often assumed that these guidelines should be generalized to include LPIs as well, especially with respect to the avoidance of formula or donor milk supplements. Whereas routine supplementation of breastfeeding is inappropriate for LPIs, the clinician must be alert to the possibility that supplements may be medically necessary to prevent or treat hypoglycemia, hypothermia, hyperbilirubinemia, or other morbidities. Similarly, LPIs and their mothers often need to use temporary lactation aids such as breast pumps, nipple shields, and bottle units, which are unnecessary for healthy term infants and mothers, and are inconsistent with select steps in the BFHI.[27]

Initiatives that focus on exclusive breastfeeding in the immediate postbirth period have been crafted from a substantial body of evidence about the interplay between infant intake and mammary physiology during this critical period. An understanding of this mother-infant synchrony is necessary to understand the inappropriateness of these guidelines for LPIs. Healthy term infants are born with adequate fat and glycogen stores so that they do not need more milk than the approximately 15 mL they consume during the entire first 24 hours of life.[63,75] Furthermore, during this time they breastfeed 10 to 11 times on average, transferring only about 1.5 mL of milk each feeding.[63] This frequent, unrestricted feeding in the first 24 hours means the breast is stimulated by the infant so that additional milk is available in the next 24 hours as the infants need additional fluid and calories.[76] This mother-infant synchrony is imbalanced following LPI birth, in that fat and glycogen stores are added exponentially between 34 weeks and term gestation.[12] This immaturity means that the LPI is at risk not only for metabolic complications as a function of preterm birth but also because of minimal milk availability in the first 24 to 48 hours of breastfeeding.[27] Thus, the "supply and demand" explanation that underpins these BFHI and Joint Commission breastfeeding initiatives is inconsistent with the evidence about LPIs and their mothers.

Similarly, strategies used by clinicians to encourage frequent breastfeeding in healthy term infants are often ineffective and can exacerbate morbidities in LPIs. For example, the most consistently reported characteristic of LPIs is sleepy behavior that compromises the frequency and duration of breastfeedings.[27,32] In healthy term infants who demonstrate sleepy behavior, mothers are encouraged to wake infants frequently and to remove the infant's clothing and blankets because the infant has become "too comfortable." Although skin-to-skin care, whereby the unclothed infant is held in immediate contact with the mother's breasts, is appropriate for LPIs, removing clothing to stimulate wakefulness exacerbates the risk of metabolic morbidities. Similarly, frequent waking not only is ineffective but can also compromise the infant's energy stores and growth.

New parents also frequently have unrealistic expectations for their LPIs. There are few resources specifically about breastfeeding LPIs for parents, so they rely on written materials for uncomplicated breastfeeding situations along with the advice of friends and family members that is not specific to LPIs. These mothers fail to recognize excessive sleepiness and short, ineffective breastfeeds in their infants as a sign of immaturity and inadequate intake, and interpret these behaviors to mean that the infants are satiated and sleep well. These parents need information about breastfeeding that is specific to LPIs and includes clear guidelines about adapting basic lactation principles to the needs of their immature infants. One evidence-based booklet available for new parents, *Breastfeeding Your Late Preterm Infant*, details reasons why their LPIs do not breastfeed in the same way as healthy term infants, as well as specific plans to protect the maternal milk supply and ensure adequate intake for infants.[77] This booklet also includes 3 real-life case studies of LPIs, which help parents understand that the immaturity-related feeding issues they observe in their own LPIs are common in this population.

MANAGEMENT OF BREASTFEEDING FOR LATE PRETERM INFANTS AND MOTHERS

There are 2 key objectives in managing breastfeeding for this population: protecting the maternal milk supply and ensuring that the infant is adequately nourished. In healthy term populations, unrestricted and effective feedings at the breast accomplish both objectives. For LPIs, separate strategies for each objective are needed until the infant is able to consume all feedings directly from the breast without the additional stimulation provided by the breast pump.[27] Although there is considerable variability as to when LPIs actually accomplish this outcome, parents can be told that it occurs at approximately the infant's expected birth date. Until this time, the use of evidence-based lactation technologies, such as breast pumps, specialized breast-pump suction patterns, nipple shields, and in-home test-weights and bottle units help the clinician individualize a safe and effective breastfeeding plan with families of LPIs.[27]

The Maternity Hospital Stay

In general, the infant should be able to feed effectively (eg, awake and feeding eagerly) for at least 15 minutes, each of 8 times daily during the maternity stay. Most LPIs and many ETIs are unable to maintain this regimen consistently. If the LPI cannot provide this stimulation to the mammary gland, the mother should use a hospital-grade electric breast pump. The pump will provide necessary breast stimulation during this critical period for lactogenesis II, and remove available milk that can be fed to the infant. One randomized clinical trial reported that the use of a breast-pump suction pattern that mimics the uniquely human infant suck during this critical period resulted in mothers' producing significantly more milk in less time spent pumping by day 14 post birth in breast-pump–dependent mothers with premature ($\leq$34 weeks of gestation) infants.[56] Thus, when possible, mothers should be encouraged to use this suction pattern in the breast pump until the onset of lactogenesis II, changing to a maintenance suction pattern in the pump thereafter.

Often mothers are instructed to try to breastfeed their infants before each pumping, and become exhausted and discouraged with the extra effort involved. A more effective approach helps the mother understand that her LPI's sleepy behavior is normal, and encourages her to breastfeed when the infant is awake, and pump when the infant is unable to awaken and feed eagerly. She can substitute the breastfeeding for skin-to-skin care with her infant before or after the pumping session.[32] Many LPIs will require additional milk during the maternity hospitalization because of concerns about hypoglycemia, hypothermia, and hyperbilirubinemia.[12] If the mother is able to remove milk with the breast pump, it can be fed to the infant. If no mother's milk is available, donor milk or formula must be supplemented. In general, the smallest volume of supplement that will prevent or treat morbidity in the LPI is indicated. In animal and human studies, large amounts of milk administered rapidly in the early days after birth results in a different pattern of feeding-induced hormone release, which may have longer-term implications and should be avoided if possible.[78]

Preparing for Hospital Discharge

The clinician should work with the family to develop a strategy that permits as much direct feeding at breast as possible, while still ensuring that the maternal milk supply is protected and that the infant receives sufficient hydration and nutrition. Often a strategy called "triple feeding" is recommended, which involves attempting to feed the infant at breast followed by use of a breast pump and feeding any expressed milk (or formula supplement) to the infant by bottle.[32] New families are often sent home with these generic instructions, and the resulting fatigue contributes to the high rates of breastfeeding failure in this population. **Box 2** summarizes an alternative plan that protects the maternal milk supply with routine use of a breast pump, and ensures the infant receives sufficient milk by substituting some breastfeedings with bottle feedings of the freshly pumped milk. The use of select lactation technologies can help make this plan even more individualized for the family of the LPI. These interventions are also suitable for MPIs and ETIs as hospital discharge approaches.

Lactation Technologies Suitable for Mothers and LPIs

Several evidence-based lactation technologies can help mothers transition from a mixture of bottle and breastfeedings to exclusive breastfeeding during the first weeks after hospital discharge. A brief review of each device and a description of the ways in which it protects maternal milk volume or ensures adequate infant intake are summarized here.

Protecting milk volume

Without an adequate milk supply, the mother cannot breastfeed exclusively. This fact must guide the clinician's recommendations for securing an effective hospital-grade electric breast pump, and for using it until the infant is gaining weight consistently on exclusive feedings at the breast without the assistance of a nipple shield or bottle supplements (unless these are a choice of the mother). Although new mothers will want to discontinue routine breast-pump use as soon as possible, they must be reminded that the pump is doing the work of maintaining the milk supply because their LPIs are incapable of doing so. Initially most LPIs will require some bottle supplements of expressed milk in addition to the amount they consume at the breast, because they are unable to remove all of the available milk from the breast.[50,51] As the infants mature, they progressively consume more milk at the breast and require less supplemented volume. Regular (2–4 times daily) breast-pump use is critical to this transition because the pump serves as the entity that "creates and maintains" the extra milk, which flows more readily to the infant despite immature sucking patterns.[50,51] Thus, the LPI "gets enough" milk partly because the pump is providing extra stimulation to the mother's breasts. Even when the LPI has made the transition to exclusive feedings at the breast and is growing appropriately, the pump must be discontinued

---

Box 2
Alternative to triple feeding as breastfeeding is advanced

- Separate the day into stretches of time for feedings at the breast and stretches of time for feedings pumped milk by bottle:

  1. Select daytime hours when the mother and infant are rested for breastfeeding and nighttime hours for pumping and feeding milk by bottle

  2. Pump both breasts thoroughly 4 to 5 times daily during the first week at home

  3. If the infant consumes at least half of the feeding volume at breast, he or she can receive fewer (eg, 4 or fewer) bottle feedings of pumped milk

  4. If the infant consumes less than one-fourth of the feeding volume at breast, as many as 6 bottle feedings of pumped milk may be indicated

- During breastfeeding stretches:

  1. Start the breastfeeding as soon as the infant shows wakeful signs. Do not wait for crying. Do not change clothing or the diaper with the intent of making the baby "more awake"

  2. Use the cross-cradle or football hold to provide head and neck support

  3. Use the nipple shield and test-weights as indicated

  4. If the baby falls asleep early in the feeding, change the diaper and clothing to see if the activity increases wakefulness

  5. Do not routinely offer a bottle after each breastfeeding

  6. Do not routinely pump after each breastfeeding

  7. Feed the baby immediately when he or she awakens again (eg, "on cue")

  8. Pump and offer a bottle every 4 to 6 hours, depending on infant's intake (eg, more intake = longer stretch without pumped milk)

- During bottle feeding stretches:

  1. When the infant awakens, the mother can use the breast pump to completely remove available milk while the father or other designated helper changes the infant's clothing (eg, ensuring breast emptying)

  2. The helper can feed the pumped milk by bottle, allowing the infant to consume as much as he or she is able (eg, ensuring adequate intake)

  3. Everyone returns to sleep quickly

  4. Repeat this pattern throughout the nighttime hours, reducing the frequency (and substituting feedings at breast) as the infant matures

Adapted from Meier PP. Breastfeeding your late preterm infant. McHenry (IL): Medela, Inc; 2010; with permission.

---

slowly, and only after the LPI no longer needs the assistance of the nipple shield to transfer sufficient amounts of milk.

The data in **Fig. 2** exemplify this progression, and can be used by the clinician to reinforce the importance of continued breast-pump use with family members for both LPIs and MPIs. These findings are a secondary analysis of one group of mothers and their premature infants from a randomized clinical trial of in-home measurement of milk intake following NICU discharge.[50,51] In this study, 24 mothers of premature infants (mean postconceptional age [PCA] 36 ± 2 weeks and weight at NICU discharge 2248 ± 97 g) measured milk intake during breastfeeding in the home for 1 month after NICU discharge.[51] All of the mothers had an adequate milk supply, and all extra milk

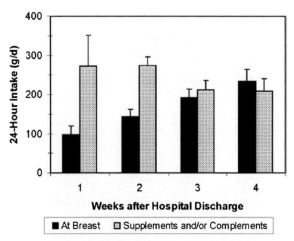

Fig. 2. Volume of milk consumed at the breast and as extra milk (supplements and complements of pumped mothers' milk) during the first 4 weeks at home in premature infants discharged from the neonatal intensive care unit. (*Courtesy of* N. Hurst, PhD, Houston, TX; P. Meier, PhD, Chicago, IL; and J. Engstrom, PhD, Chicago, IL.)

consumed by the infants was pumped milk. Although the infants had access to a sufficient amount of milk in the breast, they could not ingest all of the available milk during breastfeedings, and required bottle supplementation of expressed milk until approximately 42 weeks PCA. Breastfeeding progression continued and maternal milk supply was protected because of the mothers' routine use of the breast pump. Thus, it is critical that the mother does not discontinue the extra pumpings too soon.

Facilitating milk intake during breastfeeding
LPIs frequently do not consume an adequate volume of milk during breastfeeding because of weak suction pressures, evidenced by slipping off of the nipple and falling asleep early in the feeding. Breastfeeding positions that support the head and neck (**Fig. 3**) can be used to facilitate milk intake, but many LPIs will benefit from temporary use of an ultrathin nipple shield (**Fig. 4**).[79,80] The nipple shield creates the nipple shape so that suction pressure is not necessary. Similarly, once the infant is properly placed on the breast with the shield, strong negative pressure within the tunnel of the shield facilitates milk transfer to the infant, provided that the maternal milk supply is adequate. A study in premature infants of PCAs similar to those of LPIs revealed that infants consume significantly more milk with the shield than without it, and that the shield was necessary until approximately the infant's expected birth date.[79]

Ensuring adequate milk intake during breastfeeding
A major safety concern during the early weeks after birth for breastfeeding LPIs is whether they consume an adequate amount of milk at breast to remain hydrated and grow.[28–31] For this reason, many families are advised to routinely supplement feedings at breast with formula or pumped milk, a practice that is time-consuming and inexact. By contrast, in-home measurement of milk intake is easy, accurate, and effective for this population, and helps families achieve their breastfeeding goals, with more confidence that their LPIs are consuming an adequate volume of milk.[50,51] Also referred to as test-weighing, whereby the clothed infant is weighed on an accurate and reliable electronic scale, this technology takes the guesswork out of "getting

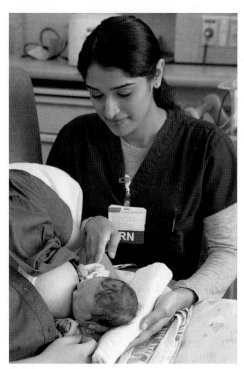

Fig. 3. Use of breastfeeding positions that support the head and neck of the LPI (and MPI and ETI) facilitate milk intake during breastfeeding. (*Source:* Copyright © 2010 Medela, Inc.)

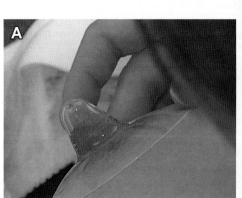
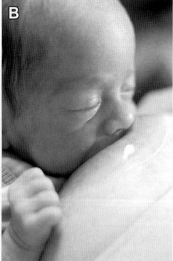

Fig. 4. Use of a nipple shield creates the nipple shape for the infant and helps compensate for weak, immature suction pressures that develop with increasing maturity. (*A*) Close-up of shield. (*B*) Close-up of infant positioned on shield. (*Source:* Copyright © 2005 Medela, Inc.)

enough," providing extra milk only when it is necessary.[51–54,81] Several studies have shown that commonly used clinical indicators of breastfeeding effectiveness, such as audible swallows, visualizing milk in the infant's mouth, and postfeed satiety, are not accurate indicators of intake in premature and LPIs. By contrast, the in-home rental scale to measure milk intake during breastfeeding (BabyWeigh; Medela, Inc, McHenry, IL) weighs to the nearest 2 g, is portable and easy to use, and has been studied extensively.[50–53] Measuring milk intake in the home helps parents learn to recognize a "good" feeding with respect to milk intake, helps them determine when to provide extra milk, and highlights the LPI's progress in consuming more milk at breast each week during the early postbirth period.[50,51]

Discontinuing Lactation Technologies for Mothers and LPIs

Because there is so little evidence-based information available for parents with respect to breastfeeding their LPIs, they are often told to discontinue all of the technologies and feed their infants as if they were healthy term infants before the LPIs are ready to make this transition.[77] Although the final cessation of lactation technologies will occur between approximately 40 and 42 weeks PCA, most LPIs will demonstrate inconsistency in staying awake and feeding eagerly before this time.[50,51] For example, the LPI may be able to consume some daily feedings without the nipple shield, but require it for others. Other LPIs demonstrate eager feeding and adequate milk transfer for the first 5 minutes of a feeding without the nipple shield, then fall asleep without completing the feeding. The nipple shield can be introduced midway through the feeding to help the infant take a full feeding.

The pump should be gradually discontinued after the nipple shield is no longer needed and the infant is gaining weight adequately on exclusive feedings at breast. For example, if a mother is currently pumping 3 times daily at this time, she should decrease the frequency of pumping, with a goal of discontinuing pumping over a 10-day period. This slow cessation of extra pumping is important because the LPI may be consuming sufficient milk during breastfeeding because the pump has created the extra milk volume that flows readily and easily to the infant.[50,51] In-home measurement of milk intake validates that the infant is transitioning from "milk remover" to "milk maintainer" as pumping is discontinued.

Most families who use lactation technologies to guide the transition to exclusive feedings at breast relinquish the in-home rental scale after breastfeeding is effective and efficient, and the pump is no longer needed to maintain an adequate maternal milk supply.[50,51] Along this trajectory, the families cease the measurement of milk transfer, and simply measure daily nude weights for a week or two to reassure themselves that milk intake is adequate for infant growth.

Adequacy of Exclusive Human Milk for MPIs, LPIs, and ETIs

Although there is some evidence that providing a nutrient-enriched formula supplement of human milk is beneficial for short-term growth in very low birth weight (VLBW) and/or extremely premature infants, there are few data about the safety and efficacy of this practice with more mature preterm infants.[1,82–84] In the absence of evidence-based guidelines, many clinicians elect to supplement human milk feedings with powdered formulas or to replace some daily breastfeedings with enriched formula "to be on the safe side." However, there is compelling evidence about the detrimental impact of bovine-based formulas in the early postbirth period with respect to the developing gut microbiota, the upregulation of inflammatory processes, and interference with the bioactive components in human milk.[17–26] These practices shorten the lifetime dose of human milk for the recipient infant, increasing the risk of later-childhood and adult-onset morbidities such as obesity, hypertension, diabetes, inflammatory bowel disease, and atopic illness.[7,8] With this evidence, supplementation of exclusive human milk feedings, whether at the breast or bottle, should not be routine, but based instead on the individual infant's nutritional risk factors and growth rates.[85] All MPIs and LPIs should receive multivitamins with iron. Unless there is a specific indication, ETIs should not be supplemented with iron owing to its interference with lactoferrin, which is a potent anti-inflammatory and anti-infective component of human milk.[6,86–89] All MPIs, LPIs, and ETIs who are feeding at the breast should be seen by the pediatrician within 2 days after hospital discharge, and should be monitored frequently by the primary health care provider until acceptable growth patterns on exclusive breastfeeding are well established.[90]

Key to the decision about replacing or enriching human milk with powdered formulas is knowledge of the infant's intake of human milk.[85] Only a handful of recent studies about postdischarge nutrition with VLBW infants has actually measured milk intake during breastfeeding using test-weighing techniques.[1,51,82–84] Thus, if infants fail to grow properly it is assumed that the quality rather than the quantity of the milk is inadequate.[51–53] In-home test-weighing procedures using scales designed for the rental market (eg, BabyWeigh) measure milk intake to the nearest 2 mL, are accurate, and are easily performed in the home by caregivers.[51–54,81,82]

SUMMARY

Human milk is especially important for infants who are born before the final maturation of body organs and systems, including MPIs, LPIs, and ETIs. However, management of lactation and breastfeeding for these populations has not been evidence based, as reflected in the high rates of breastfeeding failure and lactation-associated morbidities, especially for LPIs who are cared for in the maternity setting with their mothers. LPIs are at risk for underconsumption of milk during feedings at the breast because of immature suction pressures and sleepy behavior, and their mothers are at risk for delayed onset of lactation. In-hospital management strategies should focus on protecting the maternal milk volume and ensuring that the infant is fed appropriately, and may be inconsistent with the BFHI's Ten Steps for Successful Breastfeeding, which were intended for healthy term infants. During and after the maternity hospitalization, breastfeeding management for the LPI and mother should incorporate evidence-based lactation technologies, including the breast pump, in-home test-weighing, and the nipple shield, until the infant approximates term corrected age and can remove milk from the breast effectively. Many of the management strategies outlined for the LPI can be adapted to the MPI and ETI.

REFERENCES

1. Meier PP, Engstrom JL, Patel AL, et al. Improving the use of human milk during and after the NICU stay. Clin Perinatol 2010;37(1):217–45.
2. Jeurink PV, van Bergenhenegouwen J, Jimenez E, et al. Human milk: a source of more life than we imagine. Benef Microbes 2013;4(1):17–30.
3. Riskin A. Changes in immunomodulatory constituents of human milk in response to active infection in the nursing infant. Pediatr Res 2012;71(2):220–5.
4. Newburg DS, Walker WA. Protection of the neonate by the innate immune system of developing gut and of human milk. Pediatr Res 2007;61(1):2–8.
5. Lucas A. Long-term programming effects of early nutrition—implications for the preterm infant. J Perinatol 2005;25(Suppl 2):S2–6.

6. Lonnerdal B. Bioactive proteins in human milk: mechanisms of action. J Pediatr 2010;156(Suppl 2):S26–30.

7. Chen A, Rogan WJ. Breastfeeding and the risk of postneonatal death in the United States. Pediatrics 2004;113(5):e435–9.

8. Ip S, Chung M, Raman G, et al. Breastfeeding and maternal and infant health outcomes in developed countries (Prepared by Tufts-New England Medical Center Evidence-based Practice Center, under Contract No. 290-02-0022). AHRQ Publication No. 07-E007. Evid Rep Technol Assess (Full Rep) 2007;(153):1–186.

9. Bartick M, Reinhold A. The burden of suboptimal breastfeeding in the United States: a pediatric cost analysis. Pediatrics 2010;125(5):e1048–56.

10. Billiards SS, Pierson CR, Haynes RL, et al. Is the late preterm infant more vulnerable to gray matter injury than the term infant? Clin Perinatol 2006;33(4):915–33.

11. Darnall RA, Ariagno RL, Kinney HC. The late preterm infant and the control of breathing, sleep, and brainstem development: a review. Clin Perinatol 2006;33(4):883–914.

12. Raju TN. Developmental physiology of late and moderate prematurity. Semin Fetal Neonatal Med 2012;17(3):126–31.

13. Raju TN. Late-preterm births: challenges and opportunities. Pediatrics 2008;121(2):402–3.

14. Watchko JF. Hyperbilirubinemia and bilirubin toxicity in the late preterm infant. Clin Perinatol 2006;33(4):839–52.

15. Amaizu N, Shulman R, Schanler R, et al. Maturation of oral feeding skills in preterm infants. Acta Paediatr 2008;97(1):61–7.

16. Abe K, Shapiro-Mendoza CK, Hall LR, et al. Late preterm birth and risk of developing asthma. J Pediatr 2010;157(1):74–8.

17. Taylor SN, Basile LA, Ebeling M, et al. Intestinal permeability in preterm infants by feeding type: mother's milk versus formula. Breastfeed Med 2009;4(1):11–5.

18. Claud EC, Walker WA. Hypothesis: inappropriate colonization of the premature intestine can cause neonatal necrotizing enterocolitis. FASEB J 2001;15(8):1398–403.

19. Walker WA. Development of the intestinal mucosal barrier. J Pediatr Gastroenterol Nutr 2002;34(Suppl 1):S33–9.

20. Penn AH. Digested formula but not digested fresh human milk causes death of intestinal cells in vitro: implications for necrotizing enterocolitis. Pediatr Res 2012;72(6):560–7.

21. Sangild PT. Gut responses to enteral nutrition in preterm infants and animals. Exp Biol Med 2006;231(11):1695–711.

22. Sangild PT, Siggers RH, Schmidt M, et al. Diet- and colonization-dependent intestinal dysfunction predisposes to necrotizing enterocolitis in preterm pigs. Gastroenterology 2006;130(6):1776–92.

23. Thymann T, Burrin DG, Tappenden KA, et al. Formula-feeding reduces lactose digestive capacity in neonatal pigs. Br J Nutr 2006;95(6):1075–81.

24. Jensen AR, Elnif J, Burrin DG, et al. Development of intestinal immunoglobulin absorption and enzyme activities in neonatal pigs is diet dependent. J Nutr 2001;131(12):3259–65.

25. van Haver ER, Oste M, Thymann T, et al. Enteral feeding reduces endothelial nitric oxide synthase in the caudal intestinal microvasculature of preterm piglets. Pediatr Res 2008;63(2):137–42.

26. Bjornvad CR, Schmidt M, Petersen YM, et al. Preterm birth makes the immature intestine sensitive to feeding-induced intestinal atrophy. Am J Physiol Regul Integr Comp Physiol 2005;289(4):R1212–22.

27. Meier PP, Furman LM, Degenhardt M. Increased lactation risk for late preterm infants and mothers: evidence and management strategies to protect breast-feeding. J Midwifery Womens Health 2007;52(6):579–87.

28. Tomashek KM, Shapiro-Mendoza CK, Weiss J, et al. Early discharge among late preterm and term newborns and risk of neonatal morbidity. Semin Perinatol 2006;30(2):61–8.

29. Shapiro-Mendoza CK, Tomashek KM, Kotelchuck M, et al. Risk factors for neonatal morbidity and mortality among "healthy," late preterm newborns. Semin Perinatol 2006;30(2):54–60.

30. Shapiro-Mendoza CK, Tomashek KM, Kotelchuck M, et al. Effect of late-preterm birth and maternal medical conditions on newborn morbidity risk. Pediatrics 2008;121(2):e223–32.

31. Young PC, Korgenski K, Buchi KF. Early readmission of newborns in a large health care system. Pediatrics 2013;131(5):e1538–44.

32. Walker M. Breastfeeding the late preterm infant. J Obstet Gynecol Neonatal Nurs 2008;37(6):692–701.

33. Hurst NM. Recognizing and treating delayed or failed lactogenesis II. J Midwifery Womens Health 2007;52(6):588–94.

34. Dewey KG, Nommsen-Rivers LA, Heinig MJ, et al. Risk factors for suboptimal infant breastfeeding behavior, delayed onset of lactation, and excess neonatal weight loss. Pediatrics 2003;112:607–19.

35. Nommsen-Rivers LA, Dolan LM, Huang B. Timing of stage II lactogenesis is pre-dicted by antenatal metabolic health in a cohort of primiparas. Breastfeed Med 2012;7(1):43–9.

36. Marshall AM, Nommsen-Rivers LA, Hernandez LL, et al. Serotonin transport and metabolism in the mammary gland modulates secretory activation and involu-tion. J Clin Endocrinol Metab 2010;95(2):837–46.

37. Nommsen-Rivers LA, Chantry CJ, Peerson JM, et al. Delayed onset of lactogen-esis among first-time mothers is related to maternal obesity and factors associ-ated with ineffective breastfeeding. Am J Clin Nutr 2010;92(3):574–84.

38. Neville MC. Anatomy and physiology of lactation. Pediatr Clin North Am 2001; 48(1):13–34.

39. Neville MC, Morton J. Physiology and endocrine changes underlying human lac-togenesis II. J Nutr 2001;131(11):3005S–8S.

40. Neville MC, Morton J, Umemura S. Lactogenesis. The transition from pregnancy to lactation. Pediatr Clin North Am 2001;48(1):35–52.

41. Mathew OP. Science of bottle feeding. J Pediatr 1991;119(4):511–9.

42. Geddes DT, Kent JC, Mitoulas LR, et al. Tongue movement and intra-oral vac-uum in breastfeeding infants. Early Hum Dev 2008;84(7):471–7.

43. Lau C, Alagugurusamy R, Schanler RJ, et al. Characterization of the develop-mental stages of sucking in preterm infants during bottle feeding. Acta Paediatr 2000;89(7):846–52.

44. Geddes DT, Sakalidis VS, Hepworth AR, et al. Tongue movement and intra-oral vacuum of term infants during breastfeeding and feeding from an exper-imental teat that released milk under vacuum only. Early Hum Dev 2012;88(6): 443–9.

45. Smith WL, Erenberg A, Nowak A. Imaging evaluation of the human nipple during breast-feeding. Am J Dis Child 1988;142(1):76–8.

46. Mizuno K, Ueda A. Changes in sucking performance from nonnutritive sucking to nutritive sucking during breast- and bottle-feeding. Pediatr Res 2006;59(5): 728–31.

47. Colley JR, Creamer B. Sucking and swallowing in infants. Br Med J 1958; 2(5093):422–3.
48. Mizuno K, Ueda A. The maturation and coordination of sucking, swallowing, and respiration in preterm infants. J Pediatr 2003;142(1):36–40.
49. Lau C. The development of oral feeding skills in infants. Int J Pediatr 2012;2012: 572341–4.
50. Meier PP, Engstrom JL. Test weighing for term and premature infants is an accurate procedure. Arch Dis Child Fetal Neonatal Ed 2007;92(2):F155–6.
51. Hurst NM, Meier PP, Engstrom JL, et al. Mothers performing in-home measurement of milk intake during breastfeeding of their preterm infants: maternal reactions and feeding outcomes. J Hum Lact 2004;20(2):178–87.
52. Meier PP, Engstrom JL, Fleming BA, et al. Estimating milk intake of hospitalized preterm infants who breastfeed. J Hum Lact 1996;12(1):21–6.
53. Meier PP, Engstrom JL, Crichton CL, et al. A new scale for in-home test-weighing for mothers of preterm and high risk infants. J Hum Lact 1994;10(3):163–8.
54. Meier PP, Lysakowski TY, Engstrom JL, et al. The accuracy of test weighing for preterm infants. J Pediatr Gastroenterol Nutr 1990;10(1):62–5.
55. McManaman JL, Neville MC. Mammary physiology and milk secretion. Adv Drug Deliv Rev 2003;55(5):629–41.
56. Meier PP, Engstrom JL, Janes JE, et al. Breast pump suction patterns that mimic the human infant during breastfeeding: greater milk output in less time spent pumping for breast pump-dependent mothers with premature infants. J Perinatol 2012;32(2):103–10.
57. Bowen-Jones A, Thompson C, Drewett RF. Milk flow and sucking rates during breast-feeding. Dev Med Child Neurol 1982;24(6):626–33.
58. Mathew OP, Bhatia J. Sucking and breathing patterns during breast- and bottle-feeding in term neonates. Effects of nutrient delivery and composition. Am J Dis Child 1989;143(5):588–92.
59. Wolff PH. Sucking patterns of infant mammals. Brain Behav Evol 1968;1:354–67.
60. Wolff PH. The serial organization of sucking in the young infant. Pediatrics 1968; 42(6):943–56.
61. Drewett RF, Woolridge M. Sucking patterns of human babies on the breast. Early Hum Dev 1979;3(4):315–21.
62. Sakalidis VS, Williams TM, Garbin CP, et al. Ultrasound imaging of infant sucking dynamics during the establishment of lactation. J Hum Lact 2013;29(2): 205–13.
63. Santoro W Jr, Martinez FE, Ricco RG, et al. Colostrum ingested during the first day of life by exclusively breastfed healthy newborn infants. J Pediatr 2010; 156(1):29–32.
64. Hill PD, Aldag JC, Chatterton RT, et al. Comparison of milk output between mothers of preterm and term infants: the first 6 weeks after birth. J Hum Lact 2005;21(1):22–30.
65. Hill PD, Aldag JC. Milk volume on day 4 and income predictive of lactation adequacy at 6 weeks of mothers of nonnursing preterm infants. J Perinat Neonatal Nurs 2005;19(3):273–82.
66. Wall EH, Crawford HM, Ellis SE, et al. Mammary response to exogenous prolactin or frequent milking during early lactation in dairy cows. J Dairy Sci 2006; 89(12):4640–8.
67. Hale SA, Capuco AV, Erdman RA. Milk yield and mammary growth effects due to increased milking frequency during early lactation. J Dairy Sci 2003;86(6): 2061–71.

68. Dewey KG, Nommsen-Rivers LA, Heinig MJ, et al. Lactogenesis and infant weight change in the first weeks of life. Adv Exp Med Biol 2002;503:159–66.
69. Chen DC, Nommsen-Rivers L, Dewey KG, et al. Stress during labor and delivery and early lactation performance. Am J Clin Nutr 1998;68(2):335–44.
70. The Joint Commission. Specifications manual for joint commission national quality measures (v2013A1) 2012. 2013 (May 30). Available at: http://manual.jointcommission.org/releases/TJC2013A/rsrc/Manual/TableOfContentsTJC/PC_v2013A1.pdf.
71. Baby-Friendly USA I. The ten steps to successful breastfeeding. 2012. 2013 (May 28). Available at: http://www.babyfriendlyusa.org/about-us/baby-friendly-hospital-initiative/the-ten-steps.
72. World Health Organization, UNICEF. Baby friendly hospital initiative. 2004. 2007 (June 15). Available at: http://www.unicef.org/programme/breastfeeding/baby.htm.
73. Centers for Disease Control and Prevention (CDC). Breastfeeding-related maternity practices at hospitals and birth centers in the United States, 2007. Morb Mortal Wkly Rep 2008;57:621–5.
74. Philipp BL, Merewood A. The baby-friendly way: the best breastfeeding start. Pediatr Clin North Am 2004;51:761–83.
75. American Academy of Pediatrics. Breastfeeding and the use of human milk. Pediatrics 2012;129(3):e827–41.
76. Neville M, Keller R, Seacat J, et al. Studies in human lactation: milk volumes in lactating women during the onset of lactation and full lactation. Am J Clin Nutr 1988;48:1375–86.
77. Meier PP. Breastfeeding your late preterm infant. McHenry (IL): Medela, Inc; 2010.
78. Lucas A, Sarson DL, Blackburn AM, et al. Breast vs bottle: endocrine responses are different with formula feeding. Lancet 1980;1(8181):1267–9.
79. Meier PP, Brown LP, Hurst NM, et al. Nipple shields for preterm infants: effect on milk transfer and duration of breastfeeding. J Hum Lact 2000;16(2):106–14.
80. Chertok IR, Schneider J, Blackburn S. A pilot study of maternal and term infant outcomes associated with ultrathin nipple shield use. J Obstet Gynecol Neonatal Nurs 2006;35(2):265–72.
81. Woolridge MW, Butte N, Dewey KG, et al. Methods for the measurement of milk volume intake of the breastfed infant. In: Jensen RG, Neville MC, editors. Human lactation: Milk components and methodologies. New York: Plenum Press; 1985. p. 5–20.
82. O'Connor DL, Khan S, Weishuhn K, et al. Growth and nutrient intakes of human milk-fed preterm infants provided with extra energy and nutrients after hospital discharge. Pediatrics 2008;121(4):766–76.
83. O'Connor DL, Jacobs J, Hall R, et al. Growth and development of premature infants fed predominantly human milk, predominantly premature infant formula, or a combination of human milk and premature formula. J Pediatr Gastroenterol Nutr 2003;37(4):437–46.
84. ESPGHAN Committee on Nutrition, Aggett PJ, Agostoni C, et al. Feeding preterm infants after hospital discharge: a commentary by the ESPGHAN Committee on Nutrition. J Pediatr Gastroenterol Nutr 2006;42(5):596–603.
85. Schanler RJ. Post-discharge nutrition for the preterm infant. Acta Paediatr Suppl 2005;94(449):68–73.
86. Sherman MP, Bennett SH, Hwang FF, et al. Neonatal small bowel epithelia: enhancing anti-bacterial defense with lactoferrin and *Lactobacillus* GG. Biometals 2004;17(3):285–9.

87. Montagne P, Cuilliere ML, Mole C, et al. Changes in lactoferrin and lysozyme levels in human milk during the first twelve weeks of lactation. Adv Exp Med Biol 2001;501:241–7.
88. Ronayne de Ferrer PA, Baroni A, Sambucetti ME, et al. Lactoferrin levels in term and preterm milk. J Am Coll Nutr 2000;19(3):370–3.
89. Bhatia J. Bovine lactoferrin, human lactoferrin, and bioactivity. J Pediatr Gastroenterol Nutr 2011;53(6):589.
90. Academy of Breastfeeding Medicine. ABM clinical protocol #10: breastfeeding the late preterm infant (34 0/7 to 36 6/7 weeks gestation). 2011. 2013 (June 2). Breastfeeding Medicine 2011;6(3):151–6.

Neuropathologic Studies of the Encephalopathy of Prematurity in the Late Preterm Infant

Robin L. Haynes, PhD[a],*, Lynn A. Sleeper, ScD[b],
Joseph J. Volpe, MD[c], Hannah C. Kinney, MD[a]

KEYWORDS

- Axonopathy - Cerebral cortex - Critical period - Periventricular leukomalacia
- Thalamus

KEY POINTS

- The encephalopathy of prematurity comprises combined gray and white matter lesions underlying preterm brain injury, including periventricular leukomalacia (PVL).
- The late preterm brain can develop PVL identical to that of the early preterm brain, and potentially with a higher incidence detected at autopsy.
- There is an increased mean density of reactive astrocytes, as well as glia with the expression of the oxidative marker, 4-hydroxynonenal, in the damaged white matter of late preterm infants in comparison with early preterm and term infants.
- Thalamic damage in the late preterm infant in comparison with the early preterm and term infant is associated with an increased prevalence of intrinsic axonal injury, as determined by the immunomarker fractin.
- The spectrum of brain injury in the late preterm infant, as determined in an autopsy population, is similar, but not identical, to that found in early preterm infants, with potential differential susceptibility for various neuronal, glial, and vascular indices.

Disclosures: The authors/editors have identified no professional or financial affiliations for themselves or their spouse/partner.
This work was supported by grants from the National Institute of Neurological Disorders and Stroke (PO1-NS38475), National Institute of Child Health and Development (P30-HD18655), and Cerebral Palsy International Research Foundation.
[a] Department of Pathology, Boston Children's Hospital, Harvard Medical School, 300 Longwood Avenue, Boston, MA 02115, USA; [b] Center for Statistical Analysis & Research, New England Research Institutes, 9 Galen Street, Watertown, MA 02472, USA; [c] Department of Neurology, Boston Children's Hospital, Harvard Medical School, 300 Longwood Avenue, Boston, MA 02115, USA
* Corresponding author. Department of Pathology, Boston Children's Hospital, Enders Building Room 1109, 61 Binney Street, Boston, MA 02115.
E-mail address: Robin.haynes@childrens.harvard.edu

Clin Perinatol 40 (2013) 707–722
http://dx.doi.org/10.1016/j.clp.2013.07.003
0095-5108/13/$ – see front matter © 2013 Elsevier Inc. All rights reserved.

perinatology.theclinics.com

INTRODUCTION

Modern neonatology no longer equates "near term" birth with "term-like" outcomes, as evidenced by the reports in this issue. Indeed, it is now recognized that premature infants born near term (ie, late preterm infants born at 34–36 gestational weeks) exhibit neurologic morbidity related to a spectrum of complications that can adversely affect the brain and its development. The complications of late preterm delivery include respiratory insufficiency, apnea, feeding difficulties and suboptimal nutrition, infection, hypoglycemia, and hyperbilirubinemia.[1–3] The major neuropathologic substrate of brain damage in premature infants in general is the encephalopathy of prematurity (EP).[4–6] This disorder comprises combined gray and white matter lesions resulting from the effects of hypoxia-ischemia, infection/inflammation, and/or other insults that lead to combined toxicities attributable to glutamate, free radicals, and cytokines.[4,6] However, it is not clear from human neuropathologic studies to date whether patterns of EP differ among early, mid, and late preterm infants. The occurrence of differential patterns of EP is certainly likely because the growth and development of the human brain change so rapidly from midgestation (~20–22 weeks) to term, the time frame of premature birth, suggesting that there are rapidly changing cellular vulnerabilities to injury across temporal epochs even as short as 2 weeks. Indeed, while the brain attains 90% of term growth in the second half of gestation, it is important to realize that within this 20-week period, brain weight in the early preterm infant (24–26 weeks) is 30% to 40% of term weight, 50% to 55% of term weight in the mid preterm infant, and 65% to 80% in the late preterm infant, with an increment of 5% to 15% between each of these 3 "epochs" (**Fig. 1**). Moreover, the brain at 34 weeks still needs to gain 35% of its overall weight to reach term weight (see **Fig. 1**). Within even these last 3 weeks of fetal life, much brain development is yet to transpire.

For this report, the authors tested the hypothesis that EP occurs in late preterm infants at autopsy, and in patterns that reflect potential differential vulnerabilities of developing gray and white matter at the temporal epoch of 34 to 36 weeks. The hypothesis was tested by reanalyzing published neuropathologic data obtained in the authors' laboratory according to late preterm age (34–36 weeks) and comparing these with data from early preterm ages (<34 weeks) and, when available, term

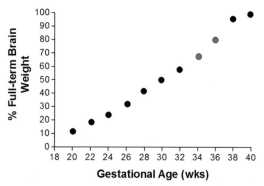

Fig. 1. Developmental changes in brain weight during the second half of gestation. The development of the brain increases dramatically over the last 20 weeks of gestation. Red circles (Gray in print) indicate gestational ages corresponding to the late preterm infant. (*Adapted from* Kinney HC. The near-term (late preterm) human brain and risk for periventricular leukomalacia: a review. Semin Perinatol 2006;30(2):81–8; with permission.)

age.[7-10] Although the authors' previously published studies did report neuropathologic findings adjusted for gestational age as well as postconceptional age, the categories of late preterm versus early preterm gestational ages were not analyzed. This latter analysis is now performed to gain potential insight into the effect of early versus late preterm birth specifically on EP. The neuropathologic findings are framed in the context of brain development in the late versus early preterm brain, as briefly summarized at the outset.

BRAIN DEVELOPMENT IN THE SECOND HALF OF HUMAN GESTATION

Brain development in the second half of human gestation, the time frame of prematurity, is nothing short of spectacular. At midgestation, the cerebrum is virtually smooth except for the indentation of the Sylvan fissure; by term, all primary, secondary, and tertiary sulci are in place, with different gyri differentiating at exquisitely timed periods over the second half of pregnancy (**Fig. 2**). The appearance of the central, cingulate, circular, calcarine, and superior temporal sulci follow on from each other from 20 to 27 weeks.[11-16] Thereafter, the transverse temporal, external occipitotemporal, and paracentral gyri form (see **Fig. 2**).[17] By term birth, the folding pattern of the brain astonishingly resembles that of the adult.[18,19] Volumetric magnetic resonance determinations during late gestation demonstrate a dramatic increase in the total gray matter volume from approximately 30 to 40 gestational weeks, with the total increase primarily reflecting a 4-fold increase in the cerebral cortical volume.[20] In addition, minimal "myelinated" white matter is present in the early preterm infant (around 29 weeks), but increases dramatically in volume as term is approached, with a 5-fold increase between 35 and 41 weeks, to obtain a total of 10% to 15% of the total unmyelinated volume.[20] Major cellular and regional events in the development of neurons, oligodendrocytes (OLs), astrocytes, microglia, and blood vessels underlie this stunning overall brain growth in the human brain across the last half of gestation, as recently reviewed.[21,22]

In considering brain injury in early versus mid versus late preterm infants, it is essential to recognize that the different cellular changes do not always progress in a linear fashion, nor directly parallel to each other. That is, there may be different "critical periods" or developmental windows during which the different neuronal, glial,

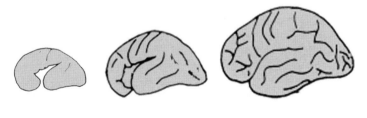

| 20-23 wks | 28-31 wks | 37-44 wks |

Fig. 2. Increasing gyration of the human cerebral cortex over the second half of gestation. At midgestation, the cerebrum is relatively smooth, except for the Sylvian fissure, central sulcus, and superior temporal sulcus. Over the second half of gestation, gyration increases dramatically until term birth when the folding pattern of the brain closely resembles that of the adult, and all primary, secondary, and tertiary sulci are in place. (*Adapted from* Dooling EC, Chi JC, Gilles FH. Telencephalic development: changing gyral patterns. In: Gilles FH, Leviton A, Dooling EC, editors. The Developing Human Brain. Littleton, MA: John Wright; 1983. p. 94–104. with permission.)

and vascular cell types are at different maturational stages, and are therefore differentially susceptible to deprivation of normal environmental influences, or to adverse insults (eg, ischemia). Because of the overall rapidity of brain growth in the second half of pregnancy (see **Fig. 1**), insults at time points separated by even 2 weeks may alter the trajectory of specific cellular programs, thereby resulting in different patterns of brain injury and, hence, different adverse neurologic outcomes. Myelination and the OL cellular differentiation illustrate this key concept. Myelination begins in different regions of the brain at different time points in the fetal or infant period, and progresses at different tempos in a hierarchal order from specific sensory and motor systems in the fetal brain to regions of higher-level associative functions in the infant brain and well beyond.[23–26] Moreover, the degree of myelination differs substantially, even within short time windows, as exemplified by the corticospinal tract.[25] Across the second half of gestation, OL maturation from an OL progenitor into a myelinating OL involves a sequence of developmental stages, each characterized by a progressively complex morphology, as well as expression of stage-specific markers. This progression includes the following OL-developmental stages in increasing order of maturation: (1) O4-expressing late OL progenitors; (2) O1-expressing immature OLs; and (3) myelin basic protein (MBP)-expressing mature OL.[27] Between approximately 20 and 30 gestational weeks, O4-positive OLs are the predominant OL population in the human parietal white matter[27]; around 30 gestational weeks, there is an expansion of O1-positive immature OLs, as well as an appearance of mature OLs expressing MBP.[27] Of note, little is known about the distribution of the OL lineage during brain development in all brain regions of the cerebral white matter. This distribution is likely to be different as a function of development and, therefore, vulnerability. Given that O4, O1, and MBP-producing OLs are differentially sensitive to glutamate, free radical, and/or cytokine toxicity,[28–36] the cerebral white matter is therefore differentially vulnerable to hypoxia-ischemia in EP at the different preterm epochs. Thus, it is simplistic to conceptualize brain injury in the late preterm infant as identical to that in the early or mid preterm infant, only with a lesser degree of severity. Rather, the pattern of injury between the preterm epochs may differ based on the differential stage of development of the different cell types during the epochs, and their differential vulnerabilities.

THE ENCEPHALOPATHY OF PREMATURITY FURTHER DEFINED

The term "encephalopathy of prematurity" was coined to characterize the multifaceted gray and white matter lesions in the preterm brain that reflect acquired insults, altered developmental trajectories, and reparative phenomena in various combinations.[5,6,37,38] It encompasses damage to white matter (periventricular leukomalacia [PVL] and diffuse cerebral white matter gliosis), as well as to white matter neurons, axons, and gray matter (neuronal loss and/or gliosis in the cerebral cortex, thalamus, hippocampus, basal ganglia, cerebellum, and/or brainstem), as recently reviewed.[4] The cause of EP is likely multifactorial, and includes cerebral hypoxia-ischemia and systemic infection/inflammation that results in glutamate, free radical, and/or cytokine toxicity to pre-OLs, axons, and neurons.[39] In addition, other maturation-dependent biochemical derangements likely contribute to EP caused by the multiple extrauterine insults the preterm infant experiences and is not developmentally equipped to defend against.[37] Given the heterogeneity and diverse combinations of the lesions that comprise EP, as well as the specific timing of the insult(s) in the early, mid, or late preterm epochs in the second half of gestation, it is not surprising that the spectrum of neurodevelopmental abnormalities in preterm survivors is wide, and includes, often in combination, deficits in executive functions,[40,41] autistic behaviors,[42] cerebral palsy,[43] and visual cognitive impairments.[44]

THE ENCEPHALOPATHY OF PREMATURITY IN THE LATE PRETERM INFANT

In an attempt to elucidate the neuropathology of the late preterm infant at autopsy, the authors undertook an analysis of previously published data sets concerning various aspects of EP in preterm infants autopsied at Boston Children's Hospital between 1997 and 2008.[7–10] This analysis compared several neuropathologic components of EP between early and mid preterm infants typically combined (<34 weeks at birth) and late preterm infants (34–36 weeks at birth), and, in some instances for which data were available, term infants (≥37 weeks at birth). Several neuropathologic features of EP were analyzed. It is understood in this analysis that the precise timing of the insult is typically unknown in autopsy cases, and in late preterm infants may have occurred in the early or mid term epoch during life, evolving to the point that the injury was examined at death in the late preterm epoch. The authors emphasize, however, that all of the preterm cases with EP (defined by the presence of PVL and variable gray matter injury) died in the perinatal period, with the entire window between midgestation and the first 2 to 3 postnatal months (median).

Periventicular Leukomalacia (PVL) in the Late Preterm Infant at Autopsy

PVL, the major white matter component of EP, is defined as focal periventricular necrosis associated with diffuse reactive gliosis and microglial activation in the surrounding cerebral white matter (**Fig. 3**).[37,45] The reader is referred to recent reviews relating to the cellular pathogenesis and morphologic evolution of PVL.[4,39] In a survey of the neuropathology of prematurity in 41 preterm infants born from 23 to 36 gestational weeks and dying within the perinatal period, the overall incidence of PVL was 41% (17 of 41) and that of diffuse white matter gliosis (DWMG) (defined as diffuse reactive astrogliosis without associated focal necrosis in the cerebral white matter) likewise 41% (17 of 41).[10] By design, there were no cases of term gestation in this survey. In 82% of the 17 preterm cases with PVL in this series, the periventricular necrotic foci were not grossly cystic, but rather 1 mm or less in diameter, detectable only with the light microscope and likely below the resolution of current clinical magnetic resonance imaging (MRI) scanners. In this series, 39% (16 of 41) were delivered late term (34–36 weeks), and 61% (25 of 41) early preterm (<34 weeks). PVL was more common in the late preterm group (63%) than in the early preterm group (28%) (**Table 1**). The necrotic foci demonstrated were of both the acute (coagulative necrosis with axonal spheroids) and organizing (tissue dissolution with infiltrating macrophages) types, indicating variable timing of injury. Nevertheless, the histopathology of each type (acute vs organizing) was essentially identical between the early and late preterm infants, indicating that the white matter cell types (astrocytes, microglia/macrophages, axons) respond morphologically to injury in the same way, at least as detected by anatomic microscopy in the single "snap-shot" of the tissue injury at autopsy. Specifically, these autopsy data confirm that the late preterm brain is susceptible to, and can develop, the histopathologic features of PVL identical to those in the early preterm brain, and potentially with a higher incidence detected at autopsy. Of note, the mean postconceptional age of the early preterm group was 2 weeks shorter (34 weeks) than that of the late preterm group (36 weeks), suggesting that the morphologic changes of PVL were able to evolve and become microscopically detectable with the longer survival period.

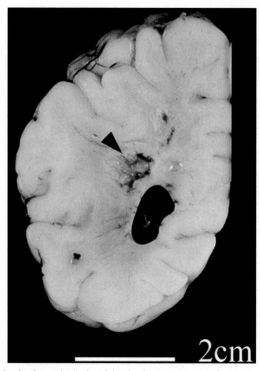

Fig. 3. Periventricular leukomalacia (PVL) in the late preterm infant. The typical appearance of PVL, with focal necrosis causing a cystic cavity (*arrowhead*) in the periventricular white matter, is seen in the brain of a late preterm infant born at 35 gestational weeks and dying at 5 postnatal (40 postconceptional) weeks. (*From* Haynes R, Folkerth R, Keefe R, et al. Nitrosative and oxidative injury to premyelinating oligodendrocytes in periventricular leukomalacia. J Neuropathol Exp Neurol 2003;62(5):441–50; with permission.)

Reactive Gliosis and Activated Microglia in the Cerebral White Matter in EP in Late Preterm Infants at Autopsy

Reactive gliosis and activated microglia are the 2 major inflammatory components of cerebral white matter injury.[37,45] Presumed to be initially protective against pre-OL cell damage, these cells can compound tissue injury when the insult is prolonged and/or severe. Both cell types produce inflammatory cytokines, and immunocytochemical studies in PVL demonstrate increased cytokine expression within them as a distinctive

Table 1
Distribution of cerebral white matter lesions in preterm infants born late preterm versus early preterm in a total cohort of 41 preterm infants

GA	Control	DWMG	PVL	Total
Early preterm (<34 wk)	7 (28%)	11 (44%)	7 (28%)	25 (100%)
Late preterm (34–36 wk)	0 (0%)	6 (38%)	10 (63%)	16 (100%)

Abbreviations: DWMG, diffuse white matter gliosis; GA, gestational age; PVL, periventricular leukomalacia.

Data from Pierson CR, Folkerth RD, Billiards SS, et al. Gray matter injury associated with periventricular leukomalacia in the premature infant. Acta Neuropathol 2007;114(6):619–31.

feature of its histopathology.[35,46] Reactive astrocytes and microglia/macrophages also help protect pre-OLs from excitotoxic injury by the upregulation of the glutamate transporter EAAT and uptake of excessive tissue glutamate.[47] Nevertheless, these cell types may contribute to free radical injury in PVL, as indicated by the expression of potential sources of reactive nitrogen and reactive oxygen species, including inducible nitric oxide synthase in reactive astrocytes of PVL[48] and 12/15-lipoxygenase in activated microglia of PVL.[49]

In archived PVL data in the laboratory,[7] the authors reanalyzed the density of reactive astrocytes (immunolabeled for glial fibrillary acidic protein [GFAP]) and activated microglia (immunolabeled with CD68), as well as immunostaining of glial cells for the oxidative stress markers 4-hydroxynonenal (HNE) and malondialdehyde (MDA) in the white matter of PVL and non-PVL cases combined, relative to late preterm versus early preterm versus term birth (**Table 2**). Original cell-density data were used, scored according to the following scale: 0 = no cells/high-powered field (hpf); 1 = 1 to 10 cells/hpf; 2 = 11 to 20 cells/hpf; and 3 = >20 cells/hpf.[7,35,48,49] Of interest was that there was a higher mean density of GFAP-positive reactive astrocytes in the cerebral white matter of the late preterm group than in both the early preterm and term groups. This finding must be considered with the caveat that the data here were not controlled for the severity of the insults (unknown) or for the postnatal age. For CD68-positive activated microglia and HNE-positive glia, the authors found marginally or statistically significantly higher density in the late preterm group compared with one or both of the early preterm and term groups (**Fig. 4**, see **Table 2**). These findings contradict, at least in autopsied infants, the notion that white matter injury is present to a less severe degree in late preterm infants than in early preterm infants, and that the degree of late preterm injury is less than that at term. The findings also suggest that the cerebral white matter at 34 to 36 weeks is potentially "more vulnerable" to reactive gliosis than in the early or later preterm epochs, and that it involves oxidative stress, as indicated by the transiently elevated density of HNE-immunopositive glia (see **Fig. 4**). The clinical significance of a peak in reactive gliosis in the late preterm white matter is unknown, as is the relationship of diffuse reactive gliosis to particular and clinically milder neurologic phenotypes in late preterm survivors. Given that the neuroimaging correlate of diffuse reactive gliosis is uncertain, it is also unclear whether diffuse reactive gliosis is a major white matter finding in living late preterm infants. Nevertheless this autopsy finding warrants further investigation in living infants to establish the ultimate role of DWMG in neurologic outcomes in later preterm survivors.

Gray Matter Lesions in EP in Late Preterm Infants at Autopsy

Neuronal loss and/or gliosis are the histopathologic hallmarks of gray matter injury in EP, and occur in virtually all gray matter sites, albeit in variable combinations.[10] In the authors' survey of the neuropathology of prematurity in 41 cases, gray matter lesions occurred in one-third or more of PVL cases (late and early preterm delivery combined), suggesting that white matter injury generally does not occur in isolation, and that the term EP does in fact best describe the scope of the neuropathology in individual preterm cases. Neuronal loss overall was almost exclusively found in association with PVL in the late and early preterm cases combined, with significantly increased incidence and severity in the thalamus (38%), globus pallidus (33%), and cerebellar dentate nucleus (29%) in comparison with DWMG cases (0% at each of the 3 listed sites).[10] Moreover, the temporospatial profile of gray matter injury varied significantly from midgestation to term: brainstem injury preceded injury in the deep gray nuclei (basal ganglia/thalamus), which preceded injury to the cerebral cortex.[10]

Table 2
Density-score[a] data as determined across different development epochs over the second half of gestation

Variable	Early Preterm (<34 wk)	Late Preterm (34–36 wk)	Term (≥37 wk)	Kruskal-Wallis P Value	P Value Early vs Late Preterm	P Value Late Preterm vs Term
RA score	1.3 ± 1.1 (9)	2.6 ± 0.5 (9)	1.7 ± 0.8 (16)	.016	.034	.019
MG score	2.0 ± 1.1 (9)	2.3 ± 0.5 (9)	1.0 ± 0.9 (15)	.006	.707	.005
HNE Score	0.9 ± 1.2 (9)	1.9 ± 1.0 (9)	1.1 ± 0.9 (16)	.058	.076	.061
MDA Score	0.8 ± 1.3 (9)	2.2 ± 1.3 (9)	1.6 ± 1.1 (16)	.050	.069	.257

Data are presented as mean ± standard deviation (n). The Wilcoxon rank-sum P values are not adjusted for multiple comparisons.

Abbreviations: HNE, 4-hydroxynonenal (oxidative stress marker); MDA, malondialdehyde (oxidative stress marker); MG, CD68-positive microglia; RA, GFAP-positive reactive astrocytes.

[a] Scoring system: 0 = no cells/hpf; 1 = 1–10 cells/hpf; 2 = 11–20 cells/hpf; 3 = >20 cells/hpf.

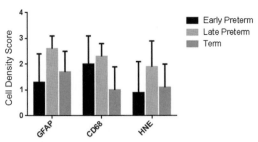

Fig. 4. Cell-density scores indicate astrocyte reactivity (GFAP), microglial activation (CD68), and oxidative damage (HNE) across different epochs of preterm brain development in PVL and control cases combined. See text for further details.

This report reanalyzes the archived gray matter data in premature infants relative to the late and early preterm categories (**Table 3**). In the original study, the authors scored neuronal loss with the following injury grades: 0, no neuronal loss/hpf; 1, mild, scattered neuronal dropout/hpf; 2, moderate, focal areas of neuronal dropout/hpf; and 3, severe, confluent areas of neuronal dropout/hpf. Neuronal loss (and gliosis) was interpreted as a marker of subacute or chronic injury, indicative of insult occurring 3 to 5 days or more before death.[6] Grade 3 neuronal loss is tabulated here, because this grade is unequivocally recognized by standard microscopic examination and therefore represents, in the authors' opinion, a substantial degree of injury (see **Table 3**). Both late and early preterm brains demonstrate neuronal loss throughout gray matter sites, and there is no significant difference between the two

Table 3		
Incidence of severe gray matter damage (Grade 3) in PVL in early versus late preterm infants		
Site	Early Preterm (n = 7)	Late Preterm (n = 10)
Frontal Cortex		
Neuronal loss	0% (0/6)	10% (1/10)
Gliosis	17% (1/6)	10% (1/10)
Thalamus		
Neuronal loss	29% (2/7)	22% (2/9)
Gliosis	29% (2/7)	11% (1/9)
Globus Pallidus		
Neuronal loss	50% (3/6)	11% (1/9)
Gliosis	17% (1/6)	11% (1/9)
Hippocampus		
Neuronal loss	14% (1/7)	25% (2/8)
Gliosis	43% (3/7)	0% (0/8)
Brainstem		
Neuronal loss	14% (1/7)	0% (0/7)
Gliosis	14% (1/7)	0% (0/7)

Because of small sample size, no significant differences were found in the overall distribution of injury grade (0–3) by Mantel-Haenszel test for linear trend or by Fisher exact test. The scoring system was: Grades: 0, no neuronal loss/high-powered field (hpf); 1, mild, scattered neuronal dropout/hpf; 2, moderate, focal areas of neuronal dropout/hpf; and 3, severe, confluent areas of neuronal dropout/hpf.
Abbreviation: PVL, periventricular leukomalacia.

groups in the distributions of grades 0 to 3 (see **Table 3**). While there was a trend toward a higher incidence of grade 3 hippocampal gliosis and grade 3 brainstem neuronal loss and gliosis in the early preterm group in comparison with the late preterm group (see **Table 3**), the differences were not significant in the overall distribution of injury (grades 0–3) by Mantel-Haenszel test for linear trend or by Fisher exact test. Thus, late and early preterm brains demonstrate the same types of gray matter lesions, possibly of the same degree of severity.

Thalamic Damage in EP in Late Preterm Infants at Autopsy

The gray matter damage in EP in regions critical to higher cognitive processing are now considered to account in large part for intellectual deficits in preterm survivors. Of gray matter structures, the thalamus, which is critically involved in cognition via extensive interconnections with the cerebral cortex, is the primary one involved in EP at autopsy (see earlier discussion).[10] MRI studies indicate a diminished volume of the thalamus in PVL.[50–54] Previously the authors found that thalamic injury in preterm infants occurs in at least 4 different patterns: (1) diffuse gliosis with or without neuronal loss; (2) microinfarcts with focal neuronal loss; (3) macroinfarcts in the distribution of the posterior cerebral artery; and (4) status marmoratus.[9] These different patterns likely each reflect separate mechanisms, including diffuse hypoxia-ischemia and focal arterial embolism, as well as potential different temporal characteristics of the responsible insults.

This report reanalyzes thalamic injury associated with PVL in preterm infants relative to early preterm, late preterm, and term gestations (total = 22 cases), with a group sample size of 11, 6, and 5, respectively.[9] In a non-PVL (normative) group in this data set, there were 16 cases, comprising 4 early preterm, 12 term, and no late preterm cases. Of note, the mean density of neurons adjusted for postconceptional age in the mediodorsal nucleus decreased significantly from 22.7 ± 2.6 neurons/hpf to 13.5 ± 1.4 neurons/hpf from the early preterm to term epochs ($P = .009$), representing a 44% cross-sectional decrease over this time frame. Given that a decrease in neuronal density in a gray matter structure reflects an increase in "spacing" between neuronal cell bodies attributable to an increase in the synapses, dendrites and their spines, and axonal arborization of the neuropil, this striking change in neuronal density in a representative subnucleus attests to the rapidly evolving changes occurring in the thalamus over the last half of gestation.

Although the late preterm group with PVL in this study comprised only 6 cases, all patterns of thalamic injury were identified except for macroinfarcts; interestingly, 2 of the 6 cases (33%) demonstrated thalamic microinfarcts, whereas this lesion was observed in only 1 of the 11 (9%) early preterm brains and in none of the 5 term brains. Moreover, the main thalamic lesion in this small study was microinfarcts in the late preterm cases (50% [2 or 4 cases with thalamic abnormalities]), but was diffuse gliosis in the early preterm cases (67% [4 of 6]), and was macroinfarcts in the term cases (67% [2 of 3]). There were no significant differences in the density of neurons and/or reactive astrocytes in the mediodorsal nucleus between the different gestational age epochs studied, nor in the prevalence of axonal damage, as assessed with positive fractin immunostaining. Nevertheless, the highest prevalence of fractin-positive axonal injury within the thalamic parenchyma was noted in the late preterm group (83% [5 of 6 cases]) compared with that in the early preterm group (36% [4 of 11]) or term group (60% [3 of 5]). The differences in the different features of thalamic abnormality observed in this study suggest the possibility that this structure, like the cerebral white matter, may be susceptible based on different developmental stages, and requires further investigation in larger sample sizes.

Deficit of Neurons in the Cerebral White Matter in EP in Late Term Infants at Autopsy

White matter neurons in the human fetal brain across the last half of gestation consist of subplate neurons and late migrating γ-aminobutyric acid (GABA)ergic neurons. Subplate neurons are among the first generated neurons of the neocortex and come to lie immediately beneath the developing cortical plate, where they form part of the early neocortical circuitry.[55,56] In the subplate stage of development (15–35 weeks), the subplate serves as a "waiting" compartment for the competition, segregation, and growth of afferents originating from the thalamus, brainstem, basal forebrain, and ipsilateral and contralateral cerebral hemisphere.[55,57] After the incoming fibers enter the cortical plate around 32 weeks, the subplate zone almost completely disappears, leaving only a "vestige" of neuronal cells scattered throughout the subcortical white matter, so-called interstitial neurons, which nevertheless contribute to the modulation of adult cortical processing.[58] Because there is no available immunomarker that specifically labels human subplate neurons in tissue sections, their phenotype is defined by morphology, location, and connectivity with the cortical plate. In the

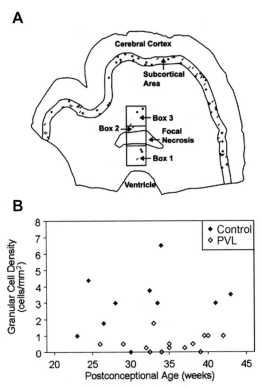

Fig. 5. Loss of white matter neurons in PVL during the second half of gestation. (*A*) This representative Neurolucida drawing indicates the methodology of white matter quantitation in a PVL case at 29 postconceptional weeks. White matter neurons were counted in 3 boxes within the periventricular and central white matter, including in the area of the focal necrosis, as well as the subcortical area underlying the cortex. (*B*) There is a significant reduction of white matter neurons with granular morphology in PVL (age-adjusted and postmortem interval–adjusted mean, 0.51 ± 0.31) compared with controls (mean, 3.02 ± 0.37) (*P*<.001). (*From* Kinney HC, Haynes RL, Xu G, et al. Neuron deficit in the white matter and subplate in periventricular leukomalacia. Ann Neurol 2012;71(3):397–406; with permission.)

human cerebral white matter, fusiform, granular, unipolar, bipolar, multipolar, and inverted pyramidal neurons have been observed.[54,56] In addition to subplate neurons, white matter neurons are composed of late migrating GABAergic neurons over the second half of human gestation.[8,59] In humans, approximately one-third of these GABAergic neurons arise from the ganglionic eminence.[60] The granular subtype expresses GAD67/65, a marker of the GABAergic phenotype, but not markers of neuronal and glial immaturity (Tuj1, doublecortin, or NG2).[8]

Previously the authors reported that the density of granular neurons was significantly reduced by 54% to 80% in the periventricular and central white matter and subplate region in 15 PVL cases in a comparison with 10 non-PVL controls,[8] a finding supported by an independent study reporting a loss of GABAergic neurons in the white matter of perinatal brains with white matter lesions in comparison with controls.[61] In the authors' study, the deficit in the granular neurons distant from the focally necrotic lesions (ie, in the subplate region) is of major interest because it occurs presumably in zones of less severe insult. In contrast to granular neurons, there is not a consistent deficit in unipolar, bipolar, multipolar, or inverted pyramidal neurons in the white matter or subplate region in PVL.[8] The preferential damage to granular neurons, including those distant from the necrotic foci, suggests that this particular subtype is exquisitely sensitive to hypoxia-ischemia. Of note, the deficit of white matter neurons occurs at all postconceptional ages, without a preference for the early preterm, late preterm, or term epochs (**Fig. 5**).

SUMMARY

At 34 gestational weeks, the late preterm brain has attained approximately two-thirds of term weight, underscoring the distance yet to reach term maturation. This study attempts to begin to define the neuropathology of EP in the late preterm infant. In autopsied late preterm infants, the spectrum of brain damage has been found to be virtually the same as that found in early preterm infants (<34 weeks at birth), suggesting that if the insult(s) is severe enough, the same histopathologic changes can result in gray and white matter. The authors propose that the lesions are severe enough in the autopsy population of late preterm infants because of the severity of the systemic disorders that have proved lethal, for example, hyaline membrane disease, necrotizing enterocolitis, and sepsis. Because these studies involve only autopsied cases, it is not possible to verify the widely held concept that brain damage in survivors of late preterm deliveries is similar to that in early preterm infants, but only less severe in degree. The likelihood that this formulation is not completely accurate is supported by the finding of a greater incidence of fractin-immunostaining axons in the thalamus in late preterm infants when compared with early preterm infants, as well as a significant peak in the density of reactive astrocytes in the cerebral white matter in the late preterm infant. These findings together suggest a differential age-related vulnerability of different cell types in EP. Further research with larger sample sizes at each preterm epoch is needed to define the role of critical periods, however short, in patterns of brain injury that potentially define the early, mid, and late preterm windows of development, and hence may be responsible for the different patterns of neurologic outcomes seen in survivors of these different epochs. Finally, it must be understood that several of the neuropathologic findings in the late preterm brain, for example, white matter neuronal loss, axonal injury, and reactive gliosis, may be difficult to detect by routine neuroimaging. Consequently, their role in defining adverse neurologic outcomes in survivors of late preterm deliveries may be clinically underappreciated.

REFERENCES

1. Raju TN, Higgins RD, Stark AR, et al. Optimizing care and outcome for late-preterm (near-term) infants: a summary of the workshop sponsored by the National Institute of Child Health and Human Development. Pediatrics 2006; 118:1207.
2. Amiel-Tison C, Allen MC, Lebrun F, et al. Macropremies: underprivileged newborns. Ment Retard Dev Disabil Res Rev 2002;8:281.
3. Davidoff MJ, Dias T, Damus K, et al. Changes in the gestational age distribution among U.S. singleton births: impact on rates of late preterm birth, 1992 to 2002. Semin Perinatol 2006;30:8.
4. Kinney HC, Volpe JJ. Modeling the encephalopathy of prematurity in animals: the important role of translational research. Neurol Res Int 2012;2012:295389.
5. Volpe JJ. Encephalopathy of prematurity includes neuronal abnormalities. Pediatrics 2005;116:221.
6. Volpe JJ. Brain injury in premature infants: a complex amalgam of destructive and developmental disturbances. Lancet Neurol 2009;8:110.
7. Haynes RL, Folkerth RD, Keefe RJ, et al. Nitrosative and oxidative injury to pre-myelinating oligodendrocytes in periventricular leukomalacia. J Neuropathol Exp Neurol 2003;62:441.
8. Kinney HC, Haynes RL, Xu G, et al. Neuron deficit in the white matter and subplate in periventricular leukomalacia. Ann Neurol 2012;71:397.
9. Ligam P, Haynes RL, Folkerth RD, et al. Thalamic damage in periventricular leukomalacia: novel pathologic observations relevant to cognitive deficits in survivors of prematurity. Pediatr Res 2009;65:524.
10. Pierson CR, Folkerth RD, Billiards SS, et al. Gray matter injury associated with periventricular leukomalacia in the premature infant. Acta Neuropathol 2007; 114:619.
11. Fogliarini C, Chaumoitre K, Chapon F, et al. Assessment of cortical maturation with prenatal MRI. Part I: normal cortical maturation. Eur Radiol 2005; 15:1671.
12. Levine D, Barnes PD. Cortical maturation in normal and abnormal fetuses as assessed with prenatal MR imaging. Radiology 1999;210:751.
13. Cohen-Sacher B, Lerman-Sagie T, Lev D, et al. Sonographic developmental milestones of the fetal cerebral cortex: a longitudinal study. Ultrasound Obstet Gynecol 2006;27:494.
14. Abe S, Takagi K, Yamamoto T, et al. Assessment of cortical gyrus and sulcus formation using MR images in normal fetuses. Prenat Diagn 2003;23:225.
15. Toi A, Lister WS, Fong KW. How early are fetal cerebral sulci visible at prenatal ultrasound and what is the normal pattern of early fetal sulcal development? Ultrasound Obstet Gynecol 2004;24:706.
16. Rolo LC, Araujo Junior E, Nardozza LM, et al. Development of fetal brain sulci and gyri: assessment through two and three-dimensional ultrasound and magnetic resonance imaging. Arch Gynecol Obstet 2011;283:149.
17. White T, Su S, Schmidt M, et al. The development of gyrification in childhood and adolescence. Brain Cogn 2010;72:36.
18. Armstrong E, Schleicher A, Omran H, et al. The ontogeny of human gyrification. Cereb Cortex 1995;5:56.
19. Naidich TP, Grant JL, Altman N, et al. The developing cerebral surface. Preliminary report on the patterns of sulcal and gyral maturation—anatomy, ultrasound, and magnetic resonance imaging. Neuroimaging Clin N Am 1994;4:201.

20. Huppi PS, Warfield S, Kikinis R, et al. Quantitative magnetic resonance imaging of brain development in premature and mature newborns. Ann Neurol 1998;43:224.

21. Billiards SS, Pierson CR, Haynes RL, et al. Is the late preterm infant more vulnerable to gray matter injury than the term infant? Clin Perinatol 2006;33:915.

22. Kinney HC. The near-term (late preterm) human brain and risk for periventricular leukomalacia: a review. Semin Perinatol 2006;30:81.

23. Brody BA, Kinney HC, Kloman AS, et al. Sequence of central nervous system myelination in human infancy. I. An autopsy study of myelination. J Neuropathol Exp Neurol 1987;46:283.

24. Volpe JJ. Neurology of the newborn. 5th edition. Philadelphia: WB Saunders Company; 2008.

25. Gilles FH. Myelination in the neonatal brain. Hum Pathol 1976;7:244.

26. Yakovlev PI, Lecours AR. The myelogenetic cycles of regional maturation of the brain. In: Minkowski A, editor. Regional Development of the Brain in Early Life. Oxford: Blackwell Scientific Publications; 1967. p. 3–70.

27. Back SA, Luo NL, Borenstein NS, et al. Late oligodendrocyte progenitors coincide with the developmental window of vulnerability for human perinatal white matter injury. J Neurosci 2001;21:1302.

28. Jantzie LL, Talos DM, Selip DB, et al. Developmental regulation of group I metabotropic glutamate receptors in the premature brain and their protective role in a rodent model of periventricular leukomalacia. Neuron Glia Biol 2010; 6:277.

29. Desilva TM, Kinney HC, Borenstein NS, et al. The glutamate transporter EAAT2 is transiently expressed in developing human cerebral white matter. J Comp Neurol 2007;501:879.

30. Deng W, Rosenberg PA, Volpe JJ, et al. Calcium-permeable AMPA/kainate receptors mediate toxicity and preconditioning by oxygen-glucose deprivation in oligodendrocyte precursors. Proc Natl Acad Sci U S A 2003;100:6801.

31. Follett PL, Deng W, Dai W, et al. Glutamate receptor-mediated oligodendrocyte toxicity in periventricular leukomalacia: a protective role for topiramate. J Neurosci 2004;24:4412.

32. Back SA, Gan X, Li Y, et al. Maturation-dependent vulnerability of oligodendrocytes to oxidative stress-induced death caused by glutathione depletion. J Neurosci 1998;18(16):6241.

33. Rosenberg PA, Dai W, Gan XD, et al. Mature myelin basic protein-expressing oligodendrocytes are insensitive to kainate toxicity. J Neurosci Res 2003;71:237.

34. Wang H, Li J, Follett PL, et al. 12-Lipoxygenase plays a key role in cell death caused by glutathione depletion and arachidonic acid in rat oligodendrocytes. Eur J Neurosci 2004;20:2049.

35. Folkerth RD, Keefe RJ, Haynes RL, et al. Interferon-gamma expression in periventricular leukomalacia in the human brain. Brain Pathol 2004;14:265.

36. Pang Y, Cai Z, Rhodes PG. Effect of tumor necrosis factor-alpha on developing optic nerve oligodendrocytes in culture. J Neurosci Res 2005;80:226.

37. Kinney HC, Volpe JJ. Perinatal Panencephalopathy in Premature Infants: Is It Due to Hypoxia-Ischemia? In: Haddad GG, Ping YS, editors. Brain hypoxia and ischemia. New York: Humana Press; 2009. p. 153–86.

38. Kinney HC. The encephalopathy of prematurity: one pediatric neuropathologist's perspective. Semin Pediatr Neurol 2009;16:179.

39. Volpe JJ, Kinney HC, Jensen FE, et al. The developing oligodendrocyte: key cellular target in brain injury in the premature infant. Int J Dev Neurosci 2011; 29:423.
40. Peterson BS, Vohr B, Staib LH, et al. Regional brain volume abnormalities and long-term cognitive outcome in preterm infants. JAMA 2000;284:1939.
41. Isaacs EB, Lucas A, Chong WK, et al. Hippocampal volume and everyday memory in children of very low birth weight. Pediatr Res 2000;47:713.
42. Limperopoulos C, Bassan H, Sullivan NR, et al. Positive screening for autism in ex-preterm infants: prevalence and risk factors. Pediatrics 2008; 121:758.
43. Lee JD, Park HJ, Park ES, et al. Motor pathway injury in patients with periventricular leucomalacia and spastic diplegia. Brain 2011;134:1199.
44. Fazzi E, Bova S, Giovenzana A, et al. Cognitive visual dysfunctions in preterm children with periventricular leukomalacia. Dev Med Child Neurol 2009;51:974.
45. Folkerth RD, Kinney HC. Perinatal Neuropathology. In: Love S, Louis DN, Ellison DW, editors. Greenfield's Neuropathology. Vol. 1. 8th edition. London, UK: Arnold; 2009. p. 241–334.
46. Kadhim HJ, Tabarki B, Verellen G, et al. Inflammatory cytokines in the pathogenesis of periventricular leukomalacia. Neurology 2001;56:1278.
47. Desilva TM, Billiards SS, Borenstein NS, et al. Glutamate transporter EAAT2 expression is up-regulated in reactive astrocytes in human periventricular leukomalacia. J Comp Neurol 2008;508:238.
48. Haynes RL, Folkerth RD, Trachtenberg FL, et al. Nitrosative stress and inducible nitric oxide synthase expression in periventricular leukomalacia. Acta Neuropathol 2009;118(3):391–9.
49. Haynes RL, Van Leyen K. 12/15-Lipoxygenase expression is increased in oligodendrocytes and microglia of periventricular leukomalacia. Dev Neurosci 2013;35(2–3):140–54.
50. Ricci D, Anker S, Cowan F, et al. Thalamic atrophy in infants with PVL and cerebral visual impairment. Early Hum Dev 2006;82:591.
51. Zubiaurre-Elorza L, Soria-Pastor S, Junque C, et al. Thalamic changes in a preterm sample with periventricular leukomalacia: correlation with white-matter integrity and cognitive outcome at school age. Pediatr Res 2012;71:354.
52. Nagasunder AC, Kinney HC, Bluml S, et al. Abnormal microstructure of the atrophic thalamus in preterm survivors with periventricular leukomalacia. AJNR Am J Neuroradiol 2011;32:185.
53. Lin Y, Okumura A, Hayakawa F, et al. Quantitative evaluation of thalami and basal ganglia in infants with periventricular leukomalacia. Dev Med Child Neurol 2001;43:481.
54. Yokochi K. Thalamic lesions revealed by MR associated with periventricular leukomalacia and clinical profiles of subjects. Acta Paediatr 1997;86:493.
55. Kostovic I, Rakic P. Developmental history of the transient subplate zone in the visual and somatosensory cortex of the macaque monkey and human brain. J Comp Neurol 1990;297:441.
56. Kanold PO, Luhmann HJ. The subplate and early cortical circuits. Annu Rev Neurosci 2010;33:23.
57. Kostovic I, Judas M. Correlation between the sequential ingrowth of afferents and transient patterns of cortical lamination in preterm infants. Anat Rec 2002; 267:1.

58. Suarez-Sola ML, Gonzalez-Delgado FJ, Pueyo-Morlans M, et al. Neurons in the white matter of the adult human neocortex. Front Neuroanat 2009;3:7.

59. Xu G, Broadbelt KG, Haynes RL, et al. Late development of the GABAergic system in the human cerebral cortex and white matter. J Neuropathol Exp Neurol 2011;70:841.

60. Letinic K, Rakic P. Telencephalic origin of human thalamic GABAergic neurons. Nat Neurosci 2001;4:931.

61. Robinson S, Li Q, Dechant A, et al. Neonatal loss of gamma-aminobutyric acid pathway expression after human perinatal brain injury. J Neurosurg 2006;104:396.

Neurologic and Metabolic Issues in Moderately Preterm, Late Preterm, and Early Term Infants

Abbot R. Laptook, MD

KEYWORDS

- Neurologic morbidities • Intracranial hemorrhage • Periventricular leukomalacia
- Apnea • Feeding ability • Suck-swallow-breathing coordination

KEY POINTS

- The frequency of germinal matrix hemorrhage–intraventricular hemorrhage and white matter injury are low in moderately preterm and late preterm infants.
- Apnea of prematurity decreases in frequency as gestational age increases among moderately and late preterm infants.
- Coordination of suck, swallow, and breathing is the major neurologic problem for moderately and late preterm infants.
- Central nervous system integration is essential for coordination of breathing with sucking and swallowing to facilitate safe oral feeding.
- Successful feeding is one of the most important determinants of the duration of hospitalization for moderately preterm and late preterm infants.

Moderately preterm and late preterm infants are generally considered to be low-risk groups of premature infants because they are compared with very preterm or extremely preterm infants. Major morbidities of prematurity reflect both organ-system immaturity and trigger events (infection, inflammation, nutritional state, and so forth), and are the basis of multiple medical problems that very preterm and extremely preterm infants encounter and need to navigate for survival. Fortunately there are prominent gradients in preterm births characterized by marked decreases in the number of infants as gestational age approaches viability. Similarly these same gradients of preterm births have an underappreciated impact on more mature gestational age strata, given the large number of moderately and late preterm births. Late preterm infants are notable for their lower rates of neonatal morbidities compared with more premature infants. However, late preterm infants cannot be considered

A.R. Laptook has nothing to disclose.
Department of Pediatrics, Women & Infants Hospital of Rhode Island, The Warren Alpert Medical School of Brown University, 101 Dudley Street, Providence, RI 02905, USA
E-mail address: alaptook@wihri.org

Clin Perinatol 40 (2013) 723–738
http://dx.doi.org/10.1016/j.clp.2013.07.005   **perinatology.theclinics.com**
0095-5108/13/$ – see front matter © 2013 Elsevier Inc. All rights reserved.

equivalent to term infants because multiple morbidities of prematurity and neonatal mortality are more frequent than in term infants.[1] Moderately preterm infants also have a distinction of low risk when compared with very preterm and extreme preterm infants; however, the morbidity and mortality of moderately preterm infants lies between those of late preterm and very preterm infants.[2] The overall impact of moderately and late preterm infants is the potential for a large effect on public health problems, as noted in the emerging data on the long-term consequences of preterm birth.[3] Specifically there was a stepwise increase in disability among young adults with increasing degrees of preterm birth; however, 74% of the total disability was accounted for by infants born between 33 and 38 weeks. This article focuses primarily on clinical neurologic problems of moderately and late preterm infants, and provides information on early term infants where available. The interface between central control of ventilation, metabolic rate, and temperature regulation is also discussed. This review seeks to identify knowledge gaps in our present state of understanding of moderately preterm and late preterm cohorts.

INTRACRANIAL HEMORRHAGE

For very preterm and extremely preterm infants a common serious neurologic morbidity is intracranial hemorrhage; specifically, germinal matrix hemorrhage–intraventricular hemorrhage (GMH-IVH). Rates of IVH increase with decreasing gestational age[4] and are of a frequency that merit performance of scheduled screening cranial ultrasonography for surveillance of this morbidity.[5] For the late preterm infant, data on the occurrence of GMH-IVH are sparse. Meta-analysis indicates that the frequency of GMH-IVH is very low in late preterm infants.[6] Multiple reports have documented the clinical morbidities manifested by late preterm infants in single centers,[7,8] multicenter consortiums,[9] and population-based cohorts,[10] and do not list GMH-IVH as an assessed morbidity. McIntire and Leveno[1] performed a retrospective cohort study of births at Parkland Hospital, the sole county hospital in Dallas, Texas, over an 18-year period from 1988 to 2005. The study included all live born singleton infants without anomalies born to mothers with prenatal care between 34 and 40 weeks (N = 213,277) and used deliveries at 39 weeks as a reference point. There were 21,771 infants included between 34^0 and 36^6 weeks. Similar to other studies of late preterm infants, multiple morbidities (respiratory distress, transient tachypnea, culture proven sepsis) and mortality decreased progressively from 34 to 39 weeks. GMH-IVH grades 1 and 2 (Papile classification[11]) also decreased with advancing gestational age from 0.5% at 34 weeks to 0.2% at 35 weeks, 0.06% at 36 weeks, and 0.01% at 39 weeks. Severe GMH-IVH (grade 3 and 4) was documented in only 6 infants between 34 and 39 weeks. There were no differences in the frequency of GMH-IVH for early term infants (37 weeks) relative to 39 weeks. Because cranial ultrasonography is not routinely performed in late preterm and term infants, these estimates of GMH-IVH are subject to selection bias and may underestimate the true incidence of GMH-IVH in late preterm and early term infants. By contrast, the incidence of GMH-IVH has been examined in 2675 full-term newborns (gestational age 39.1 $\pm$ 1.2 weeks) between 2003 and 2005 in Poland.[12] Surprisingly, 14.6% of infants had GMH-IVH, and grades 1 and 2 represented 72% and 27%, respectively, of the infants with GMH-IVH. These observations are difficult to reconcile with the reduction in germinal matrix across the third trimester, which presumably is a critical variable in the low rates of GMH-IVH with advancing gestational age.

For the moderately preterm infant there is less systematic assessment of clinical morbidities in comparison with the late preterm infant, which may reflect attention to late preterm infants following the 2005 National Institute of Child Health and Human Development (NICHD) workshop. The latter effort delineated consistent terminology and gestational age of late preterm infants (34^0–36^6 weeks)[13] and identified knowledge gaps that have triggered multiple studies in this area. A similar effort for moderately preterm infants has not occurred. However, there is increasing literature on moderately preterm infants as recognition of the scope of this cohort is appreciated. The most comprehensive data are derived from a population-based analysis of neonatal morbidity in moderately preterm infants (30–34 weeks, N = 6674 infants) using the Swedish Perinatal Quality Registrar for births between 2001 and 2008.[14] Infants born at 30, 31, and 32 weeks were actively screened for GMH-IVH, but not at 33 or 34 weeks. The percentage of infants with any GMH-IVH was 8.3%, 6.2%, and 3.5% for 30, 31, and 32 weeks, respectively, and the rates at 30 and 31 weeks differed from those at 32 weeks. The percentage of infants with grade 3 or 4 IVH was 1.6%, 1.1%, and 1.1% for 30, 31, and 32 weeks, respectively, and the rates at 30 and 31 weeks did not differ from those at 32 weeks. Rates of any GMH-IVH at 33 and 34 weeks were 0.2% and less than 0.1%, and there was less than 0.1% of infants at 34 weeks with grades 3 or 4 IVH. Similar low rates of severe GMH-IVH have been reported in a prospective cohort study using 10 birth hospitals in California and Massachusetts, which examined morbidities among moderately preterm infants of 30 to 34 weeks' gestation admitted to a Neonatal Intensive Care Unit (NICU) between 2001 and 2003.[2] The sample size was 1250 infants and the percentage of infants with grade 3 or 4 GMH-IVH was 1.2% among infants at 30 to 32^6 weeks compared with no severe GMH-IVH among infants at 33 to 34^6 weeks. It is not clear whether routine surveillance using cranial ultrasonography was in place for GMH-IVH and whether there were site differences. Clinical outcomes of 4932 moderately preterm infants (between 32 and 34 weeks) born between 2001 and 2004 have been reported for infants cared for by Paradigm Health, a care management company (453 NICUs in the United States).[15] Grades 3 and 4 GMH-IVH occurred in less than 0.5% of infants at 32 and 33 weeks, and did not occur at 34 weeks. No information was provided on cranial ultrasonography surveillance practices. Similar retrospective data have been reported for a single institution for infants born at 30 to 34 weeks' gestation, but only 38% of infants in this gestational age window underwent cranial ultrasonographys.[16] Analysis of neonatal morbidities of twin pregnancies delivered moderately and late preterm suggest similar low rates of cranial ultrasonographic abnormalities, although no information is provided on ultrasonography screening practices.[17]

Based on the available literature, any GMH-IVH or severe GMH-IVH occurs infrequently in moderately preterm and late preterm infants. Most published reports of the incidence of GMH-IVH in these gestational age strata are subject to selection bias because screening was typically not performed. Given the latter, it could be questioned whether screening should be done for this morbidity. In 2002, a report from the American Academy of Neurology and the Child Neurology Society issued a practice parameter on neuroimaging of the neonate.[5] Routine screening cranial ultrasonography was recommended for all infants of less than 30 weeks' gestation once between 7 and 14 days, optimally to be repeated between 36 and 40 weeks postmenstrual age. The target group for screening cranial ultrasonography is based on a higher incidence of severe GMH-IVH, which could affect clinical management (eg, post-hemorrhagic hydrocephalus). Studies that used gestational age as an inclusion criterion and contributed to this practice guideline reported that severe GMH-IVH (Papile grades 3 or 4) occurred in 1% to 2% of infants with a gestational age greater than 30 weeks.[18,19] A more recent retrospective review of 486 infants with a gestational age of 30 to 33 weeks and born between 1999 and 2004 determined the number of infants with clinically important abnormal screening cranial ultrasonograms at 7 to 10 days.[20] GMH-IVH occurred in 4.3% of infants, and grades 3 or 4 GMH-IVH occurred in 0.8% of infants (all 30–31 weeks). In addition to supporting the 2002 practice guideline, the investigators noted that infants with grades 3 or 4 GMH-IVH had symptoms or a clinical history that would have prompted neuroimaging.

PERIVENTRICULAR LEUKOMALACIA

Relative to GMH-IVH there are even fewer data on periventricular leukomalacia (PVL) in late preterm infants from single-center reports,[1,7,8] multicenter consortiums,[9] or meta-analysis.[6] There are limited data on moderately preterm infants. In the population-based Swedish study,[14] cystic PVL occurred in 1.6%, 1.1%, and 1.0% of infants at 30, 31, and 32 weeks' gestation, respectively. The incidence did not differ across these 3 weeks of gestation. At 33 weeks (n = 1564) and 34 weeks (n = 2620), cystic PVL was reported in 0.3% and 0.1% of infants, but systematic cranial ultrasonography screening was not used. The practice parameter on neuroimaging[5] also noted that cystic PVL was detected in 5% to 26% of infants with a birth weight less than 1 kg, compared with 1% to 5% of infants with a birth weight greater than 1 kg. Screening guidelines for cystic PVL are similar to those for GMH-IVH.[5] In view of the prognostic importance of white matter injury, clinicians need to maintain an index of suspicion to guide the use of neuroimaging for infants at or beyond 30 weeks' gestation. In an analysis of 486 infants born between 30 and 33 weeks and undergoing cranial ultrasonography at 7 to 10 days and at 40 weeks postmenstrual age, abnormalities were found in 9%.[20] The latter included GMH-IVH, cystic PVL, intraparenchymal hemorrhage, lissencephaly, agenesis of the corpus callosum, colpocephaly, and choroid plexus cyst. Of the 7 infants with cystic PVL, 5 had a birth weight greater than 1500 g. Townsend and colleagues[21] also reported the occurrence of cystic PVL in infants between 30 and 32 weeks, and noted that clinical characteristics were not helpful in guiding who to image. The importance of the diagnosis of cystic PVL is based on analysis of neurodevelopmental outcomes of extremely low birth weight infants; the odds ratio for neurodevelopmental impairment (any one of Bayley Scales of Infant Development <70, cerebral palsy, or sensory deficits) was highest for cystic PVL, in contrast to all other neonatal morbidities.[22]

Factors that contribute to the putative low rates of PVL in moderately preterm, late preterm, and early term infants reflect the developmental origin of PVL. PVL is a complex process, which fundamentally reflects a loss of early differentiating oligodendrocytes, premyelinating oligodendrocytes (pre-OLs), which lead to astrogliosis and microgliosis.[23,24] The injury and loss of the pre-OLs ultimately contribute to a diffuse myelinating disturbance, which is accompanied by neuronal and axonal abnormalities in the subplate neurons, thalamus, basal ganglia, cerebral cortex, brainstem, and cerebellum.[25] Inciting mechanisms that initiate injury to the pre-OLs are multiple and include hypoxia-ischemia (altered hemodynamics, hypocarbia) and infection/inflammation. These events trigger cellular mechanisms (microglial activation, excitotoxicity, and free radical injury), leading to loss of the pre-OLs.[24] PVL is of greatest risk to infants who are born before 32 weeks' gestation, and reflects developmental processes related to (1) the time of appearance and regional distribution of oligodendrocyte progenitors,[23] and (2) a maturation-dependent window of vulnerability to mechanisms of injury most prominent before 32 weeks. Examples of the latter include the propensity for oxidative injury secondary to delayed development of antioxidant enzymes at gestations before moderately preterm birth.[26]

An important issue affecting the frequency of PVL is the neuroimaging mode of detection. PVL can result in focal necrosis with loss of all cellular elements or a more diffuse injury with loss of specific cells (pre-OLs), leading to astrogliosis and microgliosis.[24] When the focal component is of a critical size, cysts can be detected using cranial ultrasonography. By contrast, diffuse involvement does not culminate in cysts, but rather glial scars; the latter cannot be detected by cranial ultrasonography. Noncystic PVL is currently considered the dominant form of PVL, and cystic PVL may only account for approximately 10% of infants with PVL.[27] Although cranial ultrasonography is the primary imaging modality for premature infants, its limitations are recognized. Studies that have compared detection of brain injury using cranial ultrasonography and magnetic resonance imaging (MRI) are consistent in their conclusion that MRI is better than cranial ultrasonography at detecting white matter injury.[28,29] Much of this reflects the inability of cranial ultrasonography to detect diffuse PVL. Whether the prognostic value of predicting neurodevelopment by MRI is superior to that by cranial ultrasonography remains unclear, because the specific abnormalities detected by either modality have wide confidence limits in the prediction of outcome.[30] There are currently no specific recommendations for neuroimaging of moderately preterm, late preterm, or early term infants.

APNEA

Apnea is a common problem among premature infants, although precise estimates of incidence are difficult to obtain because of differences in definition, acquisition, and documentation of events, and uncertainties in distinguishing bradycardic episodes with shallow breathing from true apnea. Among 450 infants born between 30^0 and 34^6 weeks, nearly all infants born at 30 weeks had apneic episodes (92%), with progressive decreases in the prevalence with advancing gestational age (30% at 34 weeks).[31] Among 264 infants born between 33^0 and 34^6 weeks' gestation, 49% were diagnosed with apnea.[32] Using a meta-analysis of studies of late preterm infants (34^0–36^6 weeks at delivery), apnea occurred in 0.9% of infants with progressive decreases (2.1%, 0.7%, and 0.4%) across the gestational ages of 34, 35, and 36 weeks, respectively.[6] Even though the frequency of apnea among late preterm infants is low, it represents a 15.7-fold increase in relative risk (95% confidence interval 11.8–20.9) compared with term infants. Specific data for early term infants is not available. Eichenwald and colleagues[31] have demonstrated that the resolution of apnea among infants born at 30^0 to 34^6 weeks' gestation occurs on average between 34 and 35 weeks with a somewhat later postmenstrual age for late preterm infants. The pathogenesis of apnea of prematurity is multifactorial, and many maturational variables under central control (eg, ventilator responses to hypoxia and CO_2) are a reflection of an immature brainstem neural circuitry while others reflect upper airway and chest wall/pulmonary considerations.[33] As preterm infants approach postmenstrual ages of 34 weeks and beyond, a greater percentage of apnea episodes are associated with feeding, and represent incomplete integration of breathing with suck and swallow.

MATURATION OF FEEDING ABILITY

In contrast to the common neurologic morbidities of GMH-IVH, PVL, and apnea of prematurity encountered in very preterm and extremely preterm infants, moderately and late preterm infants have very different neurologic issues. The most common clinical problem manifested in late preterm infants is feeding difficulties. In a systematic review of medical and developmental short-term and long-term outcomes of late preterm infants, feeding difficulties were documented in 34% of late preterm infants and represented the most common short-term morbidity encountered by this cohort.[6] The absolute risk of feeding difficulties decreased from 51% to 34% to 22% at 34, 35, and 36 weeks' gestation. Compared with term infants, the relative risk for feeding difficulties was higher at each week of gestation within the late preterm window; relative risk and 95% confidence intervals were 9.6 (4.6–19.8), 6.4 (2.9–13.9), and 4.1 (1.8–9.7) for infants born at 34, 35, and 36 weeks' gestation, respectively. Similar observations were reported in the 802 late preterm infants of the Association of Women's Health, Obstetric and Neonatal Nursing (AWHONN) practice project, in which feeding difficulties were identified in 41% of late preterm infants and represented the most common morbidity (**Fig. 1**).[9] Feeding issues of late preterm infants are extensions of maturational development of feeding abilities of the moderately preterm infant. In a cohort of 435 infants born between 30 and 34 weeks to examine inter-NICU variation in time of discharge, the percentage of infants requiring orogastric or nasogastric feeds decreased from 100% at 30 weeks to 42% at 34 weeks.[31]

Feeding issues of moderately preterm and late preterm infants have a clear developmental basis that reflects maturation of sucking, swallowing, and the coordinated interface with respiratory efforts. Immaturity in these mechanisms manifests with slow feeding, choking episodes, desaturation events, bradycardia, and apnea, and represent important contributors to the length of hospital stay. Feeding is a complex activity that requires an integrated approach for efficient coordination between sucking, swallowing, and breathing. For the moderately preterm and late preterm infant such coordination may be difficult, and the demands of feeding may be in conflict with the need for proper ventilation. For example, ventilation measurements by pneumotachometer during nipple feeding among infants with a postmenstrual age of 34 to 35 weeks and 36 to 38 weeks indicated 40% to 50% reductions in minute ventilation during sucking in both gestational-age strata (**Fig. 2**).[34] The change in minute ventilation reflected a decrease in both tidal volume and respiratory frequency, and was associated with a decrease in transcutaneous oxygen tension. The extent to which

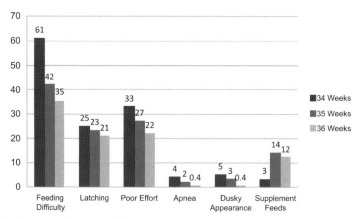

Fig. 1. Distribution of feeding difficulties among late preterm infants in the Association of Women's Health, Obstetric and Neonatal Nursing (AWHONN) report. The cohort represents 802 infants from 34[0] to 36[6] weeks from 14 hospitals. The frequency of feeding difficulties decreases as gestational age increases among late preterm infants. (*From* Medoff Cooper B, Holditch-Davis D, Verklan MT, et al. Newborn clinical outcomes of the AWHONN late preterm infant research-based practice project. J Obstet Gynecol Neonatal Nurs 2012;41(6):779; with permission.)

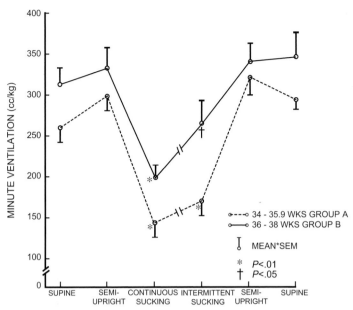

Fig. 2. Minute ventilation during continuous and intermittent sucking intervals among infants of 34 to 35 weeks and 36 to 38 weeks postmenstrual age. Both groups had reductions in minute ventilation during sucking. (*From* Shivpuri CR, Martin RJ, Carlo WA, et al. Decreased ventilation in preterm infants during oral feeding. J Pediatr 1983;103(2):286; with permission.)

early term infants manifest feeding difficulties is unclear. Moderately and late preterm infants may still have feeding problems even when the postmenstrual age is beyond 36 weeks.

The developmental pattern of suck and swallow has been serially studied among infants at a postmenstrual age of 32 to 40 weeks by recording pharyngeal and nipple pressure along with nasal thermistor and thoracic strain-gauge readings from the initiation of oral feeds to discharge.[35] The percentage of sucks aggregated into runs ($\geq$3 sucks with $\leq$2 seconds between sucks) increased with postmenstrual age. Similarly, the length of the sucking runs and the suck rate were both directly correlated with postmenstrual age, but not with postnatal age, supporting a maturational event rather than a learned effort. Swallowing may achieve stability in form and rhythm earlier than suck. Characteristics of swallow runs did not change over the postmenstrual age of 32 to 40 weeks. In moderately preterm and late preterm infants, swallowing can contribute to the reduction in minute ventilation accompanying feeding, a phenomenon known as deglutition apnea. The percentage of swallows with multiple deglutition apneas decreases with advancing postmenstrual age, but is present even in term infants.[36] Advancing neuromuscular maturation is associated with a more rapid swallow and enhanced ability to handle larger and more variable size of feeding bolus.

Sucking can be either nonnutritive or nutritive. Nutritive sucking has been defined as the rhythmic alternation between suction (negative intraoral pressure to pull milk in) with expression, which is the tongue action against the nipple to propel milk into the oral cavity.[37] During nonnutritive sucking, swallowing is not critical and only needs to clear endogenous secretions; respirations may occur independently without adverse effects. By contrast, during nutritive sucking the suck-swallow-respiration sequence must be closely interfaced. Immature nutritive sucking may reflect minimal sucking skills but also may indicate problems at the interface of these 3 critical functions.[38]

The integration of respiratory efforts with suck and swallow functions has been examined among infants at a postmenstrual age of 32 to 40 weeks using recordings of pharyngeal pressure, nasal airflow, and thoracoabdominal strain-gauge readings.[39] Multiple patterns were noted with the initiation of feedings, including breathing during swallows, alternating blocks of suck-swallow and respiratory effort, nasal airflow without thoracic movement, and paired rhythms with swallow/breath ratios greater than 1:1. With advancing postmenstrual age, coordination and phase relationships of suck-swallow and breathing stabilized as well as the percentage of synchronized nasal and thoracic respiratory efforts. Similarly, Lau and colleagues[40] reported that preterm infants swallowed preferentially at phases of respiration different to those of full-term infants. With increasing amounts of feeds taken by nipple, preterm infants shifted to swallowing more during inspiration, suggesting improvement in their ability to simultaneously breathe and feed orally. Of note, the synchronization of suck-swallow with breathing increased significantly after 36 weeks postmenstrual age in comparison with studies performed before 36 weeks (**Table 1**).[39] This potential relatively late maturation of the coordination of suck-swallow-breath is often overlooked by clinical staff.

Coordination by the central nervous system is essential for integration of breathing with sucking and swallowing to facilitate safe oral feeding. This process depends in large part on maturation of the brainstem and a complex interplay with rostral brain elements for appropriate neural control of respiration.[33] Sensorimotor control of oral feeding involves multiple central pattern generator networks, which represent an adaptive combination of neurons that activate groups of motor neurons to generate task-specific motor patterns.[38] Consistent with the clinical studies cited herein, the central pattern generators mature differentially for suck, swallow, and respiration.

The majority of moderately preterm and late preterm infants successfully manifest complete maturation of the suck-swallow-breath coordination to allow for successful oral feeding. However, there is considerable variability among preterm infants at the postmenstrual age when successful feeding is achieved; it is uncertain when feeding difficulties no longer represent a maturational delay but rather a pathologic state. Interventions to facilitate optimal feeding usually consist of simple noninvasive measures such as standardization of the feeding technique, close attention to the behavioral state and organization, and attention of the caregiver to the handling of the infant. More challenging feeding problems occur in very preterm and extremely preterm infants who have been intubated for prolonged time intervals, and may be

Table 1
Increases in respiratory synchrony between respirations and swallowing with advancing postmenstrual age

Postmenstrual Age (wk)	Apnea (% ± SD)	Unsynchronized (% ± SD)	Synchronized (% ± SD)
32^0–33^6	22.5 ± 5.2	64.3 ± 5.5	13.1 ± 6.0
34^0–35^9	21.7 ± 7.4	62.7 ± 5.8	15.8 ± 4.4
$\geq 36^0$	10.2 ± 2.7	43.0 ± 13.3	46.8 ± 15.4[a]

Abbreviation: SD, standard deviation.
[a] $P<.05$ for synchronized of ≥ 36 weeks versus both 32^0–33^6 and 34^0–35^9 postmenstrual age.
From Vice FL, Gewolb IH. Respiratory patterns and strategies during feeding in preterm infants. Dev Med Child Neurol 2008;50(6):469; with permission.

developing or have developed an oral aversion. Even short-term morbidities may affect feeding ability. Among infants with respiratory distress syndrome assessed at least 5 days following extubation and with oxygen saturation values higher than 92%, nonnutritive suck pressure amplitude is reduced compared with that in healthy preterm infants.[41] Furthermore, more extensive oxygen therapy alters the oral sensory environment, reduces motor experiences, and can disrupt the development of a coordinated nonnutritive suck in preterm infants.[42] Interventions are becoming available whereby patterned orocutaneous stimulation delivered through a pneumatic silicone pacifier can entrain preterm infants and facilitate suck development.[43]

HYPOXIC-ISCHEMIC ENCEPHALOPATHY

Neonatal encephalopathy caused by perinatal hypoxic-ischemic injury is a final common pathway for multiple perinatal conditions such as uteroplacental dysfunction, cord and/or placental accidents, acute blood loss, infection, and maternal hemodynamic compromise. It may affect fetuses and infants of all gestational ages, and is an important identifiable determinant of death and neurodevelopmental outcome. Although many interventions to ameliorate perinatal hypoxic-ischemic brain injury have been proposed and tested, only hypothermia (whole-body cooling with core temperature of 33°–34°C or head and body cooling with core temperature of 34°–35°C) has been demonstrated in multiple randomized trials to offer significant benefit in human newborns at or beyond 36 weeks' gestation.[44] Based on pooled data from 6 large randomized clinical trials, the effect size of therapeutic hypothermia is an absolute reduction of 15% (relative risk reduction 0.24) in the incidence of death or disability at 18 to 22 months.[44] These trials uniformly enrolled infants beyond 35 or 36 weeks' gestation. No interaction between gestational age and treatment effect has been reported. Although preterm infants may also suffer perinatal hypoxic-ischemic injury, systematic assessment of the safety and utility of therapeutic hypothermia in infants less than 35 to 36 weeks has not been undertaken. Application of therapeutic hypothermia in moderately and late preterm infants remains an important knowledge gap.[45] Use of therapeutic hypothermia in moderately and late preterm infants (<35–36 weeks' gestation) with encephalopathy has occurred outside of clinical trials, as documented in the registry established following the TOBY trial[46] and in the Vermont Oxford Neonatal Encephalopathy Registry.[47]

There are important challenges for rigorous evaluation of therapeutic hypothermia as neuroprotective therapy for moderately preterm and late preterm infants. All trials of therapeutic hypothermia in newborns have included a neurologic examination to confirm the presence of encephalopathy. The Sarnat criteria, as well as the modified Sarnat criteria used for neurologic qualification in the original NICHD Neonatal Research Network hypothermia study,[48] were based on findings in infants at or beyond 36 weeks gestational age at birth.[49] Even healthy preterm infants may have systematic developmental differences in primitive reflexes, tone, and posture that modify interpretation of the neurologic examination and pose challenges to determining the presence of encephalopathy. For example, hypotonia is common in premature infants and is not necessarily pathologic, and pupil reaction to light only begins to appear at 30 weeks' gestation and is not consistently present until 32 to 35 weeks.[27] The variability of primitive reflexes, tone, posture, and autonomic function in infants of less than 36 weeks' gestation will make it challenging to ensure clinical evidence of neurologic dysfunction.

Another important aspect of the application of therapeutic hypothermia for moderately preterm and late preterm infants is potential adverse effects. Hypothermia may cause many of the same medical problems that are associated with hypoxia-ischemia (eg, thrombocytopenia, disseminated intravascular coagulopathy, arrhythmias, persistent pulmonary hypertension, subcutaneous fat necrosis).[50] At present, use of therapeutic hypothermia predominantly for infants at or beyond 36 weeks' gestation has been well tolerated. The most common adverse effects of therapeutic hypothermia have included bradycardia and thrombocytopenia, which can be managed clinically and have not resulted in altering or stopping the therapy.[51] It remains unclear whether the risk/benefit ratio will change when using therapeutic hypothermia in moderately or late preterm infants with a hypoxic-ischemic injury. Prospective surveillance for adverse effects is essential, and needs to include imaging to ensure that the low prevalence of GMH-IVH is not dramatically increased by hypoxia-ischemia itself or the addition of therapeutic hypothermia. Walsh and colleagues[52] compared outcome for 48 infants of 32 to 35 weeks' gestation and 1289 infants at or beyond 36 weeks' gestation who underwent therapeutic hypothermia for encephalopathy using the combined databases of Pediatrix and the TOBY registry, and found no increase in mortality. However, the small numbers and absence of a single rigorous hypothermia protocol make it difficult to confirm the robustness of this conclusion.

A final consideration for potential application of therapeutic hypothermia in moderately preterm and late preterm infants is feasibility based on the frequency of encephalopathy to provide sufficient patients for a well-designed randomized trial. Salhab and Perlman[53] retrospectively observed that 62 of 5533 infants born between 31 and 36 weeks' gestation over 10 years at a single institution (Parkland Hospital, Dallas, Texas) had an umbilical arterial cord gas with a pH of less than 7.00, and 7 of these infants had moderate or severe encephalopathy (1.3 in 1000). Schmidt and Walsh[54] noted an incidence of 8 in 1000, based on 12 of approximately 1500 infants born at 32 to 36 weeks' gestation at a single center over a 6-year period. These preliminary reports suggest a wide range in the rate of clinically important encephalopathy in moderately and late preterm infants. It remains to be determined whether a rigorous clinical trial can be conducted, even in multicenter networks.

PERINATAL STROKE

Strokes in moderately preterm and late preterm infants are uncommon, but do occur. The incidence of vascular occlusive events, termed ischemic perinatal stroke, is estimated to range from 1 in 2300 to 1 in 5000 births, and represents an important etiologic factor in the development of neurologic sequelae such as cerebral palsy.[55] Strokes can affect the newborn with possible manifestations in utero (fetal imaging required), during the neonatal period, and after 28 days of age. However, the timing of when strokes occur remains an important unresolved issue because clinically silent strokes may not become apparent until developmental deficits are observed later in childhood. Ischemic perinatal stroke can be arterial or venous sinus in origin, although the former is more common. The incidence of arterial ischemic stroke in preterm infants remains unclear; in the Kaiser Permanente cohort study 15% were preterm,[56] and in the International Pediatric Stroke Study 8% were preterm.[57] Associated risk factors are identifiable in term infants but much less so in preterm infants.[58] The most common manifestation of arterial ischemic stroke is seizures in term infants. In preterm infants seizures appear to occur less frequently, and imaging often detects the presence of this lesion.[58,59] Whether, in comparison with term infants, preterm infants with arterial ischemic stroke have a similar vascular distribution or a potential cause (embolic event originating from the placenta and passing through the patent foramen ovale) remains unclear.

CONTROL OF BREATHING AND THERMOREGULATION

Despite limited data, it appears that brainstem development and neural control of respiration progressively matures across the moderately preterm and late preterm gestational-age strata.[33] Although respiratory drive is centrally controlled, pulmonary ventilation is responsive to changes in body temperature, which in large part can be explained by corresponding changes in metabolic rate.[60] These interrelationships have important implications for establishment of ventilation at birth and sustainment of respirations during the neonatal hospitalization. When the newborn is exposed to cold, core temperature is either maintained or drops, and ventilation follows metabolic rate.[61] Exposure to cold serves to trigger an increase in oxygen consumption (to generate heat as part of the homeothermic response of mammals), and ventilation increases secondary to changes in metabolism. Some degree of cold exposure can be viewed as a necessary prerequisite to initiate respirations at birth. The converse is also true: there is a strong association between elevated maternal temperature, poor respiratory effort at birth, and the need for positive pressure ventilation.[62] In the clinical setting, one of the first steps of newborn stabilization at birth is to minimize excessive reductions in core temperature caused by heat loss to the ambient environment.[63] When caring for moderately preterm and late preterm infants, the dramatic change in thermal conditions from in utero to the delivery room poses greater challenges in avoiding excessive heat loss relative to term infants. Because body temperature is the balance between heat production and heat loss, unless measures are taken immediately on delivery to avoid excessive heat loss, birth is associated with an inevitable decrease in temperature. Heat loss is governed by heat transfer between an infant and the environment and is composed of evaporative, convective, conductive, and radiant heat loss; these losses typically overwhelm the ability of a newborn to generate sufficient heat to maintain temperature. Thus, the physical environment and interventions to minimize heat loss are critical to the temperature on admission to the NICU.[64]

Avoidance of extreme cold stress in infants of less than 30 weeks' gestation has focused on the use of occlusive wraps and/or exothermic mattresses in addition to basic provision of heat and thorough drying when wraps are not used.[65,66] By contrast, there has been relatively little published regarding admission temperatures of moderately and late preterm and early term infants. Given the frequency of low admission temperatures for very preterm infants, surveillance of temperatures in the delivery room and on admission is an appropriate, worthwhile quality-improvement initiative for all infants triaged to an intensive care unit.[67] **Fig. 3** illustrates temperature on admission for in-born infants at the Women and Infants Hospital of Rhode Island. Infants born at less than 30 weeks are dried on exothermic mattresses under a preheated radiant warmer, and infants born at up to 26 weeks are also placed in occlusive wraps without drying the body, followed by drying of the head. Infants born at or beyond 30 weeks are dried on preheated radiant warmers with multiple warm blankets. With these interventions, admission temperatures of less than 36°C occurred in 4% of infants of less than 30 weeks, compared with 23% for infants at or beyond 30 weeks. These data indicate that measures to reduce heat loss in the delivery room (preheating the radiant warmer, use of multiple warm blankets to adequately dry, increasing the ambient room temperature) are critically important for moderately and late preterm infants. The latter reflects lower birth weight, higher surface area to weight ratios, and relatively less brown fat among these gestational-age cohorts. The data suggest that current measures to limit heat loss in infants at or beyond 30 weeks need to be performed more effectively, or other interventions to reduce heat loss may become necessary. Quality-improvement surveillance of admission

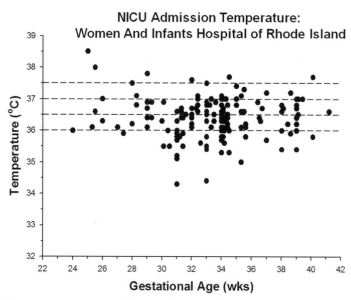

NICU Admission Temperature: Women And Infants Hospital of Rhode Island

Gestational Age (wks)

Fig. 3. Axilla temperatures on admission of in-born infants at Women and Infants Hospital of Rhode Island from December 2011 through February 2012. Time from birth to admission temperature ranged between 20 and 25 minutes. (*Data from* Women and Infants Hospital of Rhode Island, Providence, RI.)

temperatures can assist with these efforts. Once in the NICU, there are sparse data regarding hypothermia among moderately preterm infants. Meta-analysis of limited data for hypothermia among late preterm infants indicated a prevalence of 1.5% compared with 0.08% for term infants.[6] Detail regarding the clinical scenarios accompanying these percentages is limited, but presumably reflects failure to wean from isolettes and the need to return to a heated environment.

SUMMARY

Moderately preterm and late preterm infants are distinctly different from very preterm and extremely preterm infants with respect to neurologic medical problems. Moderately and late preterm infants are at low risk for serious neurologic events such as GMH-IVH and white matter disease. Apnea of prematurity is common, but the frequency decreases with advancing gestational age. The major neurologic problem encountered by moderately and late preterm infants is coordination of sucking, swallowing, and breathing to allow for successful and uneventful feeding. The complex process of feeding depends on progressive maturation of the central nervous system to provide coordination and synchronization of these functions. Successful feeding is one of the most important determinants of the duration of hospitalization among moderately and late preterm infants. Variability in the postconceptual age at which a completely integrated feeding process occurs is not uncommon, and may not occur until beyond 36 weeks postconceptual age for many moderately and late preterm infants.

REFERENCES

1. McIntire DD, Leveno KJ. Neonatal mortality and morbidity rates in late preterm births compared with births at term. Obstet Gynecol 2008;111(1):35–41.

2. Escobar GJ, McCormick MC, Zupancic JA, et al. Unstudied infants: outcomes of moderately premature infants in the neonatal intensive care unit. Arch Dis Child Fetal Neonatal Ed 2006;91(4):F238–44.
3. Lindstrom K, Winbladh B, Haglund B, et al. Preterm infants as young adults: a Swedish national cohort study. Pediatrics 2007;120(1):70–7.
4. Stoll BJ, Hansen NI, Bell EF, et al. Neonatal outcomes of extremely preterm infants from the NICHD Neonatal Research Network. Pediatrics 2010;126(3):443–56.
5. Ment LR, Bada HS, Barnes P, et al. Practice parameter: neuroimaging of the neonate: report of the Quality Standards Subcommittee of the American Academy of Neurology and the Practice Committee of the Child Neurology Society. Neurology 2002;58(12):1726–38.
6. Teune MJ, Bakhuizen S, Gyamfi Bannerman C, et al. A systematic review of severe morbidity in infants born late preterm. Am J Obstet Gynecol 2011; 205(4):374.e1–9.
7. Wang ML, Dorer DJ, Fleming MP, et al. Clinical outcomes of near-term infants. Pediatrics 2004;114(2):372–6.
8. Dimitriou G, Fouzas S, Georgakis V, et al. Determinants of morbidity in late preterm infants. Early Hum Dev 2010;86(9):587–91.
9. Medoff Cooper B, Holditch-Davis D, Verklan MT, et al. Newborn clinical outcomes of the AWHONN late preterm infant research-based practice project. J Obstet Gynecol Neonatal Nurs 2012;41(6):774–85.
10. Khashu M, Narayanan M, Bhargava S, et al. Perinatal outcomes associated with preterm birth at 33 to 36 weeks' gestation: a population-based cohort study. Pediatrics 2009;123(1):109–13.
11. Papile LA, Burstein J, Burstein R, et al. Incidence and evolution of subependymal and intraventricular hemorrhage: a study of infants with birth weights less than 1,500 gm. J Pediatr 1978;92(4):529–34.
12. Baumert M, Brozek G, Paprotny M, et al. Epidemiology of peri/intraventricular haemorrhage in newborns at term. J Physiol Pharmacol 2008;59(Suppl 4):67–75.
13. Engle WA. A recommendation for the definition of "late preterm" (near-term) and the birth weight-gestational age classification system. Semin Perinatol 2006; 30(1):2–7.
14. Altman M, Vanpee M, Cnattingius S, et al. Neonatal morbidity in moderately preterm infants: a Swedish national population-based study. J Pediatr 2011; 158(2):239–44.e1.
15. Kirkby S, Greenspan JS, Kornhauser M, et al. Clinical outcomes and cost of the moderately preterm infant. Adv Neonatal Care 2007;7(2):80–7.
16. Bhat V, Karam M, Saslow J, et al. Utility of performing routine head ultrasounds in preterm infants with gestational age 30-34 weeks. J Matern Fetal Neonatal Med 2012;25(2):116–9.
17. Refuerzo JS, Momirova V, Peaceman AM, et al. Neonatal outcomes in twin pregnancies delivered moderately preterm, late preterm, and term. Am J Perinatol 2010;27(7):537–42.
18. Batton DG, Holtrop P, DeWitte D, et al. Current gestational age-related incidence of major intraventricular hemorrhage. J Pediatr 1994;125(4):623–5.
19. Harding D, Kuschel C, Evans N. Should preterm infants born after 29 weeks' gestation be screened for intraventricular haemorrhage? J Paediatr Child Health 1998;34(1):57–9.
20. Harris NJ, Palacio D, Ginzel A, et al. Are routine cranial ultrasounds necessary in premature infants greater than 30 weeks gestation? Am J Perinatol 2007;24(1): 17–21.

21. Townsend SF, Rumack CM, Thilo EH, et al. Late neurosonographic screening is important to the diagnosis of periventricular leukomalacia and ventricular enlargement in preterm infants. Pediatr Radiol 1999;29(5):347–52.
22. Vohr BR, Wright LL, Poole WK, et al. Neurodevelopmental outcomes of extremely low birth weight infants <32 weeks' gestation between 1993 and 1998. Pediatrics 2005;116(3):635–43.
23. Back SA, Riddle A, McClure MM. Maturation-dependent vulnerability of perinatal white matter in premature birth. Stroke 2007;38(Suppl 2):724–30.
24. Volpe JJ, Kinney HC, Jensen FE, et al. The developing oligodendrocyte: key cellular target in brain injury in the premature infant. Int J Dev Neurosci 2011; 29(4):423–40.
25. Volpe JJ. Brain injury in premature infants: a complex amalgam of destructive and developmental disturbances. Lancet Neurol 2009;8(1):110–24.
26. Folkerth RD, Haynes RL, Borenstein NS, et al. Developmental lag in superoxide dismutases relative to other antioxidant enzymes in premyelinated human telencephalic white matter. J Neuropathol Exp Neurol 2004;63(9):990–9.
27. Volpe JJ. Neurology of the newborn. 5th edition. Philadelphia: Saunders Elsevier; 2008.
28. Maalouf EF, Duggan PJ, Counsell SJ, et al. Comparison of findings on cranial ultrasound and magnetic resonance imaging in preterm infants. Pediatrics 2001;107(4):719–27.
29. Inder TE, Huppi PS, Warfield S, et al. Periventricular white matter injury in the premature infant is followed by reduced cerebral cortical gray matter volume at term. Ann Neurol 1999;46(5):755–60.
30. Nongena P, Ederies A, Azzopardi DV, et al. Confidence in the prediction of neurodevelopmental outcome by cranial ultrasound and MRI in preterm infants. Arch Dis Child Fetal Neonatal Ed 2010;95(6):F388–90.
31. Eichenwald EC, Blackwell M, Lloyd JS, et al. Inter-neonatal intensive care unit variation in discharge timing: influence of apnea and feeding management. Pediatrics 2001;108(4):928–33.
32. Eichenwald EC, Zupancic JA, Mao WY, et al. Variation in diagnosis of apnea in moderately preterm infants predicts length of stay. Pediatrics 2011;127(1): e53–8.
33. Darnall RA, Ariagno RL, Kinney HC. The late preterm infant and the control of breathing, sleep, and brainstem development: a review. Clin Perinatol 2006; 33(4):883–914.
34. Shivpuri CR, Martin RJ, Carlo WA, et al. Decreased ventilation in preterm infants during oral feeding. J Pediatr 1983;103(2):285–9.
35. Gewolb IH, Vice FL, Schwietzer-Kenney EL, et al. Developmental patterns of rhythmic suck and swallow in preterm infants. Dev Med Child Neurol 2001; 43(1):22–7.
36. Hanlon MB, Tripp JH, Ellis RE, et al. Deglutition apnoea as indicator of maturation of suckle feeding in bottle-fed preterm infants. Dev Med Child Neurol 1997; 39(8):534–42.
37. Lau C. Oral feeding in the preterm infant. Neoreviews 2006;7:e19–27.
38. Barlow SM. Oral and respiratory control for preterm feeding. Curr Opin Otolaryngol Head Neck Surg 2009;17(3):179–86.
39. Vice FL, Gewolb IH. Respiratory patterns and strategies during feeding in preterm infants. Dev Med Child Neurol 2008;50(6):467–72.
40. Lau C, Smith EO, Schanler RJ. Coordination of suck-swallow and swallow respiration in preterm infants. Acta Paediatr 2003;92(6):721–7.

41. Stumm S, Barlow SM, Estep M, et al. Respiratory distress syndrome degrades the fine structure of the non-nutritive suck in preterm infants. J Neonatal Nurs 2008;14(1):9–16.

42. Poore M, Barlow SM, Wang J, et al. Respiratory treatment history predicts suck pattern stability in preterm infants. J Neonatal Nurs 2008;14(6):185–92.

43. Barlow SM, Finan DS, Lee J, et al. Synthetic orocutaneous stimulation entrains preterm infants with feeding difficulties to suck. J Perinatol 2008;28(8):541–8.

44. Tagin MA, Woolcott CG, Vincer MJ, et al. Hypothermia for neonatal hypoxic ischemic encephalopathy: an updated systematic review and meta-analysis. Arch Pediatr Adolesc Med 2012;166(6):558–66.

45. Higgins RD, Raju T, Edwards AD, et al. Hypothermia and other treatment options for neonatal encephalopathy: an executive summary of the Eunice Kennedy Shriver NICHD workshop. J Pediatr 2011;159(5):851–8.e1.

46. Azzopardi D, Strohm B, Linsell L, et al. Implementation and conduct of therapeutic hypothermia for perinatal asphyxial encephalopathy in the UK–analysis of national data. PLoS One 2012;7(6):e38504.

47. Pfister RH, Bingham P, Carpenter JH, et al. Hypothermia in practice, initial observations from the Vermont Oxford Network. Pediatric Academic Societies' Vancouver BC, Canada, Abstract# 26325. 2010.

48. Shankaran S, Laptook AR, Ehrenkranz RA, et al. Whole-body hypothermia for neonates with hypoxic-ischemic encephalopathy. N Engl J Med 2005;353(15):1574–84.

49. Sarnat HB, Sarnat MS. Neonatal encephalopathy following fetal distress. A clinical and electroencephalographic study. Arch Neurol 1976;33(10):696–705.

50. Eicher DJ, Wagner CL, Katikaneni LP, et al. Moderate hypothermia in neonatal encephalopathy: safety outcomes. Pediatr Neurol 2005;32(1):18–24.

51. Shah PS. Hypothermia: a systematic review and meta-analysis of clinical trials. Semin Fetal Neonatal Med 2010;15(5):238–46.

52. Walsh WF, Azzopardi D, Hobson A, et al. Survival of infants between 32-35 weeks gestation treated with hypothermia for hypoxic ischemic encephalopathy. Pediatric Academic Societies' Denver, CO, Abstract# 36754. 2011.

53. Salhab WA, Perlman JM. Severe fetal acidemia and subsequent neonatal encephalopathy in the larger premature infant. Pediatr Neurol 2005;32(1):25–9.

54. Schmidt JW, Walsh WF. Hypoxic-ischemic encephalopathy in preterm infants. J Neonatal Perinatal Med 2010;3:277–84.

55. Raju TN, Nelson KB, Ferriero D, et al. Ischemic perinatal stroke: summary of a workshop sponsored by the National Institute of Child Health and Human Development and the National Institute of Neurological Disorders and Stroke. Pediatrics 2007;120(3):609–16.

56. Lee J, Croen LA, Backstrand KH, et al. Maternal and infant characteristics associated with perinatal arterial stroke in the infant. JAMA 2005;293(6):723–9.

57. Kirton A, Armstrong-Wells J, Chang T, et al. Symptomatic neonatal arterial ischemic stroke: the International Pediatric Stroke Study. Pediatrics 2011;128(6):e1402–10.

58. Benders MJ, Groenendaal F, De Vries LS. Preterm arterial ischemic stroke. Semin Fetal Neonatal Med 2009;14(5):272–7.

59. Lee HJ, Lim BC, Hwang H, et al. Clinical presentations and neurodevelopmental outcomes of perinatal stroke in preterm and term neonates: a case series. J Korean Med Sci 2010;25(6):888–94.

60. Mortola JP. Influence of temperature on metabolism and breathing during mammalian ontogenesis. Respir Physiol Neurobiol 2005;149(1–3):155–64.

61. Mortola JP, Gautier H. Interaction between metabolism and ventilation: effects of respiratory gases and temperature. In: Dempsey JA, Pack AI, editors. Regulation of breathing. 2nd edition. New York: Marcel Dekker; 1995. p. 1011–64.

62. Lieberman E, Eichenwald E, Mathur G, et al. Intrapartum fever and unexplained seizures in term infants. Pediatrics 2000;106(5):983–8.

63. Kattwinkel J, editor. Neonatal resuscitation textbook. Elk Grove Village, Illinois: American Academy of Pediatrics; 2011. p. 37–70.

64. Laptook AR, Watkinson M. Temperature management in the delivery room. Semin Fetal Neonatal Med 2008;13(6):383–91.

65. Cramer K, Wiebe N, Hartling L, et al. Heat loss prevention: a systematic review of occlusive skin wrap for premature neonates. J Perinatol 2005;25(12):763–9.

66. Singh A, Duckett J, Newton T, et al. Improving neonatal unit admission temperatures in preterm babies: exothermic mattresses, polythene bags or a traditional approach? J Perinatol 2010;30(1):45–9.

67. Laptook AR, Salhab W, Bhaskar B. Admission temperature of low birth weight infants: predictors and associated morbidities. Pediatrics 2007;119(3):e643–9.

Long-Term Outcomes of Moderately Preterm, Late Preterm, and Early Term Infants

Betty Vohr, MD

KEYWORDS

- Moderate preterm • Late preterm • Early term • Neurodevelopment • Outcomes

KEY POINTS

- Brain weight at 34 weeks' gestation is 60% of the brain weight of a full-term (FT) infant.
- Moderate preterm (MPT) (32–33 weeks) and late preterm (LPT) (34–36 weeks) survivors are at increased risk of neurologic impairments, developmental disabilities, school failure, as well as behavioral and psychiatric problems from infancy to adulthood.
- MPT and LPT infants are at increased risk of having disabilities requiring early intervention, therapeutic services, and special education support services.

BACKGROUND

The National Institute of Child Health and Human Development panel reviewed the evidence of increased risk of infants with a gestation age of 34 to 36 weeks and changed the earlier definition of "near term" to "LPT" in 2006.[1] Currently, MPT infants born at 32 to 33 weeks' gestation and LPT infants born at 34 to 36 weeks' gestation make up the largest subgroup of preterm (PT) infants and contribute to more than 80% of premature births in the United States. There are increasing numbers of reports that both MPT and LPT infants are at increased risk of neonatal and postdischarge morbidity. In the United States in 2009, 12.18% of the 4,130,665 births were PT. Of these, 8.7% (357,715) were LPT. An additional 144,986 (3.5%) of births include MPT and very PT infants less than 32 weeks' gestational age (GA).[2] Multiple gestation, which comprises about 3% of births in the United States and is attributed in part to both delayed childbearing and assisted reproductive technology, contributes significantly to the MPT and LPT birth rate. Among twins, 14.5% are MPT and 49.8% are LPT, and among triplets, 35.5% are MPT and 43.6% are LPT.[3]

Financial Disclosure: Dr B. Vohr has nothing to disclose.
Department of Pediatrics, Women & Infants Hospital, 101 Dudley Street, Providence, RI 02905, USA
E-mail address: bvohr@wihri.org

Clin Perinatol 40 (2013) 739–751
http://dx.doi.org/10.1016/j.clp.2013.07.006
perinatology.theclinics.com

MATERNAL FACTORS

Mothers of PT infants are more likely to have their own medical morbidities including high blood pressure, diabetes, and obesity.[4] Some subgroups of parent-infant dyads may have greater vulnerability. Brandon and colleagues[5] reported that mothers of LPT infants have greater emotional distress (anxiety, postpartum depression, post-traumatic stress symptoms, and worry about their infant) after delivery than mothers of FT infants. In addition, their distress remained higher than that of FT mothers 1 month after delivery. The investigators concluded that multiple factors related to alterations in labor and delivery and the health status of the infant contributed to their distress.[5] Postpartum depression (PPD) is a common disorder and affects an estimated 13% of mothers.[6] Factors associated with PPD include low socioeconomic status and prior history of depression. Acute stress, posttraumatic stress disorder, and depression are common among parents in a neonatal intensive care unit (NICU).[7] The findings of Brandon and colleagues suggest that more attention needs to be shifted to monitoring and supporting the emotional distress of mothers delivering LPT infants.

NEONATAL CHARACTERISTICS

The increased neonatal and postdischarge vulnerability of MPT and particularly LPT infants has been underestimated in the past. Their level of maturation is compromised compared to an FT infant, placing them at increased risk of a spectrum of clinical medical problems including hypothermia, respiratory disorders, hypoglycemia, jaundice, immunologic problems, and increased susceptibility to infection as well as feeding problems.[8] LPT infants are also at increased risk of admission to an NICU, death, and severe neurologic morbidities when compared with FT infants.[9,10] In one large study, LPT infants were 7 times more likely to be admitted to an NICU for more than 5 nights.[11] In addition to underdevelopment of multiple organ systems, the second half of gestation is a critical period of brain development, and at 34 weeks, the brain weight is 60% of the FT brain weight.[12] Between 35 and 41 weeks, there is a 5-fold increase in brain volume.[13] Continued active brain maturation occurs during the last weeks of pregnancy with neurogenesis, synaptogenesis, and dendritic arborization. The interruption of this process by delivery removes the infant from the natural protective environment of the uterus.

POSTDISCHARGE MEDICAL PROBLEMS

After discharge from the hospital, LPT infants continue to have increased medical needs and are 2 to 3 times more likely to be rehospitalized or visit an emergency room than FT infants.[14,15] In an outcome study of 26,703 infants followed up for the first 6 months of life, rehospitalization rates between 15 and 182 days after discharge were inversely related to the GA and ranged from 3.6% for infants born at or after 41 weeks; 4.4%, for 38 to 40 weeks; 5.6%, for 37 weeks; 7.3%, for 36 weeks; 6.8%, for 35 weeks; 9.1%, for 34 weeks; to 9.3%, for 33 weeks.[14] Reasons ranged from respiratory distress, apnea, crying, fever, jaundice, vomiting, to respiratory distress. In a national cohort of commercially insured infants, 15% of LPT infants were rehospitalized in the first year of life.[16] Boyle and colleagues[17] provided population data for health outcomes from the United Kingdom including general health status, rehospitalization, and illness across the full range of GA groups and assessed outcomes of MPT (32–36 weeks) and early term (ET) (37–38 weeks) infants. The investigators reported a gradual gradient of increased risk of poor health outcomes at 3 and

5 years with decreasing GA. These data provide important population-based information that the increasing birth rate of MPT and LPT infants will potentially have a negative societal impact with increased demands of specialized health care provision and increased costs. Further study is needed to assess the relationship between neonatal and short-term health outcomes and neurodevelopmental outcomes for MPT and ET (37–38 weeks) infants.

NEURODEVELOPMENTAL OUTCOME STUDIES

Outcome studies of both MPT and LPT infants indicate that they are at increased risk of developmental disability, school failure, behavior problems, social and medical disabilities, and death.[18–23] There are, however, a limited number of neurodevelopmental studies of MPT and LPT infants, because in the past, they have been considered low risk both as neonates and postdischarge. Most NICUs have follow-up programs for very PT infants who are considered at greatest risk of postdischarge neurodevelopmental morbidity, but do not offer these services for MPT or LPT infants. A recent review of LPT and ET by Engle[24] recommended that large randomized trials are needed to test innovative diagnostic and treatment strategies to inform clinicians about optimal management of women who deliver before 39 weeks' gestation and appropriate management of their offspring. This article reviews neurodevelopmental and behavioral outcomes of MPT and LPT infants dividing them into newborn to preschool, kindergarten to middle school, and adolescence and adult categories. In addition, there is an abbreviated discussion of the outcomes of the ET infants.

Newborn to Preschool

Reports of outcomes of MPT and LPT infants may include low-risk/non-NICU infants, NICU infants only, or a combination of low- and high-risk neonates. This will be clarified if evident in the publication. This section reviews outcomes of infants aged 0 to 5 years with reports summarized in **Table 1**. The first study addresses neurobehavior in the first days of life. A neonatal study of a small cohort[25] of low-risk infants administered the NICU Network Neurobehavioral Scale (NNNS) at the age of 24 to 72 hours of age reported that the LPT (34–36 weeks) infants had decreased scores when compared with FT infants in several domains including attention, arousal, regulation, quality of movements, nonoptimal reflexes, and hypotonicity after adjustment for confounders. This is of interest because these are low-risk LPT infants who are most often considered "normal" and discharged early.

Romeo and colleagues[26] evaluated a low-risk LPT group with no evidence of brain injury compared with FT infants at 12 and 18 months of age. When comparing scores by chronological age (ChrA), the LPTs scored significantly lower; however, when comparing by corrected age (CA), there was no difference in scores compared with FT infants at either age. This raises the question of whether the examiner should be using CA for LPT infants. The findings of this study indicate that LPT infants would not be eligible for needed early intervention services if CA is used in interpreting developmental test results.

Most studies of LPT infants do not seem to use CA. A large study[27] of 1200 LPT and 6300 FT infants from the Early Childhood Longitudinal Study, Birth Cohort reported that LPTs had significantly lower mean scores and scores less than 70 on the Bayley Scales of Infant Development Short form and derived Mental Developmental Index and Psychomotor Developmental Index at 24 months of age. The report suggests that no correction was made for prematurity and that level of risk is not specifically defined.

Table 1
Newborn to kindergarten outcomes

Author	Gestation (weeks)	Age	Cognitive	Other
Barros et al,[25] 2011	36 Late PT: 34–36[6/7] wk 96 Term: 40 wk	Newborns	↓Attention $P = .04$ ↓Arousal $P = .01$ ↓Regulation $P<.001$ ↓Movements $P<.001$	↑ Nonoptimal reflexes $P<.001$ ↑ Hypotonicity $P = .029$
Romeo et al,[26] 2010	61 healthy 33–36 wk 60 healthy controls	ChrA & CA 12 and 18 mo	PT CA MDI 97 ± 9 PT ChrA MDI 88 ± 10* Term MDI 98 ± 8	NA
Woythaler et al,[27] 2011	1200 PT: 34–37 wk 6300 Term	ChrA, age 24 mo	MDI 85 vs 89 $P<.0001$ MDI <70 21 vs 16% $P<.0001$	PDI 88 vs 92 $P<.0001$

Baron et al,[28] 2009	34–36[6/7] wk
	60 NICU LPT
	35 Term
		ChrA, age
		3.5–4.1 y
			DAS scores vs term
			↓ Visuospatial: 0.005
			↓ Visuomotor: 0.12
			↓ Executive:
			   Function noun: 0.02
			   Action verb: 0.03
				NA

Baron et al,[21] 2011	34–36[6/7] wk 90 LPT-NICU 28 LPT non-NICU 100 Term	ChrA, age 3.8 y	LPT-NICU vs term ↓ DAS GCA, nonverbal reasoning, and spatial scores; ↑ rates of nonverbal reasoning and spatial impairments	NA
Baron et al,[30] 2012	52 ELBW: 23–33 wk 196 LPT: 34–36 wk 121 Term	ChrA, age 3–3 y 11 mo	Executive functions ELBW multiple weaknesses LPT↓ complex working memory	NA
Morse et al,[19] 2009	34–41 wk Low-risk singletons 164,804	ChrA, age 0–5 y	0–3 y ↑ developmental delay 4 y ↑disability in prekindergarten 5 y ↑ special education 5 y ↑kindergarten retention	
Roth et al,[31] 2004	1500–2499 g $N = 7432$	Kindergarten 5 y	11% higher rate of special services than FT controls	↑Costs per year of $11 million

Abbreviations: CA, corrected age; ChrA, chronologic age; ELBW, extremely low birth weight; GCA, General Conceptual Ability; MDI, Mental Developmental Index; PDI, Psychomotor Developmental Index; *, versus term.

The issue of degree of neonatal risk, defined as admission to a tertiary care NICU versus not admitted, was pursued in 2 studies by Baron and colleagues.[28] In the first report in which a comparison was made between high-risk LPT and FT at the age of 3 years, the LPT group had significantly lower scores than the FT comparison group on Differential Ability Scales (DAS-II) visual spatial, visuomotor, executive function noun fluency, and executive function verb fluency. In a second report, Baron and colleagues[29] reported on both high-risk LPT infants, defined as admitted to the NICU, and low-risk LPT infants (not admitted to an NICU) compared to FT infants and identified that only the high-risk LPT infants scored less than FT children on DAS-II subscores of General Conceptual Ability (GCA), nonverbal cluster, nonverbal reasoning, and spatial clusters. They concluded that the increased risk of developmental delay of the NICU-admitted infants is secondary to clinical instability, increased neonatal morbidities, gender effects, and lower birth weight. They suggest that both neonatal morbidities and male gender contribute to these early cognitive weaknesses. The sample size of the low-risk LPT infants, however, was only 28, indicating that assessment of these outcomes deserves further investigation. In a third study, Baron and colleagues[30] used computerized testing to test early executive functions in subgroups of extremely low birth weight (ELBW), LPT, and FT children at 3 years of age. Executive functions are key to more complex cognitive skills required as the child advances in school and are difficult to assess at young ages. It was not unexpected that the ELBW children would have difficulty with the tests, including lower GCA, more omissions of tasks, and worse performance with both simple and complex memory than FT children. The LPT children, however, also had lower GCA scores and more omissions of tasks. Regarding executive functions, the LPT children performed poorer than controls only in the test for complex working memory compared to the ELBW children who had difficulty with both simple and complex memory. This finding in the LPT children is of concern, because it may be an early signal for neuropsychological deficits at older ages.

In a large population-based study[19] of low-risk, defined as hospitalized for 72 hours or less, LPT (34–36 week) singleton infants and 152,661 FT infants with data from birth to the age of 5 years in the state of Florida, consistent deficits were identified. The adjusted risk for the LPT group was 36% higher for developmental delay between birth and 3 years, 15% higher for disability in prekindergarten, 12% higher for disability in kindergarten, and 13% higher for special education services in kindergarten. Although this is a retrospective analysis, it provides strong support for close surveillance and the provision of early intervention services and educational support services as needed for both low-risk and high-risk LPT infants between discharge and 5 years of age.

In a second study of the Florida birth cohort of infants born in the period September 1990 to August 1991, Roth and colleagues[31] examined maternal and infant factors associated with kindergarten costs by birth weight group. Of the total births, 3% were receiving some special education services. In addition, 23% were receiving speech/language services. Compared to FT infants, the costs of kindergarten were 60% higher for infants weighing less than1000 g, 31% higher for infants weighing 1000 to 1499 g, and 11% higher for infants weighing 1500 to 2499 g. The annual kindergarten costs for infants weighing less than 1000 g were $3150 with total cost per year for infants weighing less than 1000 g of $2.1 million. The largest number of PT children receiving special education, however, was in the 1500 to 2499 g group with an associated $900 additional cost per child per year and an additional $11 million for 1 year of kindergarten costs. Additional important contributors to total cost were complications of labor, poverty, and low maternal education. These data, however, demonstrate the increased early educational needs and costs of the MPT to LPT infant.

Early School Age

The following reports are all summarized in **Table 2**. Using the Early Childhood Longitudinal Study, Kindergarten Cohort, Chyi and colleagues[18] used US national data to compare MPT (32–33 weeks), LPT (34–36 weeks), and FT children from kindergarten to fifth grade. In standardized tests, the MPT scores were lower than FT scores for reading in kindergarten and first and fifth grades and for math in kindergarten and first, third, and fifth grades. LPT children scored lower in reading in kindergarten and first grade. In teacher rating, MPT children were less proficient in reading in kindergarten and first, third, and fifth grades and in math in first, third, and fifth grades, whereas LPT children were less proficient in reading in kindergarten and first and fifth grades and in math in kindergarten and first grade when compared with FT infants. Both groups had increased needs for an individualized education plan and special education enrollment with the greatest needs for MPT children. In multivariable analysis, the risk for special education placement remained highly significant in third and fifth grades for MPT children but was no longer statistically significant for LPT children with odds ratios (ORs) of 1.22 (confidence interval [CI] = 0.92–1.63) and 1.28 (CI = 0.95–1.74). Overall, both MPT and LPT have academic challenges that persist in the fifth grade.

A case-control study of MPT children in the first grade identified increased rates of Wechsler performance intelligence quotient (IQ) and full scale IQ but not verbal IQ less than 85 after adjustment for confounders, in addition to increased risk of borderline clinical internalizing and borderline clinical attention problems.[32] The investigators acknowledge that it is difficult to identify the mechanism involved in producing these cognitive and behavioral findings. The contribution of intrauterine exposure, neonatal morbidities, and extrauterine environment all seem to play some role. The exclusions from the data set included multiples and children with severe neurologic impairments including cerebral palsy (CP) and blindness, resulting in a baseline reduced risk cohort.

A follow-up of the Avon Longitudinal Study found lower verbal IQ, performance IQ, and total IQ scores at the age of 11 years in univariable analysis for MPT and LPT compared to FT children, which were no longer significant after adjusting for confounders.[33] However, after adjustment, 2 areas of learning difficulties (word repetition and reading accuracy) were identified. In addition, the MPT and LPT children had a 56% increased risk of needing special education services. This suggests that the MPT and LPT children may be at greater risk of more discrete learning disabilities at older ages. A limitation of this study was 49% follow-up rate.

Huddy and colleagues[34] used information obtained from parent questionnaires on health, behavior, and teacher ratings of resource needs and behavior problems with the Strengths and Difficulties Behavior Questionnaire for a cohort of combined MPT and LPT children at the age of 7 years. Approximately one-third of the children had school academic resource needs. The most commonly reported were in writing, fine motor skills, and mathematics. In addition, both teachers and parents rated about 20% of the children as having borderline or abnormal total behavior scores. The most common behavior was hyperactivity, reported by 22% of teachers and 25% of parents.

A second analysis of the Pregnancy Outcomes and Community Health (POUCH)[35] cohort reported on child outcomes of 163 LPT children of 34 to 36 weeks' gestation. The primary outcome was evidence of attention deficit disorder using the Conners' Parent Rating Scale.[36] Children with a specific diagnosis of autism were excluded. In the initial analysis of the total cohort of LPT compared to FT children, no significant

Table 2
Early school age outcomes: kindergarten to middle school

Author	Gestation	Age	Sample Size	Cognitive	School Outcomes	Behavior
Chyi et al,[18] 2008	32–36 wk	5 y	MPT 203 LPT 767 FT 13,671	MPT: ↓ reading & math in fifth grade LPT: ↓ reading fifth grade	MPT: ↑ special education in kindergarten, first, third, and fifth grades LPT: ↑ special education in kindergarten and first grade	NA
Talge et al,[32] 2010	LPT: 34–36 wk FT: 37–41 wk	6–7 y	LPT 168 FT 168	FSIQ <85 LPT: 21% FT: 12% PIQ <85 LPT: 20% FT: 13%	NA	After adjustment ↑ internalizing ↑ Attention problems
Huddy et al,[34] 2001	32–35 wk	7 y	MPT = LPT 117	NA	1/3 Resource needs	20% Behavior problems
Talge et al,[35] 2012	34–36 wk	3–9 y	LPT 152 FT610	NA	NA	↑ Attention problems on Conners
Lipkind et al,[37] 2012	MPT: 32–33 wk LPT: 34–35 wk FT: 37–42 wk	Third grade	MPT: 2332 LPT: 13,207 FT: 199,599	Math test standard deviation % vs FT MPT: 10.4% LPT: 6.7%	Special education vs FT MPT OR = 1.5 LPT OR = 1.34	NA
Odd et al,[33] 2012	32–36 wk vs 37–42 wk	8–11 y	742 Late PT Total: 8878	Similar IQ scores After adjustment for confounders ↓ Scores for one word repetition and reading accuracy	↑ Risk special education OR 1.56 (1.18–2.07)	NA

Abbreviations: FSIQ, Full Scale Intelligence Quotient; OR, odds ratio; PIQ, Performance Intelligence Quotient.

group differences in Conners' scores were found. The LPT children were then divided into a medically indicated (MI) delivery group (induced before PT labor, such as hypertension) and a spontaneous labor group. MILPT children aged 3 to 5 years had significantly higher scores for inattention and MILPT children aged 6 to 9 years had significantly higher scores for inattention, hyperactivity, and total problems. These differences compared to FT children persisted after adjustment for multiple confounders but not after mothers with hypertension or placental problems associated with hypertension were removed from the model. The investigators conclude that hypertensive disorders resulting in medical intervention may contribute to behavioral disorders in the LPT children.

A cohort[37] analysis of 215,138 children born in New York City between 1914 and 1998 compared MPT and LPT children to FT children in the third grade and found a 50% adjusted increased odds of needing special education services for MPT and a 34% increased odds of needing special education for LPT children. MPT and LPT children had adjusted English language scores 6% and 4% of a standard deviation lower than FT peers and math scores 10% and 7% of a standard deviation lower. Generalized linear models estimated increases in adjusted mean test scores for English and math of 0.73% and 0.12%, respectively, of a standard deviation for each 1 week increase in GA after adjusting for confounders. The investigators relate the continued increase in scores for children born between 37 and 41 weeks' gestation to the continued increase in brain growth and organization in the last 4 weeks of pregnancy.

An analysis of the databases of the Kaiser Permanente Medical Care Program using International Classification of Diseases (ICD) documented diagnoses of CP, mental retardation (MR), and seizure disorders at 2 visits at least 6 months apart for 141,321 children born at or before 30 weeks' gestation and identified a similar linear relationship with GA.[20] The cohort was divided into 30 to 33 weeks, 34 to 36 weeks, and 37 to 41 weeks. Decreasing GA was related to increasing rates of CP and MR for all PT children. The adjusted hazard ratios for CP and MR were 7.87 and 1.90, respectively, for 30 to 33 weeks and 3.39 and 1.25, respectively, for 34 to 36 weeks.

Adolescents and Adults

Summary data are shown in **Table 3**. There are few studies that follow-up MPT and LPT children to adolescence or adult age. The first study[38] in this review evaluated 18-year-old boys registered in the Medical Birth Registry of Norway (1967–1979) whose data were linked to the Norwegian Conscript Service for 1984 to 1999. Intelligence scores increased with each year of GA. After adjusting for social confounders and adult body size, the OR for low adult intelligence scores for LPT versus FT 19-year-olds remained significant (OR = 1.21 [CI ±1.15–1.27]).

In a large Swedish register study[39] of 119,664 boys aged 18 to 19 years conscripted for military service, mean cognitive test scores decreased in a stepwise manner for GA groups of 39 to 41, 37 to 38, 35 to 36, 33 to 34, and 24 to 32 weeks. Units of decrease in stanine test scores for the GA categories 24 to 32, 33 to 34, 35 to 36, and 37 to 38 weeks relative to 39 to 41 weeks were −0.42, −0.17, −0.11, and −0.02, respectively, after adjusting for multiple confounders. A stanine score is the equivalent of 7 points of standard score, so the effects of GA are modest at best for the MPT and ET subjects. Socioeconomic status was a significant modifier, and effects of GA were reduced by 26% to 33% after adjustment. This study and the prior Norwegian cohort reflect boys only and boys with no significant disabilities. Both studies stress the importance of adjusting for social and environmental factors. On the other hand, the data support a role for the long-term effects of GA at birth.

Table 3
Adolescents and adult outcomes

Author	Gestation	Age	Sample Size	Cognitive	School Outcomes	Behavior
Eide et al,[38] 2007	26–29 wk 30–33 wk 34–36 wk 37–38 wk	Norway 19 y	34–36 wk: 10,836 37–38 wk: 37,484	OR for ↓ IQ vs T 39–41 wk 26–29 wk: 2.19 30–33 wk: 1.44 34–36 wk: 1.21	NA	NA
Ekeus et al,[39] 2010	24–32 wk 33–34 wk 35–36 wk 37–38 wk 39–41 wk	Swedish 18–19 y	MPT: 1088 LPT: 3918 FT: 94821	↓ Cognition scores with ↓ GA	NA	NA
Lindstrom et al,[40] 2009	24–28 wk 29–32 wk 33–36 wk	Adolescents/young adults up to 29 y	Sweden 545,628	NA	NA	Hazard ratio for psychiatric disorders 24–32 wk: 1.68 33–36 wk: 1.21 37–38 wk: 1.08 30% ↑ risk of psychiatric disorders
Moster et al,[41] 2008	25–27$^{6/7}$ wk 28–30$^{6/7}$ wk 31–33$^{6/7}$ wk 34–36$^{6/7}$ wk ≥37 wk	Adults born in the period 1967–1983	Norway 867,692	↑OR for MR MPT 2.1 LPT 1.6	Any disability affecting work capacity 25–27$^{6/7}$ wk: 10.6% 28–30$^{6/7}$ wk: 8.2% 31–33$^{6/7}$ wk: 4.2% 34–36$^{6/7}$ wk: 2.4% ≥37 wk: 1.7%	30% ↑ risk schizophrenia & 40%–50% ↑ risk psychiatric disorders
Dalziel et al,[42] 2007	32–35 wk	Adults born in the period 1969–1974 31 y	MPT/LPT-112	No differences in cog function, working memory, or attention	NA	No differences in anxiety or schizoid behavior

A Swedish national cohort of 545,628 births in the period 1973 to 1979 was used to estimate the hazard ratios of hospital admissions for psychiatric disorders and alcohol/illicit drug use for a cohort consisting primarily of adolescents and young adults.[40] A total of 5.2% of subjects having GA 24 to 28 weeks and 3.5% having GA 29 to 32 weeks were hospitalized for a psychiatric disorder. The hazard ratios for hospitalization for a psychiatric disorder were 1.68 at 24 to 28 weeks, 1.21 at 33 to 36 weeks, and 1.08 at 37 to 38 weeks (ET), resulting in an increasing rate of psychiatric disorders with decreasing GA. MPT and ET births accounted for 85% of the risk.

Data from a national compulsory database in Norway examined the relationship between GA and outcomes of 867,692 adults.[41] There was a significant inverse relationship between GA and a spectrum of medical disabilities including CP, MR, autism spectrum, other psychological disorders, other major disabilities, and any medical disability affecting working capacity. In all analyses, MPT and LPT had increased odds of the adverse outcome. This extended to decreased rates of graduating from high school, graduating from college, holding a high-income job, achieving biologic parenthood, and several additional demographic variables.

Dalziel and colleagues[42] completed a comprehensive evaluation on 126 MPT adults (median gestation 34 weeks) at 31 years of age in New Zealand and found no differences compared to FT adults in cognitive function, educational achievement, marital status, working memory, attention, anxiety, or schizoid behaviors. Limitations in these findings were the 69% follow-up rate and small sample size.

EARLY TERM INFANTS

ET gestation is defined as deliveries occurring at 37 to 38 weeks of gestation. Although FT deliveries have traditionally been defined as births after 36 weeks, the FT category has been further divided to include ET (37–38 weeks), term (39–41 weeks), and late term or postterm (42–44 weeks). The focus of recent reports has been on the increased vulnerability of ET infants. A report on US births between 1992 and 2002 indicated an 8.9% increase in ET births over a 10-year period, with the increase attributable to elective deliveries.[43] Infants born ET are at increased risk of neonatal morbidities.[44] There is limited information on long-term outcomes of these infants. A large population-based study linked school census data to birth data registries that included maternal characteristic and birth data to determine the association between GA at birth and special education needs for children between 4 and 19 years.[45] As expected, below 36 weeks, the lower the GA, the greater the percentage of children receiving special services. Of interest, however, is that this increased rate, which was inversely related to gestation, extended to infants at 39, 38, and 37 weeks. The multivariable ORs, compared to delivery at 40 weeks, were as follows: for 24 to 27 weeks, 6.92 (CI, 5.58–8.58); for 28 to 32 weeks, 2.66 (CI, 2.38–2.97); for 33 to 36 weeks, 1.53 (CI, 1.43–1.63); for 37 weeks, 1.36 (CI, 1.27–1.45); for 38 weeks (CI, 1.19; CI, 1.14–1.25), and for 39 weeks, 1.09 (CI, 1.04–1.14). Because of the substantial number of deliveries at ET within this cohort, the ET infants accounted for 39.6% of special education services at school age. In the United States, there is currently a nationwide effort to decrease elective deliveries at 37 to 39 weeks gestation.[46,47]

SUMMARY

There is increasing evidence that MPT infants are at increased risk of a spectrum of developmental and behavioral morbidities that extend from birth to adult age. There is also an increasing body of evidence of the vulnerability of the LPT infant, particularly those who require NICU care, for postdischarge sequelae. The data on increased risk of behavioral and psychiatric morbidities for both MPT and LPT infants are of particular concern. Current evidence indicates that close surveillance of medical status, growth, neurologic status, behavior, and development, in conjunction with family-centered support after discharge and referral to early intervention, behavioral, and support services is needed. Because of the level of risk, NICUs should consider referring MPT and selected LPT infants for high-risk follow-up evaluation. Further investigation is needed to identify the most vulnerable infants and to provide the appropriate support for the infant and family.

REFERENCES

1. Raju TN, Higgins RD, Stark AR, et al. Optimizing care and outcome for late-preterm (near-term) infants: a summary of the workshop sponsored by the National Institute of Child Health and Human Development. Pediatrics 2006;118:1207–14.
2. Kochanek KD, Kirmeyer SE, Martin JA, et al. Annual summary of vital statistics: 2009. Pediatrics 2012;129:338–48.
3. Refuerzo JS. Impact of multiple births on late and moderate prematurity. Semin Fetal Neonatal Med 2012;17:143–5.
4. Laughon SK, Reddy UM, Sun L, et al. Precursors for late preterm birth in singleton gestations. Obstet Gynecol 2010;116:1047–55.
5. Brandon DH, Tully KP, Silva SG, et al. Emotional responses of mothers of late-preterm and term infants. J Obstet Gynecol Neonatal Nurs 2011;40(6):719–31.
6. Gibson J, McKenzie-McHarg K, Shakespeare J, et al. A systematic review of studies validating the Edinburgh Postnatal Depression Scale in antepartum and postpartum women. Acta Psychiatr Scand 2009;119:350–64.
7. Lefkowitz DS, Baxt C, Evans JR. Prevalence and correlates of posttraumatic stress and postpartum depression in parents of infants in the Neonatal Intensive Care Unit (NICU). J Clin Psychol Med Settings 2010;17:230–7.
8. Raju TN. Developmental physiology of late and moderate prematurity. Semin Fetal Neonatal Med 2012;17:126–31.
9. Hibbard JU, Wilkins I, Sun L, et al. Respiratory morbidity in late preterm births. JAMA 2010;304:419–25.
10. Gouyon JB, Vintejoux A, Sagot P, et al. Neonatal outcome associated with singleton birth at 34-41 weeks of gestation. Int J Epidemiol 2010;39:769–76.
11. Shapiro-Mendoza CK, Tomashek KM, Kotelchuck M, et al. Effect of late-preterm birth and maternal medical conditions on newborn morbidity risk. Pediatrics 2008;121:e223–32.
12. Kinney HC. The near-term (late preterm) human brain and risk for periventricular leukomalacia: a review. Semin Perinatol 2006;30:81–8.
13. Huppi PS, Warfield S, Kikinis R, et al. Quantitative magnetic resonance imaging of brain development in premature and mature newborns. Ann Neurol 1998;43:224–35.
14. Escobar GJ, Clark RH, Greene JD. Short-term outcomes of infants born at 35 and 36 weeks gestation: we need to ask more questions. Semin Perinatol 2006;30(1):28–33.
15. Lainwala S, Perritt R, Poole K, et al. Neurodevelopmental and growth outcomes of extremely low birth weight infants who are transferred from neonatal intensive care units to level I or II nurseries. Pediatrics 2007;119:e1079–87.
16. McLaurin KK, Hall CB, Jackson EA, et al. Persistence of morbidity and cost differences between late-preterm and term infants during the first year of life. Pediatrics 2009;123(2):653–9.

17. Boyle EM, Poulsen G, Field DJ, et al. Effects of gestational age at birth on health outcomes at 3 and 5 years of age: population based cohort study. BMJ 2012;344: e896.
18. Chyi LJ, Lee HC, Hintz SR, et al. School outcomes of late preterm infants: special needs and challenges for infants born at 32 to 36 weeks gestation. J Pediatr 2008;153:25–31.
19. Morse SB, Zheng H, Tang Y, et al. Early school-age outcomes of late preterm infants. Pediatrics 2009;123:e622–9.
20. Petrini JR, Dias T, McCormick MC, et al. Increased risk of adverse neurological development for late preterm infants. J Pediatr 2009;154:169–76.
21. Baron IS, Erickson K, Ahronovich MD, et al. Cognitive deficit in preschoolers born late-preterm. Early Hum Dev 2011;87:115–9.
22. Baron IS, Litman FR, Ahronovich MD, et al. Late preterm birth: a review of medical and neuropsychological childhood outcomes. Neuropsychol Rev 2012;22:438–50.
23. Bhutta AT, Cleves MA, Casey PH, et al. Cognitive and behavioral outcomes of school-aged children who were born preterm: a meta-analysis. JAMA 2002; 288:728–37.
24. Engle WA. Morbidity and mortality in late preterm and early term newborns: a continuum. Clin Perinatol 2011;38:493–516.
25. Barros MC, Mitsuhiro S, Chalem E, et al. Neurobehavior of late preterm infants of adolescent mothers. Neonatology 2011;99:133–9.
26. Romeo DM, Di Stefano A, Conversano M, et al. Neurodevelopmental outcome at 12 and 18 months in late preterm infants. Eur J Paediatr Neurol 2010;14:503–7.
27. Woythaler MA, McCormick MC, Smith VC. Late preterm infants have worse 24-month neurodevelopmental outcomes than term infants. Pediatrics 2011; 127:e622–9.
28. Baron IS, Erickson K, Ahronovich MD, et al. Visuospatial and verbal fluency relative deficits in 'complicated' late-preterm preschool children. Early Hum Dev 2009;85:751–4.
29. Baron IS, Erickson K, Ahronovich MD, et al. Spatial location memory discriminates children born at extremely low birth weight and late-preterm at age three. Neuropsychology 2010;24:787–94.
30. Baron IS, Kerns KA, Muller U, et al. Executive functions in extremely low birth weight and late-preterm preschoolers: effects on working memory and response inhibition. Child Neuropsychol 2012;18:586–99.
31. Roth J, Figlio DN, Chen Y, et al. Maternal and infant factors associated with excess kindergarten costs. Pediatrics 2004;114:720–8.
32. Talge NM, Holzman C, Wang J, et al. Late-preterm birth and its association with cognitive and socioemotional outcomes at 6 years of age. Pediatrics 2010;126: 1124–31.
33. Odd DE, Emond A, Whitelaw A. Long-term cognitive outcomes of infants born moderately and late preterm. Dev Med Child Neurol 2012;54:704–9.
34. Huddy CL, Johnson A, Hope PL. Educational and behavioural problems in babies of 32-35 weeks gestation. Arch Dis Child Fetal Neonatal Ed 2001;85:F23–8.
35. Talge NM, Holzman C, Van Egeren LA, et al. Late-preterm birth by delivery circumstance and its association with parent-reported attention problems in childhood. J Dev Behav Pediatr 2012;33:405–15.
36. Conners CK. Connors parent rating scales revised. San Antonio (TX): Psychological Corp; 1996.
37. Lipkind HS, Slopen ME, Pfeiffer MR, et al. School-age outcomes of late preterm infants in New York City. Am J Obstet Gynecol 2012;206:222.e1–6.

38. Eide MG, Oyen N, Skjaerven R, et al. Associations of birth size, gestational age, and adult size with intellectual performance: evidence from a cohort of Norwegian men. Pediatr Res 2007;62:636–42.
39. Ekeus C, Lindstrom K, Lindblad F, et al. Preterm birth, social disadvantage, and cognitive competence in Swedish 18- to 19-year-old men. Pediatrics 2010;125: e67–73.
40. Lindstrom K, Lindblad F, Hjern A. Psychiatric morbidity in adolescents and young adults born preterm: a Swedish national cohort study. Pediatrics 2009;123: e47–53.
41. Moster D, Lie RT, Markestad T. Long-term medical and social consequences of preterm birth. N Engl J Med 2008;359:262–73.
42. Dalziel SR, Lim VK, Lambert A, et al. Psychological functioning and health-related quality of life in adulthood after preterm birth. Dev Med Child Neurol 2007;49: 597–602.
43. Davidoff MJ, Dias T, Damus K, et al. Changes in the gestational age distribution among U.S. singleton births: impact on rates of late preterm birth, 1992 to 2002. Semin Perinatol 2006;30:8–15.
44. Yoder BA, Gordon MC, Barth WH Jr. Late-preterm birth: does the changing obstetric paradigm alter the epidemiology of respiratory complications? Obstet Gynecol 2008;111:814–22.
45. MacKay DF, Smith GC, Dobbie R, et al. Gestational age at delivery and special educational need: retrospective cohort study of 407,503 schoolchildren. PLoS Med 2010;7:e1000289.
46. ACOG Committee on Practice Bulletins – Obstetrics. ACOG practice bulletin no. 107: induction of labor. Obstet Gynecol 2009;114:386–97.
47. Ashton DM. Elective delivery at less than 39 weeks. Curr Opin Obstet Gynecol 2010;22:506–10.

Hospital Readmissions and Emergency Department Visits in Moderate Preterm, Late Preterm, and Early Term Infants

Michael W. Kuzniewicz, MD, MPH[a,b,*], Sarah-Jane Parker, BA[a],
Alina Schnake-Mahl, BA[a], Gabriel J. Escobar, MD[a]

KEYWORDS

- Preterm • Rehospitalization • Readmission rate • ED utilization
- Readmission diagnosis

KEY POINTS

- This review notes that there is limited literature describing health care utilization in moderate preterm, late preterm, and early term infants after their birth hospitalization.
- The primary data analysis demonstrates that late preterm infants and early term infants were at a greater risk for rehospitalization and that the overwhelming reasons for rehospitalization were jaundice and feeding problems.
- Temporal trends in readmission rates in late preterm and early term infants have been increasing despite increased awareness and changes in inpatient practices.
- Emergency department (ED) visit rates do not show a strong correlation with gestational age (GA) after controlling for other risk factors, although there is a slight increase among late preterm infants.
- Moderate preterm, late preterm, and early term infants all show increased rates of hospital readmission in the first 30 days after birth hospitalization discharge.

The increased vulnerability of late preterm infants is no longer a novel concept in neonatology. A substantial literature now documents that these infants have excess mortality[1-4] and morbidity.[5-9] This excess morbidity extends beyond the initial birth hospitalization. Readmission rates of late preterm infants are 1.5 to 3 times that of

Disclosure Statement: The authors have no conflicts of interest to declare.
[a] Division of Research, Kaiser Permanente Northern California, 2000 Broadway Avenue (2101 Webster Annex), Oakland, CA 94612, USA; [b] Division of Neonatology, University of California, San Francisco, 505 Parnassus Avenue, San Francisco, CA 94143, USA
* Corresponding author. Perinatal Research Unit, Division of Research, Kaiser Permanente Northern California, 2000 Broadway Avenue (2101 Webster Annex), Oakland, CA 94612.
E-mail addresses: Michael.W.Kuzniewicz@kp.org; KuzniewiczM@peds.ucsf.edu

Clin Perinatol 40 (2013) 753–775
http://dx.doi.org/10.1016/j.clp.2013.07.008
0095-5108/13/$ – see front matter © 2013 Elsevier Inc. All rights reserved.

term infants.[10–13] Because outcomes related to GA constitute a continuum, it is also important to analyze data from the GA groups that bookend late preterm infants–moderate preterm infants (31–32 weeks' gestation) and early term infants (37–38 weeks' gestation). Clinicians need to be cognizant of any increased vulnerability in these infants as well as the underlying pathophysiologic and developmental factors that lead to this increased vulnerability. Understanding the health care utilization patterns of moderate preterm, late preterm, and early term infants could help define what constitutes optimum health care delivery and may lead to the development of strategies that could mitigate or eliminate the adverse consequences of delivery prior to term.

The literature is limited in describing outcomes of these infants after discharge from the hospital and almost solely focuses on late preterm infants. In the past 10 years, only 13 primary data collection/analysis articles could be found to describe health care utilization after birth hospitalization (**Table 1**). In addition to limited data availability, studies not using standard GA ranges often make it difficult to disaggregate outcomes. Moderate preterm infants are especially overlooked because they are frequently grouped with extremely premature infants. The lack of a consistent observational period from delivery or from discharge also limits comparisons between studies.

The most widely studied metric of health care utilization in late preterm infants is short-term readmission after birth hospitalization. Escobar and colleagues[14] examined rehospitalization of infants discharged from level III neonatal intensive care units (NICUs) and found that infants 33 to 36 weeks' gestation with a length of stay (LOS) of less than 4 days had an odds ratio (OR) of 2.94 (95% CI, 1.87–4.62) compared with term infants with a NICU stay of less than 4 days. In this group, 71% were rehospitalized because of jaundice. Infants of 33 to 36 weeks' gestation with a stay of greater than or equal to 4 days were not at an increased risk. In a follow-up study, Escobar and colleagues[10] found that late preterm infants never admitted to a NICU were at increased risk for readmission compared with term infants never admitted to the NICU. Excluding jaundice-only admissions, late preterm infants were still at higher risk than term infants for readmission, but that risk was almost halved. Among infants with less than a two-night hospital stay at birth, Tomashek and colleagues[21] showed late preterm infants were 1.8 times more likely to be readmitted than term infants. Jaundice and infection accounted for the majority of readmissions. Only breastfed late preterm infants were at increased risk for readmission. No difference was found in readmission rates between late preterm and term infants who were not breastfed. In a related population, Shapiro-Mendoza and colleagues[13] found that risk factors for subsequent readmission or observational stay were late preterm infants with stays less than 4 days, breastfeeding, Asian/Pacific Islanders, firstborn infants, and public payers at the time of delivery.

In the United Kingdom, Oddie and colleagues[16] also found an almost 2-fold higher risk of readmission in 35- to 37-week infants compared with term infants. In contrast to other studies, infectious disease was the leading reason for readmission and jaundice accounted for few readmissions, which the investigators attributed to a differing approach to management of jaundice in the United Kingdom.[22]

Examining late rehospitalizations (after the first 2 weeks), Escobar and colleagues[17] found 36-week gestation infants at higher risk for readmission compared with term infants (although 34- and 35-week gestation infants were not). McLaurin and colleagues[11] demonstrated increased late rehospitalization rates in late preterm infants compared with term infants and found that the subset of late preterm infants with prolonged birth hospitalizations (≥4 days) had the highest rates of rehospitalization and hospitalization costs. The most common cause of readmission was respiratory disease (bronchiolitis and pneumonia). This pattern was also

Table 1
Postdischarge health care utilization (rehospitalization, ED visits, prescriptions, clinic visits, and cost) among preterm infants

Study	Years (Subjects)	Study Population and Outcome of Interest	Rehospitalization Outcomes	Notable Results
Escobar et al,[14] 1999	1992–1995	Northern California births discharged from the NICU; N = 6054. Outcome: rehospitalization within 2 wk of discharge	≥37 wk (2.4%) 33–36 wk, LOS <96 h (5.7%) 33–36 wk, LOS ≥96 h (2.2%) <32 wk (3.4%) 33–36 wk (1.8%)	Highest rate of rehospitalization found among 33–36 wk infants with <4 d LOS. In all groups except <32 wk GA, jaundice and feeding difficulties were most common rehospitalization diagnosis. For <32-wk infants, bronchiolitis was most common.
Underwood et al,[15] 2007	1992–2000	California births <36 wk GA; N = 263,883. Outcome: rehospitalization incidence and cost within 1 y of birth	<31 wk (23%) 31–33 wk (14%) 34–35 wk (13%)	Rehospitalization rates increased as GA decreased; however, the largest cohort, 35-wk GA infants, had the highest total cost of rehospitalization. The most common cause of rehospitalization was acute respiratory disease.
Martens et al,[12] 2004	1997–2001	Discharged alive in Manitoba, Canada; N = 68,321. Outcome: rehospitalization within 6 wk of discharge	<37 wk Compared with all other infants AOR^a: 1.80 (1.55–2.10)	Risk of rehospitalization was higher for infants born preterm. Breastfeeding was found protective against rehospitalization, most likely associated with the major cause of rehospitalization being respiratory illness.

(continued on next page)

Table 1
(continued)

Study	Years (Subjects)	Study Population and Outcome of Interest	Rehospitalization Outcomes	Notable Results
Oddie et al,[16] 2005	1998	Infants ≥35 wk born in northern United Kingdom; N = 32,015 Outcome: rehospitalization within 28 d of birth	35–37 wk Compared with all other infants AOR[a]: 1.72 (1.15–2.57)	Infections accounted for the largest number of rehospitalizations. Results from this study may reflect differential maternal services provided in UK that are not routine in the US: early discharge home was not associated with rehospitalization and jaundice underlay few rehospitalizations.
Escobar et al,[10] 2005	1998–2000	Northern California births; N = 33,276 Outcome: rehospitalization within 2 wk of discharge	34–36 wk, in NICU ≥24 h, AOR[a]: 0.89 (0.54–1.46) 34–36 wk, never in NICU, AOR[a]: 3.10 (2.38–4.02)	The most common reason for rehospitalization was jaundice. Among infants ≥34 wk, most important factor with respect to rehospitalization was use of home phototherapy. Factors associated with increased risk included being small for GA, 34–36 wk GA without admission to the NICU, score for Neonatal Acute Physiology, increased illness severity, male gender, having both a home and a clinic visit within 72 h of discharge, and birth facility.

Escobar et al,[7] 2006	2001–2003	California and Massachusetts births 30–34 wk GA; N = 1250 Outcome: rehospitalization within 3 mo of discharge	30-32 wk (12.5%) 33–34 wk (10.5%)	Overall rehospitalization rate was 11.3%. In unadjusted comparisons, infants who experienced assisted ventilation for at least 72 h, African American infants, male infants, and infants with chronic lung disease were more likely to be readmitted.
Tomashek[21]	1998–2002	Massachusetts vaginal births, discharged early (LOS<2); N = 1004 Outcome: rehospitalization within 28 d of birth	34–36 wk (3.5%) Compared with term infants: ARR[b] 1.8 (1.3–2.5)	In adjusted analyses, preterm infants were 1.5 times more likely than term infants be readmitted to a hospital or have observational stays in the first 28 d of life. Breastfeeding at discharge was a predictor of rehospitalization in late preterms. Jaundice was the most common rehospitalization diagnosis, followed by infection. Rehospitalization for jaundice was highest in the first 5 d of life, whereas infection accounted for 69% of admissions in the second week of life for late preterms.

(continued on next page)

Table 1
(continued)

Study	Years (Subjects)	Study Population and Outcome of Interest	Rehospitalization Outcomes	Notable Results
Shapiro-Mendoza et al,[13] 2006	1998–2002	Massachusetts singletons 34–36 wk GA, born vaginally and healthy appearing[c]; N = 9522 Outcome: rehospitalization within 28 d of delivery	34–36 wk (6.1%) 34 wk (5.5%) 35 wk (6.9%) 36 wk (5.8%)	Three-fourths of rehospitalizations had a principal diagnosis of jaundice or infection; 95% of rehospitalizations occurred on or before 7 d of age, and most between 3–5 d. An increasing proportion of rehospitalization for infection occurred after 7 d. Breastfeeding at discharge, Asian/Pacific Islander mothers (in comparison to non-Hispanic white), public payer source (in comparison to private), low parity, and complications of labor and delivery predicted rehospitalization, whereas non-Hispanic African American race was a protective.

Escobar et al,[17] 2006	1998–2004	Northern California births ≥33 wk and surviving ≥2 h; N = 47,495 Outcome: rehospitalization within 15–182 d of discharge	33 wk (9.3%) 34 wk (9.1%) 35 wk (6.8%) 36 wk (7.3%) 37 wk (5.6%)	Rehospitalization rate increased as GA decreased. There were significantly elevated hazard ratios for rehospitalization for the following predictors: 36-wk GA, male gender, use of assisted ventilation. GA 41+ wk was protective.
Dietz et al,[18] 2012	1998–2007	Californian healthy,[d] singleton births 37–42 wk GA; N = 22,420 Outcome: health care utilization, including rehospitalization, ED visits, and nonroutine outpatient visits within 2 wk and 3–52 wk of birth	Within 2 weeks of delivery: 37 wk (3.7%) with OR[e] 2.6 (1.9–3.6) Between 3–52 weeks of delivery: 37 wk (4.6%)	Infants born at 37 wk had an elevated risk of rehospitalization within 2 wk of delivery in comparison with other term infants, but there was no association with rehospitalization and GA in the 3–52 wk range. The mean ED visits/y (after adjusting for Medicaid + mental health) were higher for those born at 37–38 wk than those born 39–40 wk.

(continued on next page)

Table 1
(continued)

Study	Years (Subjects)	Study Population and Outcome of Interest	Rehospitalization Outcomes	Notable Results
Bird et al,[19] 2010	2001–2005	Arkansas singleton healthy[f] infants 34 ≤GA <42 with Medicaid as the primary payer; N = 20,419 Outcomes: care utilization and cost within 1 y of birth	34–36 wk AOR 1.11 (1.01–1.23)	After propensity score matching, preterm infants had higher odds of rehospitalization in comparison to term infants. Hospital costs in the first year were significantly higher among late preterm infants than among term infants, although magnitude of increase (~ $600) was relatively small.
McLaurin et al,[11] 2009	2004	US commercially insured births; N = 35,428 Outcomes: health care utilization and costs within 1 y of birth	33–36 wk (15.2%) 33–36 wk, LOS <96 h (14.7%) 33–36 wk, LOS ≥96 h (15.4%)	Late-preterm infants had almost 2 times the rehospitalization rate of term infants. These rates were higher in the first 15 d and throughout the first year of life. The primary rehospitalization diagnosis was respiratory syncytial virus. Late preterm infants had higher costs across every type of service category compared with term infants.

| Jain & Cheng,[20] 2006 | 2005–2006 | Infants age 0–31 d presenting in 2 EDs at tertiary care pediatric hospitals; N = 1596 Outcomes: observed GA and associated diagnosis among ED visits and ED visits with admission to the hospital | — | Proportion of visits by late preterm infants (17.7%) was double the rates reported nationally, which may reflect the institutions' status (tertiary care centers). More term infants presented in the 2nd wk of life whereas more preterm late preterm infants presented in their 4th wk of life. Among late preterm infants, a majority were 36-wk GA at presentation. The most common diagnoses for late preterm infants were the same as term in infants: feeding problems, respiratory, fever, and jaundice. |

Unless otherwise specified, all studies involve patients discharged alive.
[a] Adjusted OR and 95% CI.
[b] Adjusted RR and 95% CI.
[c] Healthy-appearing infants were defined as those who (1) were discharged home before a fourth-night hospital stay, (2) weighed at least 2000 g at birth, and (3) did not have any significant health problems or procedures.
[d] Healthy births defined as without major birth defects, fetal growth restriction, or exposure to diabetes or hypertension in utero.
[e] Unadjusted OR (95% CI).
[f] Healthy infants defined as those weighing ≥1500 g at birth and without major birth defect.

found in a study of recurrent wheezing, which found higher rates of readmission in late preterm infants.[23]

Dietz and colleagues[18] specifically evaluated health care utilization in early term infants during the first year of life. Compared with term infants, infants born at 37 weeks had an OR of 2.6 (95% CI, 1.9–3.6) and those born at 38 weeks, an OR of 1.7 (95% CI, 1.3–2.2), with jaundice present in greater than or equal to 70% of these readmissions. Rehospitalizations within 3 to 52 weeks of delivery were not associated with GA. The mean number of sick/ED visits was also higher in early term infants.

Data on ED utilization are limited to a single-center study by Jain and Cheng[20] of infants presenting to the ED in the first month of life, of whom 17.7% were preterm. The primary ED diagnoses were gastrointestinal, respiratory, and fever. Late preterm infants were more likely than term infants to be admitted after their ED visit, with 36.9% of their visits resulting in hospitalization.

KAISER PERMANENTE—PRIMARY DATA COLLECTION

To address gaps in the literature, primary data collection was used from an integrated health care delivery system, Kaiser Permanente Northern California (KPNC). Data collection methods for the analyses involving the Kaiser Permanente cohort have been described elsewhere.[10,14,24] This cohort was linked to the Virtual Data Warehouse, a resource that holds electronic records of all patient encounters (inpatient and outpatient) at KPNC facilities and enables the sharing of compatible data in multisite studies.[25] Eligible infants met the following criteria: born in KPNC birth facilities between January 1, 2003, and November 30, 2012; GA greater than or equal to $31^{0/7}$ weeks; and discharged alive. Infants with major congenital anomalies were excluded from the analysis using *International Classification of Diseases, Ninth Revision (ICD-9)* codes and chart review. The objectives of these analyses were to (1) determine the rate of hospital readmissions and ED visits in the first 30 days after birth hospitalization discharge in moderate preterm (31–33 weeks), late preterm (34–36 weeks), early term (37–38 weeks), and term infants (39+ weeks); (2) identify the major diagnoses during those encounters; (3) characterize the timing of those encounters; (4) evaluate temporal trends in readmissions; and (5) identify risk factors for readmission and ED visits.

GA was determined from the maternal record and obstetrically assigned estimated date of confinement (EDC) based on last menstrual period (LMP) and/or fetal ultrasounds and assisted reproductive technology (if used). For women with regular menstrual cycles, EDC was based on LMP if in 7-day agreement with a first-trimester ultrasound. For women with irregular menstrual cycles, EDC was determined from first-trimester ultrasound results. Small/large for GA was determined by plotting an infant's weight and GA on the Fenton growth curve, using less than 5th% as a cutoff for SGA and greater than 95th% for LGA.[26] The authors tracked all hospital admissions or ED visits that occurred within 30 days of their birth hospitalization discharge. Diagnoses were assigned to readmissions and ED visits from their discharge diagnosis *ICD-9* codes. The *ICD-9* diagnoses were grouped into 6 categories: infection/rule-out sepsis; respiratory; gastrointestinal; apparent life-threatening event/seizure; jaundice/feeding problems; and other (see Appendix Table 1). Diagnoses were not mutually exclusive. Infants with a diagnosis of "other" did not have a diagnosis in any of the other 5 categories. If an infant had multiple readmissions or ED visits, data were used from the first encounter.

Descriptive statistics were used to characterize the readmission and ED visit rates. Relative risks (RRs) and 95% CIs were used for pairwise comparisons of rates between GA categories. Multivariate logistical regression was used to evaluate risk factors for hospital readmission and ED visits. The KPNC Institutional Review Board for the Protection of Human Subjects approved the study.

KPNC COHORT

During the study period, a total of 309,736 infants were born without major congenital anomalies and survived to discharge home. The cohort consisted of 3696 (1.2%) moderate preterm infants; 19,494 (6.3%) late preterm infants; 74,023 (23.9%) early term infants; and 212,523 (68.6%) term infants. Characteristics of the cohort are presented in **Tables 2** and **3**.

HOSPITAL READMISSIONS AND DIAGNOSES

Readmission rates by GA are presented in **Fig. 1**. Compared with term infants, late preterm infants (RR 2.41; 95% CI, 2.29–2.55) and early term infants (RR 2.05; 95% CI, 1.98–2.12) were at higher risk for being readmitted. Moderate term infants were not at higher risk, for being readmitted (RR 0.88; 95% CI, 0.74–1.07) compared with term infants. Examining readmission rates by week of GA, a peak in readmission rates was found between 35 and 38 weeks. The highest readmission rate (9.8%) was among 37-week infants. In late preterm, early term, and term infants, the predominant readmission diagnosis is jaundice/feeding problems, present in 68% to 84% of readmissions (**Fig. 2**). In contrast, jaundice/feeding problems are present in only 19% of readmissions in moderate preterm infants. Moderate preterm infants are not discharged until at least 1 to 2 weeks of life, so issues surrounding jaundice are likely dealt with during the birth hospitalization.

Table 2
Birth cohort, KPNC 2003–2012

	Gestational Age			
	31–33 wk	34–36 wk	37–38 wk	39 wk+
n	3696	19,494	74,023	212,523
Male	53%	54%	53%	50%
C section	57%	39%	26%	24%
SGA—<5th%[a]	3.30%	3.60%	2.00%	1.60%
LGA—>95th%[b]	2.30%	5.00%	5.70%	3.70%
Race				
White	37%	38%	35%	41%
Black	10%	9%	8%	7%
Asian	22%	22%	24%	19%
Hispanic	23%	23%	25%	24%
Other/unknown	8%	8%	8%	8%
LOS—days (vaginal)[c]	20.9 ± 10.6	4.5 ± 4.4	1.8 ± 1.5	1.7 ± 1.2
LOS—days (C section)[c]	23.2 ± 10.7	6.3 ± 5.3	3.1 ± 1.9	2.9 ± 1.5
LOS <48 h	0%	12%	56%	60%

Abbreviations: C section, cesarean section; LGA, large for gestational age; SGA, small for gestational age.
[a] <5%, below fifth percentile on Fenton growth curve.
[b] >95%, above ninety-fifth percentile on Fenton growth curve.
[c] Mean ± SD.

Table 3
Readmissions and emergency department visits, KPNC 2003–2012

	Gestational Age			
	31–33 wk	34–36 wk	37–38 wk	39 wk+
n	3696	19,494	74,023	212,523
Readmissions	108 (2.9%)	1549 (8.0%)	4996 (6.8%)	6993 (3.3%)
Multiple readmissions	10 (0.27%)	74 (0.38%)	150 (0.2%)	169 (0.08%)
Age at readmit (d)[a]	39 (30,47)	4 (3,7)	4 (3,5)	4 (3,12)
ED visit	201 (5.4%)	909 (4.7%)	3030 (4.1%)	8241 (3.9%)
Multiple ED visits	14 (0.38%)	56 (0.29%)	179 (0.24%)	402 (0.19%)
% Admitted after ED visit	23%	22%	17%	17%
Age at ED visit (d)[a]	37 (29,47)	17 (9,26)	12 (6,21)	11 (5,20)

[a] Median (interquartile range).

Excluding admissions where the only diagnosis was jaundice or a feeding problem, the peak in readmissions seen in late preterm and early term infants is substantially reduced (**Fig. 3**). After excluding these admissions, late preterm infants (RR 1.66; 95% CI, 1.50–1.83) and early term infants (RR 1.15; 95% CI, 1.08–1.23) remained at a higher risk for being readmitted compared with term infants, although less so. In addition, moderate preterm infants (RR 1.99; 95% CI, 1.64–2.42) were now at higher risk of readmission compared with term infants. The most common reason for a non-jaundice readmission in all GA categories was infection/rule-out sepsis (**Fig. 4**).

The high rates of jaundice/feeding problem admissions in late preterm and early term infants is consistent with their underlying pathophysiology. Late preterm infants have been shown to have a decreased capacity to handle unconjugated bilirubin, placing them at higher risk for neonatal jaundice.[27–29] Additionally, late preterm infants demonstrate delayed postnatal maturation of hepatic bilirubin uptake and bilirubin conjugation.[29,30] This hepatic immaturity leads to a greater prevalence of jaundice, with bilirubin levels that may peak after being discharged home. The risk of jaundice

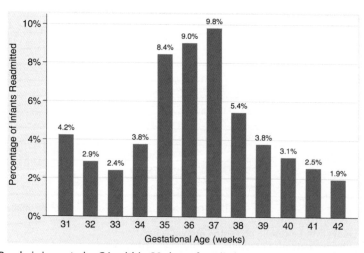

Fig. 1. Readmission rate by GA within 30 days after discharge, KPNC 2003–2012.

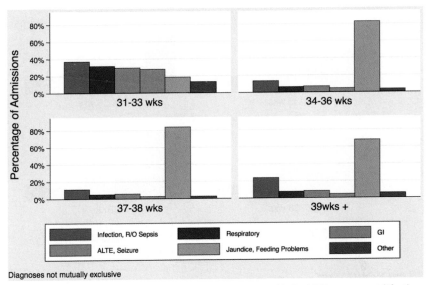

Fig. 2. Readmission diagnoses by GA group, KPNC 2003–2012. ALTE, apparent life-threatening event; GI, gastrointestinal; R/O Sepsis, rule-out sepsis.

is further exacerbated by delayed lactogenesis in mothers of preterm infants.[31–33] Late preterm infants also have an increased prevalence of oromotor dysfunction, having a further impact on oral intake.[6,34,35] These factors may create a perfect storm that manifests after an infant is discharged home and has greater feeding requirements coupled with rising bilirubin levels, ultimately resulting in readmission for jaundice. This underscores the need for enhanced outpatient lactation support in these infants as well as thoughtful formula supplementation, when appropriate, to reduce the risk of jaundice readmissions.

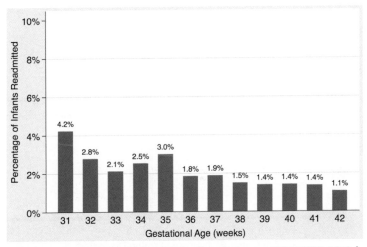

Fig. 3. Readmission rate by GA within 30 days after discharge, KPNC 2003–2012 (excluding jaundice/feeding problem–only admits).

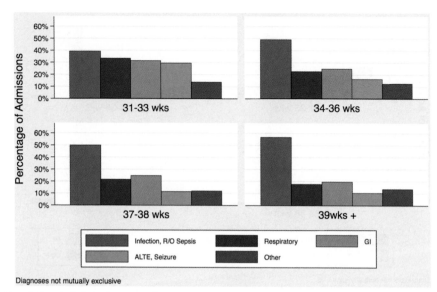

Fig. 4. Readmission diagnoses by GA group excluding jaundice/feeding problem-only admissions, KPNC 2003–2012. ALTE, apparent life-threatening event; GI, gastrointestinal; R/O Sepsis, rule-out sepsis.

READMISSION AGE

Readmissions in moderate preterm infants were relatively evenly distributed among the first 30 days after discharge (**Fig. 5**). In the other GA groups, readmissions occurred largely in the first 5 days after discharge (late preterm infants 80%, early term infants 83%, and term infants 70%). The timing of the readmissions is consistent with the finding that a majority of the readmissions were secondary to jaundice/

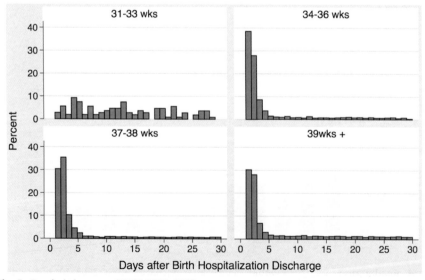

Fig. 5. Readmission age, KPNC 2003–2012.

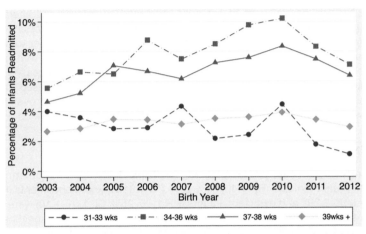

Fig. 6. Readmission rate by year within 30 days after discharge, KPNC 2003–2012.

feeding problems, because serum bilirubin would likely peak in these infants in this time frame.

TEMPORAL TRENDS IN READMISSION RATES

Because considerable effort has been made both in the research and clinical community in recent years, to highlight the increased vulnerability in late preterm infants, the authors sought to evaluate if rates of readmission were decreasing over time.[36,37] **Fig. 6** shows that from 2003 to 2010, readmission rates increased for late preterm and early term infants, before trending lower in 2011 and 2012. For moderate preterm infants, readmission rates trended lower over the time period. The readmission rates for term infants were stable over this time period. Excluding admissions where the only diagnosis was jaundice or a feeding problem, readmission rates were stable for both late preterm and moderate preterm infants (**Fig. 7**).

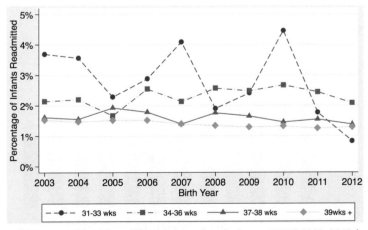

Fig. 7. Readmission rate by year within 30 days after discharge, KPNC 2003–2012 (excluding jaundice/feeding problem–only admits).

These findings demonstrate that despite increased awareness and alterations in care during the birth hospitalization, readmissions in late preterm infants have risen. This may point to a need to further address postdischarge care in order to decrease readmissions. The increased readmission rates are also consistent with changing attitudes toward jaundice in KPNC over this time, which resulted in increased bilirubin testing and phototherapy for the population as a whole.[38] The increased rates also coincide with increased breastfeeding rates (internal data) in KPNC over the time period, which may have put infants at higher risk for hyperbilirubinemia as well.[39]

EMERGENCY DEPARTMENT VISITS AND DIAGNOSES

ED visit rates by GA category are presented in **Table 1**. Compared with term infants, moderate preterm infants (RR 1.40; 95% CI, 1.22–1.61), late preterm infants (RR 1.20; 95% CI, 1.12–1.29), and early term infants (RR 1.06, 95% CI, 1.01–1.10) were all more likely to have an ED visit. Although statistically significant, the magnitude of the increased risk was small. Examining ED visit rates by week of GA (**Fig. 8**), the highest percentage of infants with an ED visit were the 31- and 33-week GA infants. ED visit rates were similar for infants from 38 to 41 weeks' gestation. Compared with term infants, ED visits were more likely to result in an admission in the moderate preterm infants (RR 1.35; 95% CI, 1.04–1.74) and late preterm infants (RR 1.29; 95% CI, 1.13–1.47). Early term infants were at no greater risk of admission after an ED visit (RR 1.01; 95% CI, 0.92–1.11).

ED visit diagnoses by GA are displayed in **Fig. 9**. Compared with reasons for hospital admission, diagnoses in the ED were much more varied. Gastrointestinal diagnoses were the most common specific diagnosis category in all GA categories. In infants who were admitted to the hospital from the ED, infection/rule-out sepsis was the most common diagnosis in all GA categories, except moderate preterm infants (**Fig. 10**).

ED VISIT AGE

A high percentage of ED visits occurred in the first 3 days after discharge in all GA categories (moderate preterm 15%, late preterm 20%, early term 24%, and term 29%).

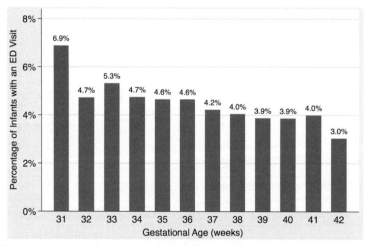

Fig. 8. ED visits by GA within 30 days after discharge, KPNC 2003–2012.

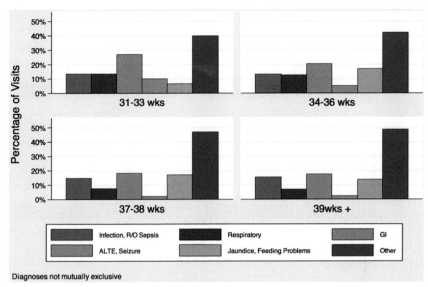

Fig. 9. ED visit diagnoses by GA group, KPNC 2003–2012. ALTE, apparent life-threatening event; GI, gastrointestinal; R/O Sepsis, rule-out sepsis.

Among moderate preterm infants, the age of ED visit was more evenly distributed (**Fig. 11**).

RISK FACTORS FOR HOSPITAL READMISSIONS AND ED VISITS

Multivariate logistic regression was used to evaluate the association between GA and hospital readmission and ED visit while controlling for other risk factors (**Table 4**). Late

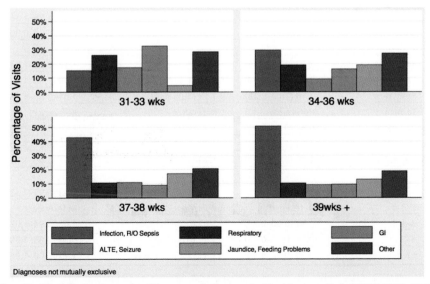

Fig. 10. ED visit diagnoses by GA group (infants admitted to hospital), KPNC 2003–2012. ALTE, apparent life-threatening event; GI, gastrointestinal; R/O Sepsis, rule-out sepsis.

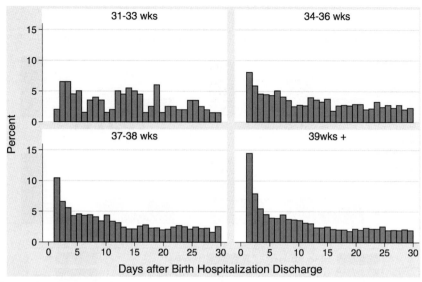

Fig. 11. ED visit age, KPNC 2003–2012.

Table 4
Multivariate models for hospital readmission and ED visit

	Outcome		
	Any Readmission	Nonjaundice Readmissions	Any ED Visit
Predictor	OR (95% CI)	OR (95% CI)	OR (95% CI)
Male	1.25 (1.21–1.30)	1.26 (1.19–1.34)	1.11 (1.07–1.15)
Race			
White	Reference	Reference	Reference
Asian	1.72 (1.65–1.80)	1.05 (0.97–1.14)	1.08 (1.02–1.13)
Black	0.94 (0.87–1.01)	1.22 (1.09–1.36)	1.81 (1.70–1.92)
Hispanic	1.24 (1.19–1.30)	1.23 (1.14–1.32)	1.32 (1.26–1.38)
Other	0.83 (0.77–0.89)	0.67 (0.59–0.77)	0.84 (0.77–0.90)
GA			
Moderate preterm	2.53 (2.02–3.16)	1.55 (1.22–1.98)	1.12 (0.95–1.33)
Late preterm	3.88 (3.64–4.14)	1.50 (1.33–1.69)	1.08 (1.00–1.17)
Early term	2.10 (2.02–2.18)	1.13 (1.05–1.21)	1.04 (0.99–1.08)
Term	Reference	Reference	Reference
SGA—<5th%	0.84 (0.72–0.98)	1.17 (0.95–1.43)	1.10 (0.97–1.24)
LGA—>95th%	1.24 (1.14–1.34)	1.29 (1.13–1.47)	1.00 (0.91–1.09)
Maternal age <18 y	1.06 (0.92–1.23)	1.28 (1.04–1.58)	1.57 (1.40–1.76)
LOS			
<2 d	1.32 (1.27–1.38)	1.02 (0.95–1.09)	1.12 (0.95–1.33)
2–3 d	Reference	Reference	Reference
3–4 d	0.64 (0.60–0.69)	1.02 (0.91–1.13)	1.00 (0.94–1.07)
4–5 d	0.55 (0.48–0.62)	1.09 (0.92–1.29)	0.98 (0.88–1.09)
>5 d	0.39 (0.34–0.44)	1.31 (1.13–1.53)	1.17 (1.06–1.29)

Abbreviations: LGA, large for gestational age; SGA, small for gestational age; <5%, below fifth percentile on Fenton preterm growth; >95%, above ninety-fifth percentile on Fenton preterm growth.

preterm infants had almost 4 times the risk of readmission compared with term infants, early preterm twice the risk, and moderate preterm 2.5 times the risk. Male infants and Asians were also more likely to be readmitted, which may correlate with their increased risk for hyperbilirubinemia. Maternal age less than 18 years had no impact on risk of readmission. Infants with birth hospitalization LOS less than 2 days were at some increased risk compared with infants staying 2 to 3 days (cohort mean LOS 2.45 days). LOS over 3 days, was highly protective. A reason for this may be that longer stays may increase the likelihood of the bilirubin peaking during the birth hospitalization and may allow more time for inpatient support of breastfeeding, thus avoiding jaundice readmissions.

When examining nonjaundice readmissions as the outcome, preterm infants were at increased risk for readmission but the magnitude of the increased risk was smaller. Blacks and Hispanics were more likely to be readmitted as well as infants of mothers under 18 years of age. In contrast, only LOS greater than 5 days was a significant factor in determining readmission and increased the risk rather than being protective.

For ED visits, GA was not significantly predictive. There was a small increase in risk for late preterm infants. This may be because in KPNC, all newborns are seen within 2 days postdischarge by a pediatrician, in a group visit, or by home health services. Blacks and Hispanics were more likely to be seen in the ED as well as infants of mothers under 18 years old. LOS greater than 5 days increased the risk of an ED visit, which may imply a more complicated initial course.

Additional analyses were done in a subgroup of the cohort from 2009 to 2012 with complete data on respiratory support (none; oxygen, nasal continuous airway pressure, or high-flow nasal cannula; and mechanical ventilation) during the birth hospitalization and level of care (newborn nursery; level II NICU or stay less than 48 hours in level III NICU; or level III NICU greater than 48 hours). Neither of these factors was predictive for readmissions or ED visits.

SUMMARY

This review notes that there is limited literature describing health care utilization in moderate preterm, late preterm, and early term infants after their birth hospitalization. Most of the existing data focus on late preterm infants. Moderate preterm infants are often grouped with less mature infants and early preterm infants with term infants, making it difficult to draw inferences for these two groups.

The primary data analysis demonstrates that late preterm infants and early term infants were at a greater risk for rehospitalization and that the overwhelming reason for rehospitalization was for jaundice and feeding problems. Although moderate preterm infants were also at increased risk for readmission, their rates of readmissions were less than late preterm and term infants mainly because readmissions for jaundice/feeding problems were not prominent. This is likely because their longer initial hospital stays allow for issues around hyperbilirubinemia and feeding to be resolved prior to discharge.

Temporal trends in readmission rates in late preterm and early term infants have been increasing despite increased awareness and changes in inpatient practices. The increased rates correlate with increased bilirubin testing and phototherapy rates as well as rising breastfeeding rates. Physiologic factors may predispose these infants to develop hyperbilirubinemia after discharge. Although longer LOS is protective against readmission, it is not reasonable to prolong the birth hospitalizations of infants who meet criteria for discharge. More effort needs to be placed on outpatient lactation and feeding support and on responsible use of formula supplementation to help avoid readmissions. Future studies designed to evaluate outpatient interventions in preterm and early term infants surrounding lactation, feeding, and management of jaundice are needed.

ED visit rates do not show a strong correlation with GA after controlling for other risk factors, although there is a slight increase among late preterm infants. Given that access to care in KPNC may differ from that found in other systems, additional research in other health care settings is needed to disentangle what may be driven by biology from what may be driven by health services.

In conclusion, moderate preterm, late preterm, and early term infants all show increased rates of hospital readmission in the first 30 days after birth hospitalization discharge. The rates are the highest in late preterm and early term infants driven by an overwhelming predominance of jaundice readmissions. These infants do not show a substantial increase in the utilization of ED visits. Additional research is needed to study interventions to reduce jaundice readmissions in late preterm and early term infants, such as improved outpatient lactation support and responsible formula supplementation when lactogenesis is delayed.

REFERENCES

1. Kramer MS, Demissie K, Yang H, et al. The contribution of mild and moderate preterm birth to infant mortality. Fetal and Infant Health Study Group of the Canadian Perinatal Surveillance System. JAMA 2000;284:843–9.
2. McIntire DD, Leveno KJ. Neonatal mortality and morbidity rates in late preterm births compared with births at term. Obstet Gynecol 2008;111:35–41.
3. Yoder BA, Gordon MC, Barth WH Jr. Late-preterm birth: does the changing obstetric paradigm alter the epidemiology of respiratory complications? Obstet Gynecol 2008;111:814–22.
4. Melamed NK, Klinger G, Tenenbaum-Gavish K, et al. Short-term neonatal outcome in low-risk, spontaneous, singleton, late preterm deliveries. Obstet Gynecol 2009;114:253–60.
5. Watchko JF, Maisels MJ. Jaundice in low birthweight infants: pathobiology and outcome. Arch Dis Child Fetal Neonatal Ed 2003;88:F455–8.
6. Wang ML, Dorer DJ, Fleming MP, et al. Clinical outcomes of near-term infants. Pediatrics 2004;114:372–6.
7. Escobar GJ, McCormick MC, Zupancic JA, et al. Unstudied infants: outcomes of moderately premature infants in the neonatal intensive care unit. Arch Dis Child Fetal Neonatal Ed 2006;91:F238–44.
8. Gouyon JB, Vintejoux A, Sagot P, et al. Neonatal outcome associated with singleton birth at 34-41 weeks of gestation. Int J Epidemiol 2010;39:769–76.
9. Tsai ML, Lien R, Chiang MC, et al. Prevalence and morbidity of late preterm infants: current status in a medical center of Northern Taiwan. Pediatr Neonatol 2012;53:171–7.
10. Escobar GJ, Greene JD, Hulac P, et al. Rehospitalisation after birth hospitalisation: patterns among infants of all gestations. Arch Dis Child 2005;90:125–31.
11. McLaurin KK, Hall CB, Jackson EA, et al. Persistence of morbidity and cost differences between late-preterm and term infants during the first year of life. Pediatrics 2009;123:653–9.
12. Martens PJ, Derksen S, Gupta S. Predictors of hospital readmission of Manitoba newborns within six weeks postbirth discharge: a population-based study. Pediatrics 2004;114:708–13.

13. Shapiro-Mendoza CK, Tomashek KM, Kotelchuck M, et al. Risk factors for neonatal morbidity and mortality among "healthy," late preterm newborns. Semin Perinatol 2006;30:54–60.
14. Escobar GJ, Joffe S, Gardner MN, et al. Rehospitalization in the first two weeks after discharge from the neonatal intensive care unit. Pediatrics 1999;104:e2.
15. Underwood MA, Danielsen B, Gilbert WM. Cost, causes and rates of rehospitalization of preterm infants. J Perinatol 2007;27:614–9.
16. Oddie SJ, Hammal D, Richmond S, et al. Early discharge and readmission to hospital in the first month of life in the Northern Region of the UK during 1998: a case cohort study. Arch Dis Child 2005;90:119–24.
17. Escobar GJ, Clark RH, Greene JD. Short-term outcomes of infants born at 35 and 36 weeks gestation: we need to ask more questions. Semin Perinatol 2006;30:28–33.
18. Dietz PM, Rizzo JH, England LJ, et al. Early term delivery and health care utilization in the first year of life. J Pediatr 2012;161:234–9.e1.
19. Bird TM, Bronstein JM, Hall RW, et al. Late preterm infants: birth outcomes and health care utilization in the first year. Pediatrics 2010;126:e311–9.
20. Jain S, Cheng J. Emergency department visits and rehospitalizations in late preterm infants. Clin Perinatol 2006;33:935–45.
21. Tomashek KM, Shapiro-Mendoza CK, Weiss J, et al. Early discharge among late preterm and term newborns and risk of neonatal morbidity. Semin Perinatol 2006; 30:61–8.
22. Dodd KL. Neonatal jaundice–a lighter touch. Arch Dis Child 1993;68:529–32.
23. Escobar GJ, Ragins A, Li SX, et al. Recurrent wheezing in the third year of life among children born at 32 weeks' gestation or later: relationship to laboratory-confirmed, medically attended infection with respiratory syncytial virus during the first year of life. Arch Pediatr Adolesc Med 2010;164:915–22.
24. Escobar GJ, Fischer A, Kremers R, et al. Rapid retrieval of neonatal outcomes data: the Kaiser Permanente Neonatal Minimum Data Set. Qual Manag Health Care 1997;5:19–33.
25. Chimmula S, Dhuru R, Folck B, et al. PS2–44: VDW data sources: Kaiser Permanente Northern California. Clin Med Res 2012;10:193.
26. Fenton TR. A new growth chart for preterm babies: Babson and Benda's chart updated with recent data and a new format. BMC Pediatr 2003;3:1–10.
27. Bhutani VK, Johnson L. Kernicterus in late preterm infants cared for as term healthy infants. Semin Perinatol 2006;30:89–97.
28. Watchko JF. Hyperbilirubinemia and bilirubin toxicity in the late preterm infant [abstract ix]. Clin Perinatol 2006;33:839–52.
29. Kaplan M, Muraca M, Vreman HJ, et al. Neonatal bilirubin production-conjugation imbalance: effect of glucose-6-phosphate dehydrogenase deficiency and borderline prematurity. Arch Dis Child Fetal Neonatal Ed 2005;90:F123–7.
30. Kawade N, Onishi S. The prenatal and postnatal development of UDP-glucuronyltransferase activity towards bilirubin and the effect of premature birth on this activity in the human liver. Biochem J 1981;196:257–60.
31. Cregan MD, De Mello TR, Kershaw D, et al. Initiation of lactation in women after preterm delivery. Acta Obstet Gynecol Scand 2002;81:870–7.
32. Henderson JJ, Hartmann PE, Newnham JP, et al. Effect of preterm birth and antenatal corticosteroid treatment on lactogenesis II in women. Pediatrics 2008;121: e92–100.
33. Meier PP, Furman LM, Degenhardt M. Increased lactation risk for late preterm infants and mothers: evidence and management strategies to protect breastfeeding. J Midwifery Womens Health 2007;52:579–87.

34. DeMauro SB, Patel PR, Medoff-Cooper B, et al. Postdischarge feeding patterns in early- and late-preterm infants. Clin Pediatr (Phila) 2011;50:957–62.

35. Adamkin DH. Feeding problems in the late preterm infant [abstract ix]. Clin Perinatol 2006;33:831–7.

36. Raju TN. The problem of late-preterm (near-term) births: a workshop summary. Pediatr Res 2006;60:775–6.

37. Raju TN, Higgins RD, Stark AR, et al. Optimizing care and outcome for late-preterm (near-term) infants: a summary of the workshop sponsored by the National Institute of Child Health and Human Development. Pediatrics 2006; 118:1207–14.

38. Kuzniewicz MW, Escobar GJ, Newman TB. Impact of universal bilirubin screening on severe hyperbilirubinemia and phototherapy use. Pediatrics 2009;124: 1031–9.

39. Kuzniewicz MW, Escobar GJ, Wi S, et al. Risk factors for severe hyperbilirubinemia among infants with borderline bilirubin levels: a nested case-control study. J Pediatr 2008;153:234–40.

APPENDIX:

Table 1: *ICD-9* codes used for diagnosis and procedure grouping		
Diagnosis Group	**Subgroup**	***ICD-9* Codes**
Infection, R/O sepsis	Bacterial infection (not UTI)	032–041.9, 047–049, 460, 462, 481–486.9, 320x, 322.9, 770.0, 771.4–771.59, 771.81, 771.83, 771.89, 785.52, 790.7, 995.91, 995.92
	Suspected infection	V29.0, 780.6, 780.60, 780.61
	Viral infection	047–049, 050–066.9, 077.99, 078.89, 079.2, 079.6, 079.89, 079.99, 464.4, 465x, 480x, 487–488.9
	UTI/pyelonephritis	590.10, 590.80, 599.0, 771.82
Jaundice/feeding problems	Jaundice	773.0, 773.1, 773.2, 774.0, 774.1, 774.2, 774.31, 774.5, 774.6, 774.7, 782.4
	Dehydration/feeding problems	276.5x, 775.5, 775.6, 779.3, 779.30, 779.31, 779.34, 783.21, 783.3, 783.41
Respiratory	Respiratory problems Complaint	V29.2, 079.6, 464.4, 466.x, 518.0, 518.81, 519.11, 770.6, 770.84, 770.89, 786–786.29
ALTE/seizure	ALTE/apnea	770.81, 770.82, 770.83, 786.03, 799.82
	Seizures	345x, 780.3x, 779.0
GI	Pyloric stenosis	537.0, 750.5
	Diarrhea/GI	003.0, 008.69, 008.8, 774.3, 774.39, 774.4, 787.7, 787.99
	Emesis/vomiting	578.0, 787.01, 787.02, 787.03, 787.04, 779.32, 779.33
	Constipation	564.00, 564.09
	Esophageal reflux	530.81
	GI complaint/diarrhea	550.90, 553.9, 558.3, 558.9, 565.0, 566, 569.3, 573.8, 574.20, 575.2, 576.2, 576.8, 577.0, 578.1, 578.9, 579.3, 579.8, 772.4, 777.8, 787.3, 787.91, 789.00, 789.09

Abbreviations: ALTE, apparent life-threatening event/seizure; GI, gastrointestinal; R/O, rule-out; UTI, urinary tract infection.

Quality Initiatives Related to Moderately Preterm, Late Preterm, and Early Term Births

Andrea N. Trembath, MD, MPH[a],*, Jay D. Iams, MD[b],
Michele Walsh, MD, MSE[a]

KEYWORDS

- Quality improvement • Preterm births • Infection reduction • Delaying preterm birth
- Human milk

KEY POINTS

- The goal of quality-improvement methodology is to improve the quality and cost-effectiveness of health care.
- The care provided to moderately preterm, late preterm, and early term births is an area with significant practice variation.
- Prior quality-improvement initiatives designed to reduce nonindicated early term births and bloodstream infections may serve as models for future initiatives in more mature infants.
- Respiratory care, feeding management, and discharge planning may serve as future directions for quality improvement in moderate preterm, late preterm, and early term births.

INTRODUCTION

Prematurity is the leading cause of death for newborns in the United States and represents more than $26 billion dollars in health care expenditure costs per year.[1] Overall, most premature infants born in the United States each year are classified as either moderately preterm (MPT) or late preterm (LPT) infants, defined as birth at 31 0/7 to 33 6/7 and 34 0/7 to 36 6/7 weeks' gestation respectively.[2] Together this group accounts for more than 70% of the preterm population. Ample opportunity exists to improve care using quality improvement (QI) methodology.

Disclosures: The authors have no financial disclosures.
[a] Division of Neonatology, Department of Pediatrics, UH Rainbow Babies & Children's Hospital, 11100 Euclid Avenue, RBC Suite 3100, Cleveland, OH 44106-6010, USA; [b] Division of Maternal Fetal Medicine, The Ohio State University Medical Center, 395 West 12 Avenue, Fifth Floor, Columbus, OH 43210-1267, USA
* Corresponding author.
E-mail address: Andrea.Trembath@UHhospitals.org

Clin Perinatol 40 (2013) 777–789
http://dx.doi.org/10.1016/j.clp.2013.07.011
0095-5108/13/$ – see front matter © 2013 Elsevier Inc. All rights reserved.

The principal tenets of QI to improve and ensure the safety, quality, and cost-effectiveness of health care are particularly appropriate for application among preterm infants.[3] QI in the neonatal intensive care unit (NICU) has primarily focused on extremely low-gestational-age newborns (ELGANs) because they are at highest risk for death or morbidity. However, they represent a minority of premature infants: ~5% of premature infants born in the United States each year.[2] Therefore, MPT and LPT infants represent an important focus for QI within the United States because they are subject to a great deal of variation in care practices among individual centers as well as among practitioners. Unnecessary variation in care and lack of evidence-based practices may contribute to the morbidities of prematurity.

Over the last decade the number of QI projects involving neonatal and perinatal topics has increased substantially. As a result, the number of national collaboratives focused on the care of neonates has also increased. One of the most recognized collaboratives is the Vermont Oxford Network (VON). An international collaborative of more than 900 NICUs established in 1988, the mission of the VON is to improve the quality, safety, and efficiency of health care delivery to newborns.[4] The VON iNICU Quality Improvement Collaboratives for Neonatology works to identity and implement evidence-based practices through the creation of shared goals and measurable achievements. iNICU define 4 key habits necessary for effective QI: change, collaborative learning, evidence-based practice, and systems thinking.[5]

National and international collaboratives are an important component to improving the care delivered to newborns and provides an established platform for sharing strategies for QI. However, the scope and direction of QI initiatives must be taken in the context of the health care systems in which they will function.[6] As a result, the VON platform for QI in NICUs has now been applied to multiple regional perinatal quality collaboratives. State collaboratives such as the Perinatal Quality Collaborative of North Carolina, Tennessee Initiative for Perinatal Quality Care, New York State Perinatal Quality Collaborative, California Perinatal Quality Care Collaborative, and the Ohio Perinatal Quality Collaborative (OPQC) have built particularly active quality initiatives based on the VON platform. This article uses the experience of the OPQC to show how quality collaboratives could be applied to decreasing unnecessary variation in the care provided to MPT, LPT, and early term (ET) infants.

OPQC

OPQC is a network of Ohio institutions, hospitals, and individuals dedicated to improving perinatal health in the state. The collaborative includes 24 neonatal teams and 19 obstetric teams that represent the 6 perinatal regions of Ohio. The OPQC mission is "Through collaborative use of improvement science methods, to reduce preterm births and improve outcomes of preterm newborns in Ohio as soon as possible." OPQC uses an adapted methodology from the Institute for Healthcare Improvement's (IHI) Breakthrough Series Model (**Fig. 1**). OPQC's primary goal is to target improvements in outcome through defined shared goals based on established scientific evidence, which includes using rapid-cycle QI techniques such as Plan-Do-Study-Act.

OPQC brings together a multidisciplinary team of individuals through face-to-face sessions and webinar-based action period calls to review individual site and collaborative data, share successful QI initiatives and strategies, and plan future OPQC projects. Thus far 6 project titles have been designed: reducing late onset infections, human milk, antenatal corticosteroid (ANC), 39 weeks charter and 39 weeks/birth registry accuracy project. Three of the projects have targeted reducing preterm birth, and the other two are designed to reduce the morbidity and mortalities of preterm birth.

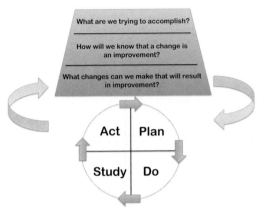

Fig. 1. IHI model for improvement (Plan-Do-Study-Act cycle). (*Adapted from* Langley GL, Nolan KM, Nolan TW, et al. The improvement guide: a practical approach to enhancing organizational performance. 2nd edition. San Francisco (CA): Jossey-Bass Publishers; 2009; with permission.)

OPQC Neonatal Initiatives

Reducing late-onset infections

Prematurity is a well-established risk factor for infection, particularly in the hospital setting. Nosocomial infections occur in 15% to 30% of extremely preterm infants and cause increased morbidity, mortality, and hospital costs. As a result, OPQC identified infection as a key target for a neonatal quality initiative. Bloodstream infection in NICUs is a multifactorial problem with several important factors playing a role in reducing infection, including appropriate use of centrally inserted catheters, hand hygiene, a culture of providing quality care, and maintaining skin integrity (**Fig. 2**). By focusing on improving the process of inserting and maintaining central lines, several of these modifying factors could be enhanced. For the insertion bundle, key measures include a focus on hand hygiene, sterile technique, and identifying problems with maintaining sterile fields during insertion. For the maintenance bundle, the primary elements identified are related to sterility during tubing changes and catheter hub care and assessing the need for the line daily.

As a result of the OPQC infection project, a 20% sustained decrease in bloodstream infections in premature infants was seen among the 24 NICUs.[7] Throughout the project it has become apparent that there are significant differences in the relative importance of each of the bundles. Among NICUs the key component to sustaining a decrease in bloodstream infections is the continued use of the maintenance bundle. As a new focus, OPQC members are working to achieve greater than 90% compliance with the catheter maintenance bundle (**Fig. 3**). OPQC anticipates this will be the most critical component to decreasing and maintaining the new baseline rate of bloodstream infections.[8,9]

Human milk

The first collaborative to reduce infection noted that 30% of late-onset infections occurred without any line in place. Thus, other measures to further reduce infection were sought. The use of human milk in preterm infants is associated with a decrease in the risk of infection.[10,11] Thus, a bundle to increase the number of infants receiving any human milk and with an emphasis on increasing the intake of each infant's mother's own milk (MOM) was created. Although targeted at the smallest and most

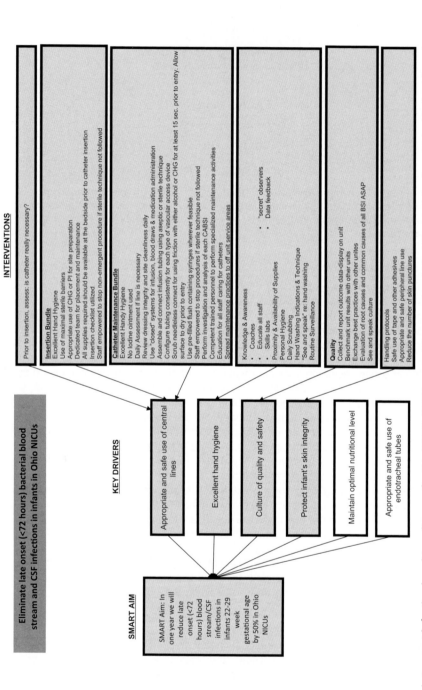

Fig. 2. Late-onset infection key driver diagram for the OPQC. CABSI, central line associated bloodstream infection; CHG, chlorhexidine gluconate; CSF, cerebrospinal fluid. (*Courtesy of* Ohio Perinatal Quality Collaborative, Cincinnati, Ohio; with permission.)

OPQC Maintenance Bundle Compliance Self Reporting Tool
This form should be completed for every patient 22-29 weeks gestation in your NICU who has a central catheter in place at the time you have elected to survey maintenance practices.

Initials of person completing form _____

Data Collection Tool Data **must** be entered into OPQC website				
Shift (select one):	☐ Day ☐ Evening/Night			
Date of Birth:	_____ (MM/DD/YYYY)			
Type of Catheter:	☐ PICC			
	☐ Umbilical			
	☐ PICC and Umbilical			
	☐ Non-Tunneled Central Line(i.e. Cook Catheter)			
	☐ Tunneled Line (i.e. Broviac)			
Date Maintenance performed:	_____ (MM/DD/YYYY)			

Daily Assessment			
Was there assessment that the baby needed the catheter (e.g. assessment whether the catheter should be retained or removed)?	Yes	No	Don't Know

Catheter Site Care			
Was dressing integrity & site cleanliness assessed during your shift?	Yes	No	Don't Know
Was a central catheter dressing change performed during your shift today?	Yes	No	N/A (Umbilical catheter)

If a dressing change was done on your shift		
• Was the site cleansed with appropriate solution (CHG, PI, or ETOH)?	Yes	No
• If yes, which cleansing solution was used? (select one)	☐chlorhexidine ☐povidone iodine ☐alcohol	
• Was cleansing solution allowed to air dry completely?	Yes	No

Catheter Entry		
Was a closed system maintained for infusion, blood draws & medication administration?	Yes	No
Was the catheter accessed or entered for any reason on your shift today?	Yes	No

If the catheter was accessed or entered on your shift today, for all accesses or entries			
• Did staff scrub needleless connector or hub using friction with alcohol or CHG for ≥ 15 sec? **	Yes	No	
• Did staff allow surface of connector or hub to dry prior to entry?	Yes	No	
• If you are not using a "closed system", did staff accessing or entering catheter wear clean gloves?	Yes	No	N/A
• Did staff accessing or entering catheter perform hand hygiene before & after access or entry?	Yes	No	
Was infusion tubing changed during your shift today?	Yes	No	
• If yes, did staff at a minimum wear clean gloves?	Yes	No	
• Did staff use a sterile or clean barrier for tubing assembly?	Yes	No	
Pre-filled, flush containing syringes were used for all catheter flushes?	Yes	No	N/A

**If SwabCap is used, it remained in place for >5 minutes prior to accessing the catheter; If SiteScrub is used, a standard 15 second friction scrub was used prior to accessing the catheter, or if another product is used all manufacturer instructions have been followed.

Rev 8/30/2012jkn

Fig. 3. Maintenance bundle data form for reducing late-onset infections among OPQC NICUs. PICC, peripherally inserted central catheter. (*Courtesy of* Ohio Perinatal Quality Collaborative, Cincinnati, Ohio; with permission.)

premature infants, this project is now being extended to include more mature infants including the MPT and LPT populations. For the human milk project, OPQC intends to reduce late-onset blood stream infections to less than 10% in Ohio NICUs. Intermediate goals include the commencement of human milk feeds within 72 hours of life and the use of greater than 100 mL/kg/d of human milk feeds by 21 days of life. In this setting the use of maternal breast milk should be maximized, donor milk minimized, and ideally the use of formula eliminated.

This project has proved particularly challenging because it requires collaboration between multiple caregivers including obstetric, labor and delivery, postpartum, and NICU staff. The key drivers on this project include education of mother and staff on the benefits of breast-feeding, provision of early pumping (<6 hours after delivery), early initiation of enteral feeds in the first 72 hours of life, and persistent advances of enteral feedings such that greater than 100 mL/kg/d of feedings is reached by day 21, and that at least half is provided as MOM. Teams created a multipronged education package that included emphasis on human milk in prenatal care with the obstetric teams; in high-risk pregnancies, antenatal consultation with a neonatologist who strongly encourages provision of maternal breast milk; and reinforcement at the time of delivery.

Teams have identified significant barriers to beginning expression of breast milk within 6 hours of birth, including lack of familiarity of obstetric nursing staff and lack of equipment. Another barrier has been identified in neonates who are transported long distances. Donor milk has been used as a substitute in this setting until MOM is available. With this combined approach, at the 23 participating level 3 NICUs 80% of neonates born between 22 and 29 weeks began enteral feeds within 72 hours of birth, and 84% were receiving more than 50% of the intake as MOM at day 21 of life.

Late-onset infections have shown a trend toward reduction from a baseline of 18% to 12% (**Fig. 4**). To avoid unintended harm, growth failure and necrotizing enterocolitis (NEC) were tracked as balancing measures. Growth failure (defined as a weight at discharge <3%) declined throughout the project period from 15% to 13%. NEC also decreased from 8% to 5.8% across this period. This finding suggests that, despite earlier introduction of feeds and progressive increases in feeds, the risk for NEC was not increased.

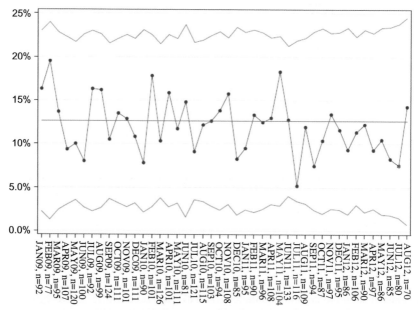

Fig. 4. Late-onset infection among extremely ELGANs at Ohio Perinatal Quality Collaborative hospitals from January 2009 to August 2012. (*Courtesy of* Ohio Perinatal Quality Collaborative, Cincinnati, Ohio; with permission.)

OPQC Obstetrics Initiatives

Thirty-nine weeks delivery project

In order to reduce the morbidities and mortalities of prematurity, delaying preterm birth when feasible remains the ultimate solution. Even among LPT and ET infants, delivery increases the risk of respiratory disease, infection, feeding issues, and death compared with infants born at 39 to 40 weeks. In 2008, OPQC launched the first state-wide initiative designed to reduce the number of non–medically indicated scheduled births between 36 0/7 to 38 6/7 weeks. The project involved 20 obstetric delivery centers throughout the state and aspired to "In one year, reduce by 60%, the number of women in Ohio of 36.1 to 38.6 weeks gestation for whom initiation of labor or caesarean section is done in absence of appropriate medical or obstetric indication." In order to achieve this goal, the primary focuses of the project involved educating consumers about the risks of early deliveries at less than 39 weeks, optimizing gestational age (GA) dating, and educating physicians on the standards of medical practice as defined by the American College of Obstetrics and Gynecology.

Between September 2008 and September 2010, the rate of scheduled (non–medically indicated) births between 36 0/7 and 38 6/7 weeks GA decreased from greater than 15% to less than 5% within the collaborative network. This decline was confirmed in the Ohio Department of Health Office of Vital Statistics data for this time period, showing a concurrent increase in the number of births between 39 and 41 weeks GA (**Fig. 5**). Since project initiation, OPQC estimates that efforts to reduce early nonindicated deliveries has resulted in ~27,000 births shifted to after 39 weeks and 180 fewer NICU admissions annually. The cost savings have been estimated at more than $10 million annually.

Thirty-nine weeks delivery/birth records accuracy

Promotion of optimal obstetric care is maximally efficient when applied to large birth hospitals, but more than half of births occur in smaller facilities. Following the successful 39 Weeks Scheduled Birth Initiative (39 weeks project), OPQC undertook a project to spread the intervention to hospitals with moderate birth volumes. A key component of this project was to improve the quality of documentation on the birth certificate, and to use the birth certificate as a QI reporting tool. In this way the project built on work that hospitals were already required to do, and it simultaneously improved the quality of birth certificate documentation.

Techniques based on IHI Breakthrough Series that were used successfully in the OPQC 39 weeks project were applied to 15 pilot hospitals chosen to represent a spectrum of locations, populations, and delivery volumes in Ohio. Local data abstractors in the initial 39 weeks project were replaced by birth certificate personnel at each site who were educated by Ohio Office of Vital Statistics staff and supported by QI experts. Ohio birth certificate data were collected and reported promptly. Rates of scheduled inductions of labor that lacked a documented medical indication were reported in monthly QI webinars. Local teams used IHI techniques to promote compliance with ACOG practice guidelines.

Rates of scheduled inductions of labor at less than 39 weeks without a medical indication in the 15 pilot sites decreased while the original OPQC project was ongoing, and declined further when Ohio began reporting hospital rates on a public Web site. Rates have continued to decline in pilot project sites since project inception, and accuracy of birth certificate information has improved.

Collaboration by clinical, administrative, and Ohio Office of Vital Statistics staff to improve the accuracy of birth certificate data has been accompanied by a decline in scheduled births at less than 39 weeks' gestation in medium-sized maternity units.

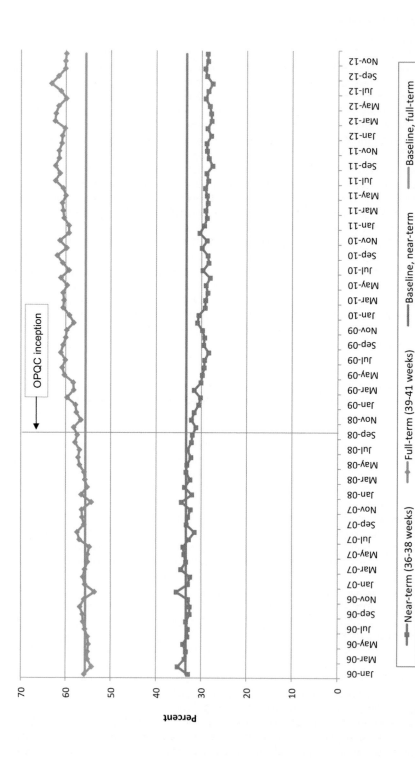

Fig. 5. Percent distribution of full-term and near-term births at the OPQC member hospitals by month from January 2006 to December 2012. Baseline averages were calculated from the initial 24 months. (*Courtesy of* Ohio Perinatal Quality Collaborative, Cincinnati, Ohio; with permission.)

Antenatal corticosteroids

Timely administration of ANCS has long been known to improve lung maturity, reduce respiratory distress syndrome, and reduce intraventricular hemorrhage in premature infants. OPQC sought to achieve optimal ANCS use in 20 large Ohio maternity hospitals. The project used modified IHI Breakthrough Series methods to improve the proportion of eligible women treated with ANCS before births at 240/7 to 340/7 weeks. A key driver diagram was used to apply interventions intended to identify all eligible women quickly, to reduce intervals from admission to assessment and from ANCS order to administration, and to document ANCS treatment accurately in hospital and birth records.

Sites selected interventions and recorded the number of eligible women who were treated with any ANCS (primary outcome), a full ANCS course, intervals from arrival to treatment and delivery, location of treatment, and reasons for failure to receive ANCS. Deidentified limited data were sent to a central repository and reviewed in monthly webinars. Techniques of maximizing appropriate ANCS treatment were shared. The goal was to achieve one or more doses of ANCS in 90% of eligible women at all sites.

From October 2011 to June 2012, 1221 (91.8%) of 1330 infants born between 240/7 to 340/7 weeks at 18 participating sites received greater than or equal to 1 dose of ANCS (all betamethasone). Documentation of ANCS administration on the birth certificates did not reflect the high rates of administration seen in the health records; education efforts directed at both clerical and medical staff improved birth certificate documentation. Even so, 109 eligible women did not receive ANCS. Delivery less than 2 hours after arrival was the most common reason (46%) for missed treatment, followed by a rapid unexpected change in clinical status. System failures to order or administer treatment accounted for 10% of missed treatment. The mean interval for all sites from first dose to delivery ranged from 190 to more than 340 hours, averaging 288 hours. Individual site intervals had wider ranges. Almost 40% of treated women received the first dose of ANCS before admission to the delivery hospital. OPQC concluded that ANCS administration at large obstetric hospitals exceeds 90% of eligible women but opportunities to improve remain to reduce system failures, optimize the treatment to delivery interval, and promote treatment in referring hospitals. Future work will expand these interventions to smaller hospitals that care for preterm pregnancies less frequently.

AREAS FOR FUTURE QI INITIATIVES

The areas for future QI initiatives parallel the need for increased evidence-based research in the common morbidities of MPT, LPT, and ET births. Practice variation in respiratory care, feeding management, and discharge planning are particularly in need of QI.

Delaying Preterm Birth

Delaying preterm birth remains the primary solution to decreasing the morbidities of prematurity. The 39-week initiative, as described previously, represents an area for ongoing focus in delaying preterm birth. However, dissemination of this initiative could improve the outcomes for LPT and ET infants nationally.

Progesterone

The use of progesterone in pregnant women at high risk of preterm birth, such as those with shortened cervix or history of preterm birth, can delay preterm birth. Evidence for the prophylactic use of progesterone has been increasing since the 1970s. Several studies suggested that the use of prophylactic progesterone (17-alpha hydroxyprogesterone or vaginal progesterone gel) was efficacious in preventing preterm birth among women with a history of preterm birth.[12,13]

In 2007, Fonseca and colleagues[14] found a 44% reduction in preterm birth before 34 weeks in asymptomatic women with shortened cervix (<15 mm) treated with vaginal progesterone. In a large multicenter randomized controlled trial of asymptomatic women designed to reduce preterm birth at less than 33 weeks' gestation, women with shortened cervix (10–22 mm) were treated with vaginal progesterone or placebo until 36 6/7 weeks, rupture of membranes, or delivery. Those treated with vaginal progesterone were significantly less likely to have preterm delivery (8.9% vs 16.1%), even after adjustment for other influential factors (Relative risk 0.55 [95% Confidence interval: 0.33, 0.92]).[15] These results suggested that identification of candidates for prophylactic progesterone administration is an important factor in delaying preterm birth. Recent economic analyses also suggest that universal cervical length measurement during pregnancy is a cost-effective screening tool.[16,17]

A statement from the American College of Obstetrician Gynecologists (ACOG) in October 2012 recommended routine cervical length screening in all pregnancies. ACOG recommends that women with a history of preterm birth, as well as those patients with shortened cervical lengths (<20 mm), before or at 24 weeks' gestation be offered vaginal progesterone therapy.[18]

In 2013, OPQC will begin a new obstetric project designed to reduce the rate of preterm births before 37, 35, and 32 weeks by increasing the proportion of women in Ohio who receive appropriate progesterone therapy. The pilot project will begin with 20 OPQC obstetric teams across the state and will disseminate the experience gained to additional centers following anticipated completion in 2015.

Admission/Level of Care

Optimizing the services available for preterm infants has been the focus of the American Academy of Pediatrics (AAP) for several decades. In 2004, in a policy statement (updated in 2012), the AAP reinforced the need for regionalized systems of perinatal care, in which both mothers and infants with complex needs should be referred to higher-level centers for specialized care and additional health resources.[19] This recommendation includes infants with congenital anomalies as well as anticipated preterm birth and the postnatal care of extremely premature infants. Meta-analysis of outcomes in both extremely low birth weight infants and ELGANs suggests an improvement in the odds of death with birth at a level III or IV neonatal center. As a result, the AAP policy statement recommends that infants less than 32 weeks and of less than 1500 g should be cared for at level III centers. Despite the AAP statement, the rate of delivery of very low birth weight infants in the United States changed little (from 74.2% to 74.9%) and remains a focus of QI initiatives for the US Department of Health and Human Services Maternal and Child Health Bureau.

For infants 32 weeks or more, the recommendations are less clear and lack sufficient evidence for more concrete guidelines. For infants 35 weeks or more who are physiologically stable, the AAP recommends delivery and management at a level I center, and, for infants 32 weeks or more, delivery and management at a level II center may be adequate. Statewide initiatives designed to improve the number of deliveries at appropriate levels of neonatal care for MPT and LPT may optimize the outcomes and services needed for this group of infants.

Respiratory Management

Preterm infants are vulnerable to long-term disturbances in lung histology, anatomy, and function, even without significant needs for respiratory support in the first days of life.[20] Multiple studies have shown that prematurity is an independent risk factor for several respiratory morbidities, including transient tachypnea of the newborn, respiratory distress syndrome, and respiratory failure, compared with term infants.[21] However, increasing evidence for alteration in lung development in the absence of respiratory symptoms has emerged. On histologic examination of lungs from LPT infants, the normal pattern of alveolarization seen after the third trimester of pregnancy in term infants is absent.[22,23] These findings suggest that the increased risk for future respiratory issues including respiratory infection and asthma for moderate preterm, LPT, and ET infants may at least in part be caused by lung dysfunction that is not readily apparent by clinical examination.

Strategies for the management of respiratory disease in preterm infants are variable and represent an ideal area for further research and QI initiatives. The early management of respiratory disease in preterm infants of MPT and LPT gestations is often characterized by the need for continuous positive airway pressure and/or supplemental oxygen, whereas ET births typically require no respiratory support. However, there remains a population of MPT and LPT infants who have significant respiratory complications that require intubation, mechanical ventilation, and possible exogenous surfactant therapy.[24] Defining guidelines for the management of these infants in the delivery room, thresholds for intubation and surfactant therapy, and using oxygen saturation targets are all possible areas for improvement.

Infection Reduction

Reducing infection among preterm infants involves multiple, complex interactions. Hand hygiene remains the most basic and effective strategy available to prevent infection. QI initiatives should at a minimum contain hand hygiene as a component. Maintenance of skin integrity is important, whether through the care of central lines, minimizing skin breakdown, or consolidating blood draws.

Feeding Management

The needs of preterm infants in terms of feeding management can be variable. Not only ELGANs but also MPT and LPT infants have different nutritional needs than their term counterparts. They are more likely to have increased needs for iron, calcium, phosphate, and micronutrients. MPT infants often require the use of nasogastric feeds and parenteral nutrition early in life. The need for intravenous nutrition is typically accompanied by the need for long-term venous access and central venous catheters, previously identified as an area for QI. For this group, a standardized approach toward feeding may be helpful and may improve the quality of care provided at an individual site. Reducing the placement and the duration of peripherally inserted central catheter lines should decrease the likelihood of infection; however, this needs to be balanced with the risks of rapid feeding advances such as intolerance or NEC.

The strategies used to feed LPT and ET infants most commonly involve nasogastric feeds and oral feeds, and there is less often a need for parental nutrition or intravenous fluids. However, initiatives designed to increase the use of maternal breast milk represent an area for QI. Goals for improving the outcomes of LPT and ET infants may include educating mothers on the importance of providing breast milk, particularly in the setting of a premature infant, as well as improving the breastfeeding resources available both in hospital and following discharge.

Discharge Planning

Prior studies have shown that LPT infants are at higher risk of multiple comorbidities as well as readmission to the hospital after discharge. For all infants, safe discharge home must be balanced with the increased risks of prolonged hospitalization and the additional costs of health care utilization. Previously identified predictors of readmission in all infants discharged from hospital (term and preterm) include first-born infants, breastfeeding, mother with postpartum complications, and public insurance. However, it is unclear whether these risk factors are specific for MPT and LPT infants. No clear evidence-based data exist to guide clinicians in determining when to discharge preterm infants home. Such data will improve care and reduce health care costs by avoiding preventable readmissions.

SUMMARY

MPT and LPT infants are subject to a great deal of variation in care practices among individual centers as well as among practitioners. Unnecessary variation in care and lack of evidence-based practices may contribute to the morbidities of prematurity. QI initiatives designed for neonates have primarily focused on ELGANs. However, the lessons learned in this group of infants could be applied to decreasing unnecessary variation among MPT and LPT infants.

ACKNOWLEDGMENTS

The authors would like to acknowledge the Ohio Perinatal Quality Collaborative for the use of the project information and figures.

REFERENCES

1. Behrman RE, Butler AS. Preterm Birth: causes, consequences and prevention. National Academy Press; 2007.
2. Martin J, Hamilton BE, Ventura SJ. Births final data for 2009. National Vital Statistics Reports 2011;60(1):1–70.
3. 2013. Available at: www.ahrq.gov. Accessed April 1, 2013.
4. The Vermont Oxford Trials Network: very low birthweight outcomes for 1990. Pediatrics 1993;91:540–5.
5. Vermont Oxford Network. 2012. Available at: www.vtoxford.org. Accessed December 1, 2013.
6. Gould JB. The role of regional collaboratives: the California perinatal quality care collaborative model. Clin Perinatol 2010;37:71–86.
7. Kaplan HC, Lannon C, Walsh MC, et al, Ohio Perinatal Quality Collaborative. Ohio statewide quality-improvement collaborative to reduce late-onset sepsis in preterm infants. Pediatrics 2011;127:427–35.
8. Niedner MF, Huskins WC, Colantuoni EP, et al. Epidemiology of central line–associated bloodstream infections in the pediatric intensive care unit. Infect Control Hosp Epidemiol 2011;32:1200–8.
9. Wheeler DS, Giaccone MJ, Hutchinson N, et al. A hospital-wide quality-improvement collaborative to reduce catheter-associated bloodstream infections. Pediatrics 2011;128:e995–1004 [quiz: e1007].
10. Furman L, Taylor G, Minich N. The effect of maternal milk on neonatal morbidity of very low-birth-weight infants. Arch Pediatr Adolesc Med 2003;157:66–71.
11. Blaymore Bier JA, Oliver T, Ferguson A, et al. Human milk reduces outpatient upper respiratory symptoms in premature infants during their first year of life. J Perinatol 2002;22:354–9.
12. Keirse MJ. Progestogen administration in pregnancy may prevent preterm delivery. Br J Obstet Gynaecol 1990;97:149–54.

13. Meis PJ, Klebanoff M, Thom E, et al. Prevention of recurrent preterm delivery by 17 alpha-hydroxyprogesterone caproate. N Engl J Med 2003;348:2379–85.
14. Fonseca EB, Celik E, Parra M, et al. Progesterone and the risk of preterm birth among women with a short cervix. N Engl J Med 2007;357:462–9.
15. Hassan SS, Romero R, Vidyadhari D, et al. Vaginal progesterone reduces the rate of preterm birth in women with a sonographic short cervix: a multicenter, randomized, double-blind, placebo-controlled trial. Ultrasound Obstet Gynecol 2011;38: 18–31.
16. Cahill AG, Odibo AO, Caughey AB, et al. Universal cervical length screening and treatment with vaginal progesterone to prevent preterm birth: a decision and economic analysis. Am J Obstet Gynecol 2010;202:548.e1–8.
17. Werner EF, Han CS, Pettker CM, et al. Universal cervical-length screening to prevent preterm birth: a cost-effectiveness analysis. Ultrasound Obstet Gynecol 2011;38:32–7.
18. Committee on Practice Bulletins—Obstetrics, The American College of Obstetricians and Gynecologists. Practice bulletin no. 130: prediction and prevention of preterm birth. Obstet Gynecol 2012;120:964–73.
19. American Academy of Pediatrics Committee on Fetus And Newborn. Levels of neonatal care. Pediatrics 2012;130:587–97.
20. Escobar GJ, Clark RH, Greene JD. Short-term outcomes of infants born at 35 and 36 weeks gestation: we need to ask more questions. Semin Perinatol 2006;30: 28–33.
21. Hibbard JU, Wilkins I, Sun L, et al. Respiratory morbidity in late preterm births. JAMA 2010;304:419–25.
22. Hjalmarson O, Sandberg K. Abnormal lung function in healthy preterm infants. Am J Respir Crit Care Med 2002;165:83–7.
23. McEvoy C, Venigalla S, Schilling D, et al. Respiratory function in healthy late preterm infants delivered at 33-36 weeks of gestation. J Pediatr 2012;162(3):464–9.
24. Bates E, Rouse DJ, Mann ML, et al. Neonatal outcomes after demonstrated fetal lung maturity before 39 weeks of gestation. Obstet Gynecol 2010;116:1288–95.

Moderately Preterm, Late Preterm and Early Term Infants: Research Needs

Tonse N.K. Raju, MD, DCH

KEYWORDS

- Preterm • Immaturity • Respiratory distress • Apnea • Hypothermia • Hypoglycemia
- Jaundice • Infection

KEY POINTS

- Maturation is a continuum, and not all newborn infants are equally mature.
- There is a need for better understanding of the epidemiology of moderate, late, and early term births, among various ethnic groups, as well as their geographic variations.
- There is a need to develop more precise measures of assessing gestational age, so that infants will be categorized into appropriate subgroups based on evidence-based risk levels.
- Many knowledge gaps in obstetric and neonatal topics need to be addressed with research to optimize the care of all preterm and term newborn infants.

INTRODUCTION

In 1969 the World Health Organization defined prematurity as childbirth occurring at less than 37 completed weeks, or 259 days of gestation, counting from the last day of the last menstrual period in women with regular (28-day) menstrual cycles.[1] Births beyond this period were implied to be term and those after 42 completed weeks, post-term births.

However, during the mid-1970s through the 1980s, for unknown reasons, the phrase near term began to appear in research publications.[2–5] The phrase referred to experimental animals that were very close to their species-specific term gestations, and preterm infants in clinical trials who were also close to term gestations with an un-defined lower boundary.[2–5] The reports did not provide data on gestational age-specific outcomes, suggesting that the investigators considered their cohorts fully mature, homogeneous, and term.

Funding Sources: None.
Conflicts of Interest: None.
Pregnancy and Perinatology Branch, Eunice Kennedy Shriver National Institute of Child Health and Human Development, National Institutes of Health, 6100 Executive Boulevard, Room 4B03, Bethesda, MD 20892-MS 7510, USA
E-mail address: rajut@mail.nih.gov

Clin Perinatol 40 (2013) 791–797
http://dx.doi.org/10.1016/j.clp.2013.07.010
0095-5108/13/$ – see front matter Published by Elsevier Inc.

perinatology.theclinics.com

Over time, the phrase near term acquired a physiologic connotation. This shift was perhaps caused by a practice recommendation that antenatal steroids to enhance fetal lung maturation are recommended for women between 24 and 33 completed weeks of gestation.[6] An unstated implication was that the lungs and the surfactant systems of infants born beyond 34 weeks of gestation would be fully mature, and hence there should be no concerns about the maturity of other organs.

However, this was not to be. An expert panel in a 2005 workshop convened by the *Eunice Kennedy Shriver* National Institute of Health and Human Development (NICHD), reviewed the literature and recommended that the vague and imprecise phrase near term be replaced with late preterm, to reflect the developmental immaturity of infants born between $34^{0/7}$ and $36^{6/7}$ weeks' gestation.[7] The new phrase and its definition were endorsed by the Committee on Fetus and Newborn (COFN) of the American Academy of Pediatrics (AAP)[8] and by other professional entities in the United States and in other countries.[9]

In recent years, many studies documented that all term infants are not equally mature. Compared with those born between $39^{0/7}$ and $40^{6/7}$ weeks' gestation, those born between $37^{0/7}$ and $38^{6/7}$ weeks of gestation were at higher risk for mortality,[10] as well as for short-term and long-term morbidities.[11–13]

In spite of these developments, there are many knowledge gaps, and addressing them could help further improve patient care. This article provides a list of possible research topics, largely based on the research agenda proposed by the NICHD expert panel,[7] and the COFN of the AAP noted earlier.[8]

SOME ASPECTS OF DEVELOPMENTAL MATURATION

Maturation is a continuous process with no specific goals to be achieved. By contrast, maturational milestones are useful signposts developed to assess the pace and the trajectory of maturation to help make clinical decisions when they deviate from normal. Milestones also define stages of maturation into concrete intervals, which provides a valuable tool for epidemiologic research and for developing treatment guidelines.

The duration of gestation (or time) is one of the many factors that influence fetal and neonatal maturational pace and its trajectory. Others include intrauterine environment, maternal health and medications, diet, nutrition, lifestyle (eg, exercise, stress, smoking, and drug abuse), the number of fetuses, fetal sex, and fetal health/diseases.

Maturation is nonlinear. It is programmed to meet the needs of the organism for an independent extrauterine existence at different stages in life. Thus, organs tend to mature at trajectories independent of each other. For instance, most late preterm infants breathe with no external support and manifest no evidence of respiratory distress at birth, which is a reflection of their mature breathing apparatus and surfactant systems. However, many of them are prone to develop hypoglycemia[14–16] coupled with difficulty in initiating and maintaining breastfeeding, which is a reflection of their immature perinatal glucose homeostasis as well as coordination of breathing, sucking, and swallowing mechanisms.[17–20]

DEFINITION AND EPIDEMIOLOGY

Large vital statistics databases, such as those in the National Center for Health Statistics of the Centers for Disease Control and Prevention,[21,22] Consortium for Safe Labor,[21] California Perinatal Quality Care Collaborative[23] are invaluable resources for epidemiologic research. Sources like these can be used to address additional areas on this topic:

- Develop a risk-based system to subclassify the heterogeneous category of pre-term and term infants to improve the precision of risk assessment and compara-bility of outcomes.
- Refine methods to assess pregnancy duration and fetal/neonatal gestational ages and maturity.
- Develop gestational age–specific anthropometric indices for singleton and mul-tiple gestations among different ethnic groups to classify infants into appropriate risk categories.
- Study the national and regional epidemiologic data on gestational age–specific birth and death vital statistics among different ethnic and sociodemographic subgroups, and their trends over time.
- Study the causes of moderate and late preterm and early term births, assessing how many were from indicated causes, and how many were possibly prevent-able. Explore their relation to the mother's payer status, and levels of hospital care in which the infant was delivered.
- Study the contribution of the gestational age–specific preterm birth rates on the overall neonatal and infant mortality and morbidity, and their regional variations.
- Study the postdischarge outcomes for all preterm and term infants treated in special care or intensive care units.

OBSTETRIC ISSUES

The management of women in labor at any preterm gestation presents many chal-lenges for the obstetrician. The best time to deliver has to be based on the anticipated risks to the mother and the fetus from expectant management, versus the risks and benefits to the mother and the newborn of early delivery. Although preterm birth increases neonatal morbidity and mortality, expectant management of the pregnancy when the fetus is in a potentially hostile intrauterine environment can lead to fetal compromise, including organ dysfunctions, neurologic injury, or death.

A panel of obstetric and neonatal experts developed specific guidelines to inform clinicians about optimal management of indicated late preterm births. However, they noted that there is a need for more evidence-based research.[13] Some research areas are as follows:

- Develop improved methods to assess pregnancy duration, enhancing the preci-sion of gestational age estimates to within 5 days.
- Assess the risks and benefits for diagnosis-specific indications for delivery at all gestations periods before 39 weeks.
- Study the factors accelerating or delaying fetal organ maturation.
- Improve the accuracy of estimating fetal well-being in the presence of maternal diseases (eg, hypertension, diabetes, prolonged rupture of membranes, and chorioamnionitis) for choosing appropriate time for and route of delivery.
- Develop strategies to identify fetuses at risk for midpregnancy and late-pregnancy stillbirth.

NEONATAL ISSUES

Compared with those born before 32 weeks of gestation, moderate and late preterm and early term infants are at lower risks for numerous medical problems, but, compared with those born at 39 and 40 weeks' gestation, they are at higher risks for mortality and morbidities.[10–13,24–30] Potential areas for research are listed later.

Cardiovascular and Pulmonary Systems

- Study the risk factors for transient tachypnea of the newborn, respiratory distress syndrome, and severe respiratory failure, and their treatment options at these gestations.
- Study the mechanisms for impaired or delayed maturation of breathing and deglutition functions (central as well as peripheral apparatus) that lead to apnea of prematurity and feeding difficulties.
- Study the epidemiology of late-onset apnea and bradycardia, paroxysmal oxygen desaturation events, their detection, and treatment.
- Study the role of caffeine therapy beyond the hospital stay to prevent unexplained oxygen desaturations and improve neurologic outcomes.
- Evaluate the risk factors for sudden infant death syndrome in preterm and early term infants.

Nervous System

- Study the nature of vulnerability of preterm and early term infants to white matter injury and evaluate their functional consequences on neurodevelopmental outcomes.
- Study the incidence and natural history of intraventricular hemorrhage, periventricular leukomalacia, periventricular leukomalacia, and perinatal stroke.
- Assess the role of routine use of standard and functional magnetic resonance imaging to understand the ontogeny of brain growth and maturation and to assess their value in identifying babies at risk for long-term poor outcomes.
- Study how the intrauterine fetal environment promotes white matter growth, synaptic growth, and arborization, potentially affecting neurobehavioral development.
- Develop strategies to improve neurologic and behavioral outcomes.

Metabolic

- Study how to prevent and treat hyperbilirubinemia and bilirubin-induced brain injury.
- Study the prevalence of hypoglycemia and its long-term consequences.
- Study the prevalence and causes of electrolyte abnormalities and their impact on water balance, with implications for fluid and nutritional therapy.

Nutrition, Breastfeeding and Lactation, and the Gastrointestinal System

- Study the optimal nutritional and feeding practices for preterm and early term infants, and their potential role in the causes of necrotizing enterocolitis.
- Study the mechanisms of acid secretion; the causes, diagnosis, and treatment of gastroesophageal reflux; the understanding of gut motility; and their impact on feeding strategies and hospital discharge practices.
- Study how to improve breastfeeding success rates, assess the role of lactation consultants during prenatal and postnatal periods, and study the health and economic impact of increased intensity of breastfeeding in this vulnerable population.
- Study the causes and treatment of lactation failure among women who delivery preterm infants.
- Continue the evolving study of the microbiome,[31–34] including assessing the development of the gastrointestinal microbiome in relation to the mode of

delivery, feeding strategies, antenatal and postnatal antibiotic use, and the influence of the microbiome on long-term immunologic functions.

Immunology and Sepsis

- Study how immune system immaturity may lead to impaired inflammation and responses to infections.
- Evaluate the effects of preterm birth on developmental immune programming and its role in allergy and asthma in later life.
- Study the temporal trends in maturation of T-cell and granulocyte functions, other immune mediators, and their roles in host-defense mechanisms in late preterm gestations.
- Continue efforts to reduce nosocomial sepsis, and develop methods to prevent excessive use of antibiotics in infants suspected of having sepsis.

Renal and Genitourinary Systems

- Study gestational age–specific definitions for acute kidney injury and biomarkers to detect them.
- Improve the timely management of acute kidney injury.
- Study the short-term and long-term consequences of acute kidney injury on the development of chronic kidney disease in later life.

Development Pharmacology

- Gestational age–specific studies are needed to understand drug disposition, maturational changes in drug metabolism and elimination, and the factors that induce or inhibit these processes.
- Drug dosing guidelines are needed that take into account the immaturity of the liver and kidney, their dysfunctions resulting from disease states, and cholestasis associated with parenteral nutrition.
- Strategies are needed to prevent medication errors during neonatal care.

MISCELLANEOUS

- Study the risk factors for readmission of preterm and early term infants.
- Educate physicians, nurses, and other health care personnel that even seemingly healthy moderate and late preterm infants, and early term infants, are physiologically immature and should be diligently evaluated, monitored, and followed.
- Make available expert health care teams in units of various levels of obstetric and neonatal care, and study their effect on obstetric and neonatal treatment practices and referral patters.
- Study the economic impact of the maternal and neonatal care of preterm and early term infants during their hospitalizations and during follow-up care; this may include the costs of early intervention and other medical and social services, and various strategies to reduce such costs.

SUMMARY

This article is not comprehensive, but is an expanded version of the template suggested by the NICHD workshop expert panel,[7] and the COFN of the AAP.[8] It is hoped that results from future research will continue to improve outcomes for women and newborn infants of all gestational age groups.

REFERENCES

1. World Health Organization. Prevention of perinatal morbidity and mortality. Public Health Papers. 42. Geneva (Switzerland): WHO; 1969.
2. Rankin JH, Phernetton TM. Circulatory responses of the near-term sheep fetus to prostaglandin E2. Am J Physiol 1976;231:760–5.
3. Junge HD, Walter H. Behavioral states and breathing activity in the fetus near term. J Perinat Med 1980;8:150–7.
4. Lange AP, Secher NJ, Nielsen FH, et al. Stimulation of labor in cases of premature rupture of the membranes at or near term: a consecutive randomized study of prostaglandin E2-tablets and intravenous oxytocin. Acta Obstet Gynecol Scand 1981;60:207–10.
5. Bartlett RH, Gazzaniga AB, Toomasian J, et al. Extracorporeal membrane oxygenation (ECMO) in neonatal respiratory failure: 100 cases. Ann Surg 1986; 204:236–45.
6. Cunningham FG, Leveno KJ, Bloom SL, et al, editors. Williams obstetrics. 23rd edition. New York: McGraw-Hill; 2010. p. 820–31.
7. Raju TN, Higgins RD, Stark AR, et al. Optimizing care and outcome for late-preterm (near-term) infants: a summary of the workshop sponsored by the National Institute of Child Health and Human Development. Pediatrics 2006;118(3):1207–14.
8. Engle WA, Tomashek KM, Wallman C. Committee on Fetus and Newborn, American Academy of Pediatrics. "Late-preterm" infants: a population at risk. Pediatrics 2007;120:1390–401.
9. Raju TN. Developmental physiology of late and moderate prematurity. Semin Fetal Neonatal Med 2012;17:126–31.
10. Reddy UM, Bettegowda VR, Dias T, et al. Term pregnancy: a period of heterogeneous risk for infant mortality. Obstet Gynecol 2011;117:1279–87.
11. Bailit JL, Gregory KD, Reddy UM, et al. Maternal and neonatal outcomes by labor onset type and gestational age. Am J Obstet Gynecol 2010;202:245.e1–12.
12. Bates E, Rouse DJ, Mann ML, et al. Neonatal outcomes after demonstrated fetal lung maturity before 39 weeks of gestation. Obstet Gynecol 2010;116:1288–95.
13. Tita AT, Landon MB, Spong CY, et al. Timing of elective repeat cesarean delivery at term and neonatal outcomes. N Engl J Med 2009;360:111–20.
14. Laptook A, Jackson GL. Cold stress and hypoglycemia in late preterm ("near term") infant: impact on nursery admission. Semin Perinatol 2006;30:24–7.
15. Tews D, Wabitsch M. Renaissance of brown adipose tissue. Horm Res Paediatr 2011;75:231–9.
16. Garg M, Devaskar SU. Glucose metabolism in late preterm infants. Clin Perinatol 2006;33:853–70.
17. Cummings KJ, Li A, Nattie EE. Brainstem serotonin deficiency in the neonatal period: autonomic dysregulation during mild cold stress. J Physiol 2011;589: 2055–64.
18. Colin AA, McEvoy C, Castile RG. Respiratory morbidity and lung function in preterm infants of 32 to 36 weeks' gestational age. Pediatrics 2010;126:115–28.
19. Darnall RA, Ariagno RL, Kinney HC. The late preterm infant and the control of breathing, sleep, and brainstem development: a review. Clin Perinatol 2006;33: 883–914.
20. Barlow SM. Oral and respiratory control for preterm feeding. Curr Opin Otolaryngol Head Neck Surg 2009;17:179–86.
21. Centers for Disease Control and Prevention, National Center for Health Statistics. Available at: http://www.cdc.gov/nchs/. Accessed April 22, 2013.

22. Consortium on Safe Labor, Hibbard JU, Wilkins I, et al. Respiratory morbidity in late preterm births. JAMA 2010;304:419–25.
23. California Perinatal Quality Care Collaborative. Available at: http://cpqcc.org/. Accessed April 22, 2013.
24. Watchko JF. Hyperbilirubinemia and bilirubin toxicity in the late preterm infant. Clin Perinatol 2006;33:839–52.
25. Kinney HC. The near-term (late preterm) human brain and risk for periventricular leukomalacia: a review. Semin Perinatol 2006;30(2):81–8.
26. Academy of Breastfeeding Medicine. ABM clinical protocol #10: breastfeeding the late preterm infant (340/7 to 366/7 weeks gestation) (first revision June 2011). Breastfeed Med 2011;6:151–6.
27. Walker JC, Smolders MA, Gemen EF, et al. Development of lymphocyte subpopulations in preterm infants. Scand J Immunol 2011;73:53–8.
28. Blumer N, Pfefferle PI, Renz H. Development of mucosal immune function in the intrauterine and early postnatal environment. Curr Opin Gastroenterol 2007;23: 655–60.
29. Newell SJ, Sarkar PK, Durbin GM, et al. Maturation of the lower esophageal sphincter in the preterm baby. Gut 1988;29:167–72.
30. Neu J. Gastrointestinal development and meeting the nutritional needs of premature infants. Am J Clin Nutr 2007;85(Suppl):629S–34S.
31. van Nimwegen FA, Penders J, Stobberingh EE, et al. Mode and place of delivery, gastrointestinal microbiota, and their influence on asthma and atopy. J Allergy Clin Immunol 2011;128:948–55.
32. Murgas Torrazza R, Neu J. The developing intestinal microbiome and its relationship to health and disease in the neonate. J Perinatol 2011;311:S29–34.
33. Mshvildadze M, Neu J, Shuster J, et al. Intestinal microbial ecology in premature infants assessed with non-culture based techniques. J Pediatr 2010;156:20–5.
34. Biasucci G, Benenati B, Morelli L, et al. Cesarean delivery may affect the early biodiversity of intestinal bacteria. J Nutr 2008;138:1796S–800S.

Index

Note: Page numbers of article titles are in **boldface** type.

A

Acid mantle, of skin, 649
Alcohol ingestion
  birth defects related to, 639
  causing early birth, 639
Amniotic fluid, excess, causing early birth, 631–632
Aneuploidy, causing early birth, 631
Apnea of prematurity, 648, 727
Association of Women's Health, Obstetric and Neonatal Nursing practice project, 728
Astrocytes, reactive, in encephalopathy of prematurity, 714
Autonomic dysregulation, 648
Avon Longitudinal Study, 744

B

Baby Friendly Hospital Initiative, 693
Behavioral factors, causing early birth, 639
Bilirubin, excess of. *See* Hyperbilirubinemia.
Bilirubin-albumin molar ratio, 683–684
BIND spectrum, in hyperbilirubinemia, 681–682
Birth defects, **629–644**
  causing early birth, 630–633
  early elective delivery with, 633–637
  historical perspective of, 629–630
  maternal conditions related to, 637–639
  stillbirth risk in, 620
Bradycardia, 732
Brain
  encephalopathy of prematurity and, **707–722**
  hyperbilirubinemia effects on, 681
  immaturity of, 657
Breakthrough Series model, for quality improvement, 778
Breast pumps, 694–697, 699
Breastfeeding, **689–705**
  advantages of, 690
  for infection reduction, 779–782
  guidelines for term infants applied to, 693–694
  importance of, 690
  management of, 694–700
  poor outcomes of, 690–693
  research needs for, 794–795
  supplementation of, 695, 699–700

Clin Perinatol 40 (2013) 799–805
http://dx.doi.org/10.1016/S0095-5108(13)00117-6
0095-5108/13/$ – see front matter © 2013 Elsevier Inc. All rights reserved.
perinatology.theclinics.com

Breastfeeding (*continued*)
    timing of, 694–695
Breathing
    coordination of, in feeding, 728–730
    immature control of, 648, 733–734

C

Cardiovascular disorders, 794
Cervical length screening, for delaying preterm birth, 786
Chorioamnionitis, 648–649
Chromosomal defects, causing early birth, 631
Collaborative Home Infant Monitoring Evaluation Study, 648
Complement system, abnormalities of, 652
Congenital abnormalities. *See also* Birth defects.
    stillbirth risk in, 620
Congenital heart disease, causing early birth, 636
Corticosteroids, for lung immaturity, 670–671, 785
Cytokines, in encephalopathy of prematurity, 712–714

D

Depression
    birth defects related to, 638
    causing early birth, 638
Developmental disabilities, 673–674
Developmental maturation, research needs for, 792–793
Diabetes mellitus
    birth defects related to, 637–638
    stillbirth risk in, 616–617
Diaphragmatic hernia, causing early birth, 635–636
Diethylstilbestrol, prematurity due to, 630
DIGITAT cohort, 618
Discharge planning, 787–788
Down syndrome, causing early birth, 631

E

Early Childhood Longitudinal Study, 741–745
Early-term deliveries and infants (37-38 weeks)
    adverse outcomes in, 607
    breastfeeding for, **689–705**
    causes of, 602
    definition of, 602
    epidemiology of, **601–610**
    implications of, 612–615
    long-term outcomes of, **739–751**
    neurologic issues in, **723–738**
    quality initiatives for, **777–789**
    research needs for, **791–797**
    respiratory disorders in, **665–678**

risk factors for, 606
Edwards syndrome, causing early birth, 631
Emergency department visits, **753–775**
Encephalopathy of prematurity, **707–722**
    autopsy findings in, 711–718
    definition of, 709–710
    developmental aspects of, 710–712
    hypoxic-ischemic, 731–732
Exchange, transfusions, for hyperbilirubinemia, 684–685
Extracorporeal membrane oxygenation, 672–673

F

FASTER (First and Second Trimester Evaluation of Risk) trial, 630–631
Feeding problems, 654–655, 727–731
    hospital readmissions and, 762–766, 771
    quality initiatives for, 787
    research needs for, 794–795
Fetal abnormalities, stillbirth risk in, 620
Fetal alcohol syndrome, 630
Fetal Lung Maturity II (TDx-FLM II) surfactant/albumin ratio, 668
Fetal testing
    abnormal results of, stillbirth risk in, 621
    for intrauterine growth restriction, 618–619
First and Second Trimester Evaluation of Risk (FASTER) trial, 630–631

G

Gastrointestinal system
    defects of, causing early birth, 635–636
    immaturity of, 654–655
    research needs for, 794–795
Gastroschisis
    causing early birth, 635–636
    stillbirth risk in, 620
Genitourinary disorders, 795
Gestational age, versus stillbirth rate, 612–615
Glial fibrillary protein, in encephalopathy of prematurity, 714
Gliosis, reactive, in encephalopathy of prematurity, 712–714
Glucose abnormalities, 653–654
Gonorrhea, causing early birth, 632–633
Gray matter pathology, in encephalopathy of prematurity, 713, 715–718

H

Hemorrhage, intracranial, 724–726
Hospital readmissions, **753–775**
Hydroxyprogesterone, for delaying preterm birth, 786
Hyperbilirubinemia, 655–657, **679–688**
    brain injury in, 681
    clinical manifestations of, 682
    complications of, 680

Hyperbilirubinemia (*continued*)
    epidemiology of, 680–681
    hospital readmissions and, 762–766, 771
    treatment of, 682–685
Hypertension, stillbirth risk in, 615–616
Hypoglycemia, 646, 653–654
Hypothermia, 646, 731–732
Hypoxic respiratory failure, 646–648
Hypoxic-ischemic encephalopathy of prematurity, 731–732

I

Immunoglobulin G, deficiency of, 652
Immunologic immaturity, 648–652, 795
Infarction, of thalamus, in encephalopathy of prematurity, 716
Infections, 648–652
    causing early birth, 632–633
    reduction of, 779–782, 787
International Pediatric Stroke Study, 732
Intracranial hemorrhage, 724–726
Intrauterine growth restriction
    causing early birth, 636–637
    stillbirth risk in, 617–618

J

Jaundice, 655–656, 762–766, 771

K

Kaiser Permanente
    hospital readmissions and emergency department visits study of, 762–771
    Medical Care Program of, 746
Kernicterus, 655–657, 681–682
Kidney disorders, 795

L

Lactogenesis, delayed, 692–693
Late-preterm deliveries and infants (34-36 weeks)
    adverse outcomes in, 606–607
    breastfeeding for, **689–705**
    causes of, 602
    clinical problems in, **645–663**
    definition of, 601
    encephalopathy of prematurity in, **707–722**
    epidemiology of, **601–610**
    implications of, 612–615
    long-term outcomes of, **739–751**
    neurologic issues in, **723–738**
    quality initiatives for, **777–789**
    recurrence of, 603, 605–606

  research needs for, **791–797**
  respiratory disorders in, **665–678**
  risk factors for, 606
Learning disability, **739–751**
Lecithin/sphingomyelin test, 668
Liver, immaturity of, 655–657
Lung, development of, 667–671

M

Maturation, developmental, 792–793
Medical Birth Registry of Norway, 746
Metabolic disorders, research needs for, 794
Microglia, activated, in encephalopathy of prematurity, 712–714
Milk removal, in breastfeeding, 691–692
Moderate-preterm deliveries and infants (32-33 weeks)
  adverse outcomes in, 606
  breastfeeding for, **689–705**
  causes of, 602
  clinical problems in, **645–663**
  definition of, 601
  emergency department visits in, **753–775**
  epidemiology of, **601–610**
  hospital readmissions in, **753–775**
  hyperbilirubinemia in, **679–688**
  long-term outcomes of, **739–751**
  neurologic issues in, **723–738**
  quality initiatives for, **777–789**
  recurrence of, 603, 605–606
  research needs for, **791–797**
  respiratory disorders in, **665–678**
  risk factors for, 606
Multiple gestations
  birth defects in, 633–634
  stillbirth risk in, 618–619

N

Necrotizing enterocolitis, 648
Neurodevelopmental outcomes, **739–751**
Neurologic disorders, **723–738**. *See also specific disorders.*
  research needs for, 794
Neurons, deficit of, in encephalopathy of prematurity, 717–718
Neutrophil abnormalities, 652
NICHD Neonatal Research Network hypothermia study, 731–732
Nipple shield, 697–698

O

Obesity, birth defects related to, 637
Obstetric issues, research needs in, 793
Ohio Perinatal Quality Collaborative, quality initiatives program of, 778–785

P

Parvovirus infections, causing early birth, 623
Patau syndrome, causing early birth, 631
Pattern recognition receptors, deficiency of, 649
Periventricular leukomalacia, 657, 711, 726–727
Persistent pulmonary hypertension of the newborn, 646–648, 666, 672
Pharmacology, developmental considerations in, 795
Phosphatidylglycerol test, 668
Phototherapy, for hyperbilirubinemia, 681–684
Placenta accreta, stillbirth risk in, 620
Placenta previa, stillbirth risk in, 619–620
Placental abnormalities, stillbirth risk in, 619–620
Pneumonia, 648
Polyhydramnios, causing early birth, 631–632
POUCH (Pregnancy Outcomes and Community Health) cohort, 744, 746
Preeclampsia, stillbirth risk in, 615–616
Pregnancy Outcomes and Community Health (POUCH) cohort, 744, 746
Premature birth, risk factors for, 630, 637–639
Preterm deliveries and infants (28-31 weeks), recurrence of, 605
Progesterone, for delaying preterm birth, 785–786
Pulmonary function tests, long-term results of, 673–674

Q

Quality initiatives, **777–789**
    collaboratives for, 778
    future plans for, 785–788
    infection reduction, 779–782
    obstetrics-related, 783–785
    tenets of, 778

R

Reactive gliosis, in encephalopathy of prematurity, 712–714
Readmissions, hospital, **753–775**
Rehospitalization, **753–775**
Research, **791–797**
Respiratory disorders, 646–648, **665–678**
    causes of, 671–673
    epidemiology of, 665–667
    long-term risk of, 673–674
    lung development and, 667–671
    neonatal respiratory transition and, 667–671
    quality initiatives for, 786–787
    research needs for, 794
    versus gestational age, 671–673
Respiratory distress syndrome, 646–647, 666–667, 671–672

S

Scale, for measuring milk intake, 699
Selective serotonin reuptake inhibitors, causing birth defects, 638

Smoking
    birth defects related to, 639
    causing early birth, 639
Sodium channels, in lung, 668–669
Stillbirth
    definition of, 611
    epidemiology of, 611–615
    prior, recurrent stillbirth risk in, 620–621
    recurrence of, risk of, 620–621
    risk factors for, 615–621
    versus gestational age, 612–615
Stroke, 732
Sucking, immature, 655, 726–731
Suction pressures, in breastfeeding, 691–692
Surfactant deficiency, 668, 671–672
Swallowing, immature, 655, 726–731
Syphilis, causing early birth, 632–633

T

TDx-FLM II (Fetal Lung Maturity II) surfactant/albumin ratio, 668
Thalamic damage, in encephalopathy of prematurity, 716
Thalassemia, stillbirth risk in, 620
Thalidomide, as teratogen, 630
Thermoregulation, ineffective, 646, 733–734
Thrombocytopenia, 743
TOBY trial, 731
Toll-like receptors, deficiency of, 649–652
Transfusions, exchange, for hyperbilirubinemia, 684–685
Transient tachypnea of the newborn, 646–647, 666–669, 672
Trisomy 13, causing early birth, 631
Trisomy 18, causing early birth, 631
Trisomy 21, causing early birth, 631
Twins
    birth defects in, 633–634
    stillbirth risk in, 618–619
Twin-to-twin transfusion syndrome, causing early birth, 634

V

Vermont Oxford Neonatal Encephalopathy Registry, 731
Vernix caseosa, protective properties of, 649

W

White matter pathology, in encephalopathy of prematurity, 712, 717–718

United States Postal Service

Statement of Ownership, Management, and Circulation
(All Periodicals Publications Except Requestor Publications)

1. Publication Title	2. Publication Number	3. Filing Date
Clinics in Perinatology	0 0 1 - 7 4 4	9/14/13

4. Issue Frequency	5. Number of Issues Published Annually	6. Annual Subscription Price
Mar, Jun, Sep, Dec	4	$273.00

7. Complete Mailing Address of Known Office of Publication *(Not printer)* *(Street, city, county, state, and ZIP+4®)*

Elsevier Inc.
360 Park Avenue South
New York, NY 10010-1710

Contact Person: Stephen R. Bushing

Telephone (Include area code): 215-239-3688

8. Complete Mailing Address of Headquarters or General Business Office of Publisher *(Not printer)*

Elsevier Inc., 360 Park Avenue South, New York, NY 10010-1710

9. Full Names and Complete Mailing Addresses of Publisher, Editor, and Managing Editor *(Do not leave blank)*

Publisher *(Name and complete mailing address)*

Linda Belfus, Elsevier, Inc., 1600 John F. Kennedy Blvd. Suite 1800, Philadelphia, PA 19103-2899

Editor *(Name and complete mailing address)*

Kerry Holland, Elsevier, Inc., 1600 John F. Kennedy Blvd. Suite 1800, Philadelphia, PA 19103-2899

Managing Editor *(Name and complete mailing address)*

Adrianne Brigido, Elsevier, Inc., 1600 John F. Kennedy Blvd. Suite 1800, Philadelphia, PA 19103-2899

10. Owner *(Do not leave blank. If the publication is owned by a corporation, give the name and address of the corporation immediately followed by the names and addresses of all stockholders owning or holding 1 percent or more of the total amount of stock. If not owned by a corporation, give the names and addresses of the individual owners. If owned by a partnership or other unincorporated firm, give its name and address as well as those of each individual owner. If the publication is published by a nonprofit organization, give its name and address.)*

Full Name	Complete Mailing Address
Wholly owned subsidiary of	1600 John F. Kennedy Blvd., Ste. 1800
Reed/Elsevier, US holdings	Philadelphia, PA 19103-2899

11. Known Bondholders, Mortgagees, and Other Security Holders Owning or Holding 1 Percent or More of Total Amount of Bonds, Mortgages, or Other Securities. If none, check box ☐ None

Full Name	Complete Mailing Address
N/A	

12. Tax Status *(For completion by nonprofit organizations authorized to mail at nonprofit rates)* *(Check one)*
The purpose, function, and nonprofit status of this organization and the exempt status for federal income tax purposes:
☐ Has Not Changed During Preceding 12 Months
☐ Has Changed During Preceding 12 Months *(Publisher must submit explanation of change with this statement)*

13. Publication Title	14. Issue Date for Circulation Data Below
Clinics in Perinatology	September 2013

15. Extent and Nature of Circulation		Average No. Copies Each Issue During Preceding 12 Months	No. Copies of Single Issue Published Nearest to Filing Date
a. Total Number of Copies *(Net press run)*		1,474	1,811
b. Paid Circulation (By Mail and Outside the Mail)	(1) Mailed Outside-County Paid Subscriptions Stated on PS Form 3541. *(Include paid distribution above nominal rate, advertiser's proof copies, and exchange copies)*	1,086	1,252
	(2) Mailed In-County Paid Subscriptions Stated on PS Form 3541 *(Include paid distribution above nominal rate, advertiser's proof copies, and exchange copies)*		
	(3) Paid Distribution Outside the Mails Including Sales Through Dealers and Carriers, Street Vendors, Counter Sales, and Other Paid Distribution Outside USPS®	303	319
	(4) Paid Distribution by Other Classes Mailed Through the USPS (e.g. First-Class Mail®)		
c. Total Paid Distribution *(Sum of 15b (1), (2), (3), and (4))*		1,389	1,571
d. Free or Nominal Rate Distribution (By Mail and Outside the Mail)	(1) Free or Nominal Rate Outside-County Copies Included on PS Form 3541	54	70
	(2) Free or Nominal Rate In-County Copies Included on PS Form 3541		
	(3) Free or Nominal Rate Copies Mailed at Other Classes Through the USPS (e.g. First-Class Mail)		
	(4) Free or Nominal Rate Distribution Outside the Mail (Carriers or other means)		
e. Total Free or Nominal Rate Distribution *(Sum of 15d (1), (2), (3) and (4))*		54	70
f. Total Distribution *(Sum of 15c and 15e)*		1,443	1,641
g. Copies not Distributed *(See instructions to publishers #4 (page #3))*		31	170
h. Total *(Sum of 15f and g)*		1,474	1,811
i. Percent Paid *(15c divided by 15f times 100)*		96.26%	95.73%

16. Publication of Statement of Ownership
☐ If the publication is a general publication, publication of this statement is required. Will be printed in the December 2013 issue of this publication. ☐ Publication not required

17. Signature and Title of Editor, Publisher, Business Manager, or Owner

Stephen R. Bushing – Inventory Distribution Coordinator

Date: September 14, 2013

I certify that all information furnished on this form is true and complete. I understand that anyone who furnishes false or misleading information on this form or who omits material or information requested on the form may be subject to criminal sanctions (including fines and imprisonment) and/or civil sanctions (including civil penalties).

PS Form 3526, September 2007 (Page 2 of 3)

PS Form 3526, September 2007 (Page 1 of 3 (Instructions Page 3)) PSN 7530-01-000-9931 PRIVACY NOTICE: See our Privacy policy in www.usps.com

Moving?

Make sure your subscription moves with you!

To notify us of your new address, find your **Clinics Account Number** (located on your mailing label above your name), and contact customer service at:

Email: journalscustomerservice-usa@elsevier.com

800-654-2452 (subscribers in the U.S. & Canada)
314-447-8871 (subscribers outside of the U.S. & Canada)

Fax number: 314-447-8029

Elsevier Health Sciences Division
Subscription Customer Service
3251 Riverport Lane
Maryland Heights, MO 63043

*To ensure uninterrupted delivery of your subscription, please notify us at least 4 weeks in advance of move.

ELSEVIER